T0231841

BIOTECHNOLOGIES APPLIED TO ANIMAL REPRODUCTION

Current Trends and Practical Applications for Reproductive Management

BIOTECHNOLOGIES APPLIED TO ANIMAL REPRODUCTION

Current Trends and Practical Applications for Reproductive Management

Edited by
Juan Carlos Gardón, MSc, PhD
Katy Satué, MSc, PhD

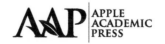

APPLE ACADEMIC PRESS

First edition published [2021]

Apple Academic Press Inc.
1265 Goldenrod Circle, NE,
Palm Bay, FL 32905 USA

4164 Lakeshore Road, Burlington,
ON, L7L 1A4 Canada

CRC Press
6000 Broken Sound Parkway NW,
Suite 300, Boca Raton, FL 33487-2742 USA

2 Park Square, Milton Park,
Abingdon, Oxon, OX14 4RN UK

First issued in paperback 2021

© 2021 Apple Academic Press, Inc.

Apple Academic Press exclusively co-publishes with CRC Press, an imprint of Taylor & Francis Group, LLC

Library and Archives Canada Cataloguing in Publication

Title: Biotechnologies applied to animal reproduction : current trends and practical applications for reproductive management / edited by Juan Carlos Gardón, PhD, Katy Satué, PhD.
Names: Gardón, Juan Carlos, editor. | Satué, Katy, editor.
Description: Includes bibliographical references and index.
Identifiers: Canadiana (print) 20200256092 | Canadiana (ebook) 20200256408 | ISBN 9781771888714 (hardcover) | ISBN 9780367817527 (ebook)
Subjects: LCSH: Livestock—Reproduction. | LCSH: Livestock—Breeding. | LCSH: Reproductive technology.
Classification: LCC SF871 .B56 2021 | DDC 636.08/24—dc23

Library of Congress Cataloging-in-Publication Data

Names: Gardón, Juan Carlos, editor. | Satué, Katy, 1958- editor.
Title: Biotechnologies applied to animal reproduction : current trends and practical applications for reproductive management / edited by Juan Carlos Gardón, Katy Satué.
Description: Palm Bay, Florida : Apple Academic Press, Inc. [2021] | Includes bibliographical references and index. | Summary: "This comprehensive volume focuses on recent trends and new technologies used in the management of reproduction in major farm animals, focusing on both males and females of bovine, equine and porcine species. With chapters written by scientists who specialize in their respective topics, the volume presents a selection of different technologies that have been developed to assure reproductive success by improving reproductive efficiency, generating germplasm banks, and maintaining genetic diversity in cattle, horses, and pigs. In the last decade, reproductive technologies in veterinary medicine have progressed considerably, providing high profitability to livestock farms. This book provides basic and applied information on the most used reproductive technologies in bovine, equine, and porcine species for academics, scientists, and veterinarians. The volume discusses reproductive and postpartum management, reproductive ultrasound, sperm management, egg retrieval, artificial insemination, embryo transfer, nutrition, genetics, and certain clinical aspects, such as endocrinology and robustness of reproductive systems. Biotechnologies Applied to Animal Reproduction: Current Trends and Practical Applications for Reproductive Management is the culmination of the efforts of several researchers and scientists from around the world who are well known and respected in their different frontiers of research in reproductive biotechnology"-- Provided by publisher.
Identifiers: LCCN 2020023857 (print) | LCCN 2020023858 (ebook) | ISBN 9781771888714 (hardcover) | ISBN 9780367817527 (ebook)
Subjects: MESH: Reproductive Techniques, Assisted--veterinary | Cattle | Horses | Sus scrofa
Classification: LCC SF201.5 (print) | LCC SF201.5 (ebook) | NLM SF 201.5 | DDC 636.2/08245--dc23
LC record available at https://lccn.loc.gov/2020023857
LC ebook record available at https://lccn.loc.gov/2020023858

ISBN: 978-1-77188-871-4 (hbk)
ISBN: 978-1-77463-901-6 (pbk)
ISBN: 978-0-36781-752-7 (ebk)

About the Editors

Juan Carlos Gardón, MSc, PhD

Juan Carlos Gardón, PhD, is currently working as a professor in the Department of Animal Medicine and Surgery, Faculty of Veterinary and Experimental Sciences of the Catholic University of Valencia San Vicente Mártir (UCV), Valencia, Spain. He also participates in academic post-graduate activities at the Veterinary Faculty of Murcia University, Spain. Since 2018, Dr. Gardón has been the Director of the UCV Veterinary Farm. He has over 30 years of teaching and research experience. He is the author of eight book chapters and has published around 200 research papers in national and international journals and conference proceedings. He has participated as principal researcher in 12 R+D projects and in the organization of seven national and international scientific events. His main research interests include animal physiology, physiology and biotechnology of reproduction either in males or females, the study of gametes under *in vitro* conditions, and the use of ultrasound as a complement to physiological studies and development of applied biotechnologies. He regularly supervises students in preparing their PhD and master theses or in final degree projects.

Katy Satué, MSc, PhD

Katy Satué, PhD, is a professor in the Department of Animal Medicine and Surgery at the Faculty of Veterinary Medicine of the CEU-Cardinal Herrera University, Valencia, Spain. She teaches courses in general pathology, integrated in the module of applied bases of the equine veterinary clinic for the 2nd, 3rd and 4th years of the degree program in veterinary sciences. Her research activity is focused in the field of hematology, biochemistry, immunology, and fundamentally in equine endocrinology in pregnant Spanish purebreed mares. Dr. Satué has directed five PhD theses and five Certificates of Advanced Studies, has participated in 10 research projects as a collaborating researcher, and has written two books and 14 book chapters published by international publishing houses related to her research areas. She has written 70 scientific publications in international journals and has attended 70 international congresses, participating with more than 125 communications. She is also a scientific reviewer for several indexed international journals (*American Journal of Obstetrics and Gynecology, Journal of Equine Veterinary Science, Veterinary Radiology & Ultrasound,* and others). Since 2014, she has been responsible for the Clinical Analysis Laboratory of the Veterinary Clinical Hospital of CEUCardinal Herrera University. She is also an honorary member of the Peloritan Academy of Pericolanti since February 2018.

Contents

Contributors

Cristina Álvarez
Chief Veterinary Officer of the Veterinary Unit, Zaragoza, Spain

Susana Astiz
Department of Animal Reproduction, INIA, Avda Pta. de Hierro s/n, 28040 Madrid, Spain

Gabriel Amilcar Bó
Institute A.P. of Basic and Applied Sciences, National University of Villa María,
Villa del Rosario, Córdoba, Argentina
Animal Reproduction Institute Córdoba (IRAC), Pozo del Tigre, Córdoba, Argentina

José Javier de la Mata
Bovine Reproduction and Biotechnology-Veterinary Services, Santa Rosa, La Pampa, Argentina
Cathedra of Animal Anatomy and Physiology, Faculty of Agronomy,
National University of La Pampa, Santa Rosa, La Pampa, Argentina
Institute A.P. of Basic and Applied Sciences, National University of Villa María,
Villa del Rosario, Córdoba, Argentina

Francisco Alberto García-Vázquez
Department of Physiology, Faculty of Veterinary Science, International Excellence Campus for
Higher Education and Research "Campus Mare Nostrum", University of Murcia, Murcia, Spain
Institute for Biomedical Research of Murcia (IMIB-Arrixaca), Murcia, Spain

Juan Carlos Gardón
Department of Animal Medicine and Surgery, Faculty of Veterinary and Experimental Sciences
Catholic University of Valencia, San Vincente Mártir, Spain

Gabriela Garrappa
Department of Physiology, Faculty of Veterinary Science, International Excellence Campus for
Higher Education and Research "Campus Mare Nostrum", University of Murcia, Murcia, Spain
Institute of Animal Research of the Semi-Arid Chaco (IIACS), Agricultural Research Center (CIAP),
National Institute of Agricultural Technology (INTA), Tucumán, Argentina

Lydia Gil Huerta
Department of Animal Pathology, Faculty of Veterinary Medicine, Agroalimentary Institute of
Aragón IA2, University of Zaragoza, Center for Agrifood Research and Technology (CITA),
Zaragoza, C/Miguel Servet 133, 50013, Zaragoza, Spain

Giovanni Gnemmi
Bovinevet Internacional, Bovine Ultrasound Services and Herd Management, Calle de la Mecanica,
9, Huesca, 22006, Huesca, Spain
Department of Animal Medicine and Surgery, Faculty of Veterinary and Experimental Sciences
Catholic University of Valencia, San Vincente Mártir, Spain

Ana Heras-Molina
Department of Animal Reproduction, INIA, Avda Pta. de Hierro s/n, 28040 Madrid, Spain

Victoria Luño Lázaro
Department of Animal Pathology, Faculty of Veterinary Medicine, Agroalimentary Institute of Aragón IA2, University of Zaragoza, Center for Agrifood Research and Technology (CITA), Zaragoza, C/Miguel Servet 133, 50013, Zaragoza, Spain

Chiara Luongo
Department of Physiology, Faculty of Veterinary Science, International Excellence Campus for Higher Education and Research "Campus Mare Nostrum", University of Murcia, Murcia, Spain

Cristina Maraboli
Bovinevet Internacional, Bovine Ultrasound Services and Herd Management, Calle de la Mecanica, 9, Huesca, 22006, Huesca, Spain

María Marcilla
Department of Animal Medicine and Surgery, Faculty of Veterinary, University CEU-Cardenal Herrera, Valencia, Alfara del Patriarca, Tirant lo Blanc, 46115 Valencia, Spain

Carmen Matás
Department of Physiology, Faculty of Veterinary Science, International Excellence Campus for Higher Education and Research "Campus Mare Nostrum", University of Murcia, Murcia, Spain Institute for Biomedical Research of Murcia (IMIB-Arrixaca), Murcia, Spain

José Luis Pesantez Pacheco
Department of Animal Reproduction, INIA, Avda Pta. de Hierro s/n, 28040 Madrid, Spain School of Veterinary Medicine and Zootechnics, Faculty of Agricultural Sciences, University of Cuenca, Avda. Doce de Octubre, Cuenca, Ecuador

Ernesto Rodríguez Tobón
Department of Physiology, Faculty of Veterinary Science, International Excellence Campus for Higher Education and Research *"Campus Mare Nostrum"*, University of Murcia, Murcia, Spain

Salvador Ruiz López
Department of Physiology, Faculty of Veterinary Science, International Excellence Campus for Higher Education and Research "Campus Mare Nostrum", University of Murcia, Murcia, Spain Institute for Biomedical Research of Murcia (IMIB-Arrixaca), Murcia, Spain

Katy Satué
Department of Animal Medicine and Surgery, Faculty of Veterinary, University CEU-Cardenal Herrera, Valencia, Alfara del Patriarca, Tirant lo Blanc, 46115 Valencia, Spain

Cristina Soriano-Úbeda
Department of Physiology, Faculty of Veterinary Science, International Excellence Campus for Higher Education and Research "Campus Mare Nostrum", University of Murcia, Murcia, Spain Institute for Biomedical Research of Murcia (IMIB-Arrixaca), Murcia, Spain

Abbreviations

ADG	average daily gain
AETE	Association of Embryo Technology in Europe
AFP	antral follicle population
AI	artificial insemination
AIJ	ampullary-isthmic junction
AI-NS	fixed time artificial insemination-natural service
AMH	anti-Müllerian hormone
AR	acrosome reaction
ARTs	assisted reproductive technologies
BCS	body condition score
BHB	β-hydroxybutyrate
BO	Brackett-Oliphant solution
BS	breeding season
BSE	breeding soundness evaluation
BTB	blood–testis barrier
CAI	cervical artificial insemination
CASA	computerized assisted sperm analysis
CIDR	progesterone-releasing intravaginal device
CL	corpus luteum
COCs	*cumulus* oocyte complexes
COX2	cyclooxygenase 2
DHA	dihydroandrosterone
DHEA	dehydroepiandrosterone
DIM	days in milk
DO	double ovsynch
DpCAI	deep cervical artificial insemination
DRF	dominant follicle removal
DUI	deep intrauterine insemination
EB	estradiol benzoate
eCG	equine chorionic gonadotrophin
ED	embryonic death
EDTA	ethylenediaminetetraacetic acid
EGF	epidermal growth factor

EGTA	ethylene glycol-bis (2-aminoethyl ether) - N, N, N'N'-tetraacetic acid
EPL	early pregnancy loss
EU	European Union
FF	follicular fluid
FPU	fetoplacental unit
FSH	follicle-stimulating hormone
FTAI	fixed-time artificial insemination
GABA	gamma-aminobutyric acid
GAS	gene assisted selection
GnRH	gonadotropin-releasing hormone
GT	genital tubercle
hCG	human chorionic gonadotropin
HD	heat detection
HOST	hypo-osmotic swelling test
HPG	hypothalamic-pituitary-gonadal
ICSI	intracytoplasmic sperm injection
IETS	International Embryo Transfer Society
IFN	interferon
ITM	inorganic trace minerals
IVD	*in vivo* derived
IVEP	*in vitro* embryo production
IVF	*in vitro* fertilization
IVM	*in vitro* maturation
IVP	*in vitro* produced
LH	luteinizing hormone
L-OPU	laparoscopic procedure of oocyte collection
LOS	large offspring syndrome
MAP	multiple angle sector
MAS	marker assisted selection
MGR	maternal recognition of pregnancy
MOET	multiple ovulation and embryo transfer
NEB	negative energy balance
NPD	nonpregnancy diagnosis
NS	natural service
NSAIDs	nonsteroidal anti-inflammatory
OEC	oviductal (isthmus) epithelial cell
OECs	oviductal epithelial cells

OF	oviductal fluid
o-FSH	ovine FSH
OIE	World Organization for Animal Health
ONS	only natural service
OPU	ovum pick-up
P/AI	pregnancy per artificial insemination
P4	progesterone
P5	pregnenolone
P5ββ	5-pregnene-3β,20β–diol
PAGS	pregnancy-associated glycoproteins
pAI	porcine artificial insemination
PCAI	post-cervical artificial insemination
p-FSH	porcine FSH
PGDH	15-hydroxyprostaglandin dehydrogenase
PGE2	prostaglandin E2
$PGF_2\alpha$	prostaglandin F2α
PGFM	13,14-dihydro-15-keto-prostaglandin F2α
PGs	prostaglandins
PLGF	placental growth factor
PMN	polymorphonuclear granulocytes
PMSG	pregnant mare serum gonadotropin
PS	presynch protocol
PS	presynch protocol
QTL	quantitative trait loci
ROS	reactive oxygen species
RR	recovery rate
RTS	reproductive tract scoring
sAC	soluble adenyl cyclase
SCNT	somatic cell nuclear transfer
SLC	single layer centrifugation
SNP	single nucleotide polymorphisms
SP	seminal plasma
SR	sperm reservoir
TAI	timed artificial insemination
TBM	tris-buffered medium
TGF-β	transforming growth factor-β
TNB	timed natural breeding
Tyr-P	tyrosine phosphorylation

UECs	uterine epithelial cells
UF	uterine fluid
UTJ	utero-tubal junction
VEGF	vascular endothelium growth factor
VWP	voluntary waiting period
ZP	zona pellucida
βα-diol	5α-pregnane-3β,20α-diol
ββ-diol	5α-pregnane-3β,20β-diol
20α5P	20α-hydroxy-5α-pregnan-3-one
3β5P	3β-hydroxy-5α-pregnan-3-one
3β-HSD	3β-hydroxideshydrogenase
5αDHP	5α-pregnane-3,20-dione

Preface

We are aware that in the last decade reproductive technologies in veterinary medicine have progressed considerably, providing high profitability to livestock farms. This book aims to provide basic and applied information on the most used reproductive technologies in bovine, equine, and porcine species for academics, scientists, and veterinarians dedicated to reproductive clinics. This work contains three main sections for each animal species and covers a wide range of applications of biotechnology in animal reproduction. Therefore, the motivation for editing a comprehensive volume on advances in biotechnology arose from a growing awareness of recent advances in reproductive and postpartum management, reproductive ultrasound, sperm management, egg retrieval, artificial insemination, embryo transfer, and certain clinical aspects, such as endocrinology and robustness of reproductive systems. The authors are recognized researchers from several countries who, beyond the theoretical foundations, have a deep practical knowledge of the topics dealt with in this work.

This volume is the culmination of the efforts of several researchers and scientific fellows from around the world, and they are all known and respected at different frontiers of research in reproductive biotechnology. We sincerely believe that the book will prove to be a useful contribution not only to science, but also to the general public interest.

We express our gratitude to all the contributing authors and to all the members of the international review panel who helped us enormously with their contributions, time, critical thoughts, and suggestions to produce this peer-reviewed and edited volume.

The editors also thank Apple Academic Press and its team members for the opportunity to publish this book.

Finally, we thank our family members for their love, support, encouragement, and patience throughout the period of this work.

Introduction

Reproductive success is a very important goal for those species destined for production, for sports, as pets, and wild animals. As a result, knowledge of the physiology and pathology of the male and female reproductive systems, obstetrics, gynecology, and andrology is expanding considerably every day. For this reason, over the years numerous interesting works have been carried out to clarify, resolve, or explain several aspects of reproduction in different animal species. In this way, different reproductive biotechnologies have been developed for both males and females in order to improve reproductive efficiency, generate germplasm banks, maintain genetic diversity, or to use them as animal models for human reproduction.

In this book we present a series of chapters dedicated to males and females of bovine, equine, and porcine cattle in which, in the last years, different technologies have been developed to assure reproductive success every time. We also present the most relevant topics of each of them, carrying out a detailed review of the knowledge communicated to the present time.

Foreword

Domestication of farm animals started 12,000–15,000 years ago in the Middle East and was a seminal achievement in human development during which agriculture as it is known today gradually emerged. Initially, domesticated animals were selected according to phenotype and/or specific traits adapted to a local climate and production system. The science-based breeding systems used today originated with the introduction of statistical methods in the 16th century, which made possible a quantitative approach to selective breeding for specific traits. Now, with the availability of accurate and reliable DNA analysis, this quantitative approach has been extended to DNA-based breeding concepts that allow a more cost-effective but still quantitative determination of a genomic breeding value (GBV) for individual animals. The accurate and reliable prediction of genetic traits made possible from this introduction revolutionized breeding practices and, together with advances in DNA technology, ultimately led to the quantitative molecular genetic selection procedures used today.

The impact of these developments is critically dependent upon the introduction of reproductive technologies that can greatly extend the genetic influence of superior individual animals. The first of these was artificial insemination (AI) that started to be developed in the late 19th century. Industry uptake of AI was initially slow, but increased rapidly following the development of semen extenders, the reduction of veneral disease risk by inclusion of antibiotics, and most significantly the development of effective freezing and cryostorage procedures in the mid 20th century. AI is now used in most livestock breeding enterprises, most notably by the dairy industry where more than 90% of dairy cattle are produced through AI in countries with modern breeding structures.

With the introduction of practical and effective embryo transfer (ET) protocols in the latter part of the 20th century, exploitation of the female genetic pool became possible for the first time. Advances in understanding of the reproductive cycle and its hormonal control, the availability of purified gonadotropins, and improved cell and embryo culture procedures all played significant roles for the rapid and worldwide use of ET, mainly in cattle. ET is now being increasingly implemented in the top 1–2% of a given cattle population and has also been developed in other farm animal species. But its real impact is yet to come as ET is the key enabler in the introduction of the next generation of enhanced breeding technologies. ET has already played a key role in advances such as *in vitro* production of embryos (IVP), including the development of techniques to retrieve oocytes repeatedly from female donors for IVF, sexing, cloning and transgenesis. Some of these technologies have been thoroughly addressed in this book.

With the birth of "Dolly," the cloned sheep, in 1996, a century-old dogma in biology that inferred that a differentiated cell cannot be reprogrammed into a pluripotent stage was abolished. Today available protocols are efficient enough to allow commercial application of somatic cloning in all the major farm animal species. This will not only further enhance the rate of genetic gain in herds and flocks but, through the recent advent of precise genome editing tools, allow the production of novel germlines for agricultural and biomedical purposes through the capacity to genetically modify farm animals with targeted modifications with high efficiency. This paves the way for the introduction of new precision breeding concepts urgently needed to respond to future challenges in animal breeding, stemming from matching the demands of the ongoing human population growth to the limited availability of arable land and environmental constraints. The implementation of these new concepts requires the application of reliable and effective reproductive technologies.

This book is designed to provide the reader with the most recent information on the practical application of a series of advanced reproductive technologies in the major farm animal species such as cattle, pigs and horses, with emphasis on female and male cattle. The readership will appreciate the detailed description of the technologies, their critical appraisal, the extensive reference lists, and the rich illustration of the book.

—**Prof. Dr. Heiner Niemann**
Hannover Medical University
Germany

SECTION I
Bovine

CHAPTER 1

Bovine Reproductive Management

JOSÉ JAVIER DE LA MATA[1,2,3*] and GABRIEL AMILCAR BÓ[3,4]

[1]Reproduction and Biotechnology-Veterinary Services, Santa Rosa, La Pampa, Argentina

[2]Cathedra of Animal Anatomy and Physiology, Faculty of Agronomy, National University of La Pampa, Santa Rosa, La Pampa, Argentina

[3]Institute A.P. of Basic and Applied Sciences, National University of Villa María, Villa del Rosario, Córdoba, Argentina

[4]Animal Reproduction Institute Córdoba (IRAC), Pozo del Tigre, Córdoba, Argentina

*Corresponding author. E-mail: javidelamata@gmail.com

ABSTRACT

Beef cattle production is a widespread industry carried out worldwide. Reproduction management is an essential tool that producers and veterinarians must realize to achieve the aim of beef production: to get pregnant high number of females, to develop and maintain gestations, to ensure easy-calving offspring and to wean healthy calves. Knowledge in the physiology of reproduction such as endocrinology of the estrus cycle and dynamics events in the reproductive tract in cattle has advanced in the last 20 years. Stages as puberty, anestrus, and cyclicity of cattle have been studied in detail after many experiments and publications from researchers from many countries, and these informations have favored for the massive application of biotechnologies of reproduction such as artificial insemination and fixed-time artificial inseminations. This chapter describes recent advances in bovine reproductive management emphasizing in different treatments for the synchronization of ovulation for natural breeding or fixed-time artificial insemination in beef cattle.

1.1 INTRODUCTION

Beef production is a huge industry worldwide, and in Europe, Australia, North America, and South America extension forage-based systems are a commonly use practice for producers. Longevity and precocity are two features pursued by producers and have an important impact in the profitability and sustainability of the business. Heifers and cows must conceive every year to wean one calf, challenging the prepuberal and postpartum anestrus, respectively. Faced with nutritional deficiency, and depending on its severity, the natural physiological response is to renounce reproduction (Meikle et al., 2018). Therefore, there are many nutritional and hormonal strategies and calf management to prevent the physiological status above mentioned that could benefit heifers and suckled cows before the breeding season initiation.

Artificial insemination (AI) treatment protocols are an alternative tool to enhance reproductive management, not only by manipulating the estrus and ovulation or by inducing cyclicity (Lucy et al., 2001), but also by producing an advanced in genetics in the future calves generation. Hormonal treatments are efficient and economical strategies that enhance reproductive responses either in natural service (NS) or in fixed-time AI programs (FTAI; Baruselli et al., 2018). Recently, new technologies in relation with sexed-sorted semen are available for commercial applications (Bó et al., 2018a). These new technologies are a milestone in the industry of the FTAI and will be an interesting option to increase superior genetic of predefined sex calves. The objective of this chapter is to review different and recent hormonal treatments strategies to avoid negative effects of anestrus and will focus in new approaches of programs for FTAI for improving reproduction managements in beef cattle.

1.2 BEEF HEIFERS AND BEEF COWS REPRODUCTIVE MANAGEMENT

In beef cattle production, the nutritional management of the herd is essential to attain cyclicity in both heifers and postpartum cows. Beef heifers must achieve puberty before breeding season (BS) and postpartum beef cows cyclicity depends on different main factors such as body condition score (BCS) at calving, body reserves (energy stores), suckling and nutrition (feed intake). BCS is an easy and quick method to predict adipose tissue reserves in animals and is useful to estimate the physiological active endocrine activity of different substances (insulin, IGF1, leptine, and adiponectin) that fine-tune the reproductive axis at central (hypothalamus-pituitary gland) and peripheral (ovaries, reproductive tract, and embryos) levels (Meikle et al., 2018). Briefly the BCS, based on a scale 1–9 score point (Herd and Sprott, 1986), in which code 1 is consider an emaciated animal (BCS 1) whereas code 9 indicates an obese animal (BCS 9). At the beginning of BS, the optimum BCS in all animal categories should be more than 5, with fluctuations lower than 1fold, to permit a normal occurrence of the estrus cycle. In beef cows if nutrition is adequate and allows for an increase gain plane, the first postpartum ovulation takes place on the third follicular wave after parturition (~30 days), but if beef cows present poor body condition and/or with undernourished conditions, ovulation is delayed (~70–100 days, reviewed by Crowe et al., 2014). Short et al. (1990) described the biological priorities for nutrient utilization by cattle, ranking in different vital physiological functions: (i) basal metabolism, (ii) motor activity, (iii) growth, (iv) basic energy reserves, (v) maintenance of pregnancy, (vi) lactation, (vii) additional energy reserves, (viii) estrus cycles and initiation of pregnancy, and (ix) excess reserves. Beef cattle have the unique ability to convert low-quality forages into meat and milk for the offspring, and in times of excess nutrition they deposit energy stores for future maintenance of bodily functions and production (Perry and Cushman, 2013).

During the postpartum period (Fig. 1.1), negative energy balance (NEB) is generated particularly by deficient nutrition and the presence of the offspring. The reproductive response increases the length of anestrus, decreased fertility and increases early embryo mortality. In cows, BCS at parturition was the most important factor that determines the period to re-conception postpartum (D'Occhio et al., 2019) and cows with high BCS synchronized with progesterone-based treatment protocols for FTAI had higher pregnancy rates than cows with poor BCS (Bó et al., 2002). Resumption of ovarian cyclicity is largely dependent on LH pulse frequency (Crowe et al., 2014) as well as the dominant follicle in the ovary should grow with the stimulation of many growth factors (e.g. IGF 1 family) and nutrients (Meikle et al., 2018). At calving, pituitary LH stores are low, because of high plasma concentration of progesterone in the early and medium gestation, and later estrogen is synthesized by placental tissue. The re-accumulation of pituitary stores of LH takes 2–3 weeks to complete (reviewed by Crowe et al., 2014). In Argentina, a common practice is to wean calves as early as ~ 60 days (early weaning), ~120 days (anticipated weaning) or later at ~150 days (traditional weaning). After the early weaning, calves are feed with high quality hay and a protein supplementation, and management must be done in a dry lot system with an intensive assistance during 40–50 days after weaning. Calf management enable to postpartum cow to return to cyclic stage between 10–20 days post weaning, preventing the maternal-offspring bonding, resulting in cyclic LH pulse frequency and periodic surge that will trigger a subsequent ovulation. First ovulation after parturition is generally silent (without behavioral estrus signs) and the first luteal phase would be, at least in 70% of cases, of short duration (short-live corpus luteum), in which oocyte can become fertilized. However, embryo arrests growing, an early luteolysis undergoes and the embryo dies prior to the maternal-embryo recognition (day 10–14 after ovulation).

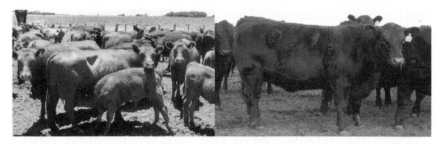

FIGURE 1.1   Left: Angus suckled beef cows and their calves at the beginning of spring breeding season (BS). Body condition score (BCS; scale 1:9) of cows in the image are among 5 to 6. Different strategies of managements, not only in cows but also in calves, can be done to enhance reproductive performance during BS. Right: 2-year old Angus beef heifers ready for breeding season. Heifers must attain at least 60% of mature body weight to be satisfactory for a breeding program.

Heifer reproductive management has been widespread studied in a large amount of research that is available in the literature (Gutierrez et al., 2014; Perry and Cushman, 2013). Beef heifers should be managed, well-nourished and selected for the reposition (Fig. 1.1). Puberty in heifers has been defined as the first ovulation that is accompanied by visual signs of estrus and normal luteal function. Selection criteria are focus in 3 basic concepts: (1) age, (2) body weight and (3) average daily gain (ADG) during rearing. Usually, the target weight considered suitable in beef heifer management practice is 65% of mature weight. The ideal developing varies among breeds, mature size, and some research works reported that puberty was obtained between 55% and 60% of mature body weight, suggesting that adequate growth and BCS are necessary for the initiation of normal estrus cycle (Perry and Cushman, 2013). Optimal timing of puberty in beef heifers requires an ADG of 0.6–0.7 kg/day (reviewed by D'Occhio et al., 2019), indicating that, similarly to postpartum cows, gain plane is essential for heifers reproduction success during the rearing period from weaning to puberty stage. In modern production systems, *Bos taurus* beef heifers might attain puberty, conceive, and achieve first calving at around 2 years, to optimize lifetime reproductive performance, and heifers that calve as early tend to calve early throughout their entire life (Reviewed by Perry and Cushman, 2013).

Previous to the BS, practitioners can examine the herd to determine if postpartum cows and/or heifers are ready, not only for natural service (NS) but also before the initiation of assisted reproductive technologies, such as estrus synchronization protocols for FTAI, superovulation protocols for *in vivo* -derived embryos and/or *in vitro* embryo production. BCS and nutrition are important factors that should be considered to evaluate, account that BCS should be 5–7 at the beginning of the season to ensure the likelihood of reproductive success.

In heifers, reproductive tract scoring (RTS) is a valid method to determine reproductive size development and maturation (Anderson et al., 1991). RTS uses rectal palpation and/or ultrasonography to determine size of the uterine horns and the structures that are present on the ovary (1 = no palpable follicles, 2 = 8 mm follicles, 3 = 8–10 mm follicles, 4 = >10 mm follicles and possibly a corpus luteum [CL], 5 =CL present; Anderson, 1991). In a recent publication (Gutierrez et al., 2014) including 15 months old Angus cross heifers (n=4041), reported the effect of RTS on reproductive efficiency in heifers bred by FTAI and NS (AI-NS) or only NS (ONS). In this study, heifers of AI-NS group were synchronized for FTAI (n=2660) and two weeks later were exposed to bulls (bull-to-heifer ratio= 1:40–1:50) for the reminder of the 85-day breeding season. Angus cross heifers (n=1381) in ONS group were submitted to bulls (bull-to heifer ratio= 1:20–1:25) for 85-day breeding season. Assessment of the reproductive tract score by palpation was done 4 weeks pre-breeding to categorize the females. Results showed that in AI-NS group pregnancy rate was significantly different per FTAI between RTS 1, 2 and 3 (44.2%) *vs.* 4 and 5 (61.9%); also, BS pregnancy rate was higher in heifers of RTS

4 and 5 than those of RTS 1 and 2 (90.4, 95.2% *vs.* 81.2%, for RTS 4, 5, and 1–2, respectively). Furthermore, BS pregnancy rate in ONS group was higher in heifers of RTS 4 and 5 (88.4 and 90.2%, respectively) than RTS 1, 2 and 3 (79.7 and 84.3%, respectively). More else, authors hypothesized that the use of synchronization protocol might have induced cyclicity in pre- and peripubertal heifers in AI-NS group and aided to achieve higher pregnancy rate.

Natural service is the most popular management for BS in beef cattle. In Argentina and Brazil, 88% of females of reproductive age are exposed to clean-up bulls for a natural breeding (Baruselli et al., 2018). The bull:cow ratio frequently used by producers in Argentina (Región Pampeana) is 3–4% (Acuña et al., 2014), for the remainder of 60–90 days of the breeding season. Bulls are evaluated before the BS for reducing the risk of using low fertility ones. Breeding soundness evaluations (BBSEs) are low-cost screening methods to ensure the bull's health and fertility (reviewed by Barth, 2018) and with this method practitioners could check maturity, BCS, physical abnormalities, scrotal circumference and risks of venereal or infectious diseases that could be present in sires.

The anestrus at the initiation of spring BS will be a negative effect to reach higher pregnancy rate and can affect the profitability of cattlemen. Exogenous administration of progesterone by insertion of intravaginal progesterone-release devices (Fig. 1.2), with or without the addition of equine chorionic gonadotropin (eCG), have demonstrated improvement in estrus synchrony and reduction in the interval parturition-conception (Lucy et al., 2001; Gutierrez et al., 2014; Baruselli et al., 2018). Recently, Ferreira et al. (2018) proposed different progesterone synchronization treatments (with or without eCG) used before a 98 day-NS, called timed natural breeding (TNB) in *Bos inducus* postpartum beef cows. In this publication, control cows (without treatment) were less likely to be pregnant the first 21 days of the NS (Table 1.1). Also, they concluded that the use of TNB, efficiently improved the early conception of postpartum beef cows, suggesting that TNB may have increased LH pulses frequency and anticipating cyclicity. Further, the association of eCG enhanced follicular growth, ovulation rate and pregnancy rate after the synchronization protocol. Similar data were reported by our group (without eCG; Pérez Wallace, et al., 2016) and by other colleges (with or without eCG; Hugenine et al., 2017), in which the TNB treatment improved reproductive efficiency in *Bos taurus* postpartum beef cows with 95% of anestrus at the beginning of the spring

BS (Table 1.1). Consequently, TNB is a recommended practice that might improve pregnancy rate not only in postpartum beef cows but also in beef heifers. These practices are especially useful in grass- feeding systems, in which low BCS generates anestrus, affecting negatively the reproductive outcomes. Moreover, higher pregnancy rates achieved during first 21 days of BS will ensure greater percentage of earlier calves calving, weaning heavier calves and helping cows to recover more rapidly after parturition for the next BS.

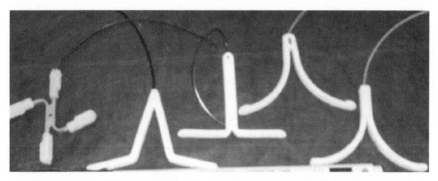

FIGURE 1.2 Five different models of intravaginal progesterone-releasing device commercially available in Argentina. From the left side to the right: Cronipres® Monodosis (0.558 g of progesterone; Biogénesis Bagó, Garín, Buenos Aires, Argentina); DIB® 1 g Syntex (1.0 g of progesterone; Zoetis, Buenos Aires, Argentina); CIDR® (1.9 g of progesterone; Zoetis, Buenos Aires, Argentina); Emefur® monodosis (0.6 g of progesterone; Boehringer Ingelheim Animal Health Argentina S.A., Buenos Aires, Argentina); and Pluselar 0.6 (0.6 g of progesterone, Laboratorio Calier de Argentina SA, Buenos Aires, Argentina).

TABLE 1.1 Pregnancy Rate During the First 21 Days of Breeding Season of Postpartum Beef Cows Treated with Progesterone-Based Protocol (TNB) or Non-Treated (control), Exposed To Natural Service.

TNB	TNB+eCG	Control	sp	Author
48.1% (26/52)[a]	-	20.0% (9/45)[b]	*Bos taurus*	Pérez Wallace et al., 2016
19.4% (13/67)[c]	43.5% (27/62)[d]	12.2% (9/74)[e]	*Bos taurus*	Hugenine et al., 2017
30.4% (35/115)[f]	51.8% (58/112)[g]	5.7% (7/123)[h]	*Bos indicus*	Ferreira et al., 2018

Timed natural breeding (TNB) and TNB + equine chorionic gonadotropin (eCG) cows received an estradiol and progesterone, based protocol treatment to synchronize follicular wave emergence and ovulation with or without eCG, respectively. Control cows received no prior protocol treatment. Different superscript letters indicate differ significant at the P value ($P < 0.05$).

1.3 ARTIFICIAL INSEMINATION IN BEEF CATTLE

Artificial insemination (AI) is an old technique used massively to disseminate genetics among beef and dairy herds. AI has many advantages compared with NS. It avoids the transmission of venereal diseases, enables the use of high merit genetic expensive sires, increases calf uniformity and increases genetic gain resulting in more productive future calves. In Argentina, AI programs based on heat detection (HD) were widely used in beef industry in the 80's and 90's in a reduced number of beef cattle, primarily in beef heifers. Traditionally, the standing estrus or "heat" (18–24 h) is recognized in postpartum cows or postpuberal heifers when sexual activity begins, that is when bull or others female is accepted for the first time. Ovulation occurs normally at 24–32 h after the onset of estrus and then a brief period begins in which the oocyte can be fertilized (Reviewed by Nebel, 2012). On account of biological events, the proper timing of insemination in cattle is associated with the moment of ovulation and the viability of gametes (Fig. 1.3). AI performed between 4–16 h after the estrus initiation results in acceptable pregnancy rates and the HD will be critical for the success of the technique (Fig. 1.3). Nevertheless, the implementation of AI programs based on HD in beef cattle is laborious and difficult and requires observation at least twice a day by experimented personnel. Although, the HD + AI is hampered by postpartum anestrous, the large size of many farms and the labor cost reduce the reproductive efficiency of the herd (Bó et al., 2007). Therefore, during the last 15 years, HD based-AI programs have been replaced by a variety of treatment strategies that allow insemination at a predetermined time (FTAI) eliminating the need for HD and allowing insemination of beef cows regardless of cyclic status (Bó et al., 2016).

1.3.1 PROGRAMS FOR FIXED-TIME ARTIFICIAL INSEMINATION IN BEEF CATTLE

Basically, there are two types of FTAI treatment protocols currently used in beef cattle: GnRH-based and estradiol-based protocols, both of which are combined with progesterone devices (Fig. 1.4). Estradiol-based protocols are used in South America and in beef herds in Australia, whereas GnRH-based protocols tend to be used in North America, Europe and New Zealand, where the use of estradiol is prohibited. In South America, FTAI programs increased dramatically and at the present ~15,000,000 FTAI have been performed in Argentina, Brazil, Paraguay and Uruguay.

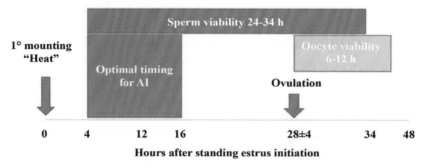

FIGURE 1.3 Biological events associated with the ideal timing for artificial insemination in the cow (adapted and modified from Nebel, 2012).

Estradiol-based treatments consist of insertion of a progesterone-releasing device and the administration of 2 mg of estradiol benzoate (EB) on Day 0, to induce follicle regression and synchronize the emergence of a new follicular wave 3–5 days later (Bó et al., 2007). On Day 7 or 8, progesterone device is withdrawal and prostaglandin $F_2\alpha$ ($PGF_2\alpha$) is administered to ensure luteolysis, and the subsequent application of 1 mg EB 24 h later (ovulation inducer) or 0.5 mg (beef heifers and cyclic cows) or 1 mg (postpartum anestrous cows) estradiol cypionate (ECP) at the time of progesterone device removal to synchronize ovulation (Colazo et al., 2003; Uslenghi et al., 2016; Fig. 4). In a recent report from Argentina, 431,008 FTAI synchronized with estradiol-based protocols, showed a mean pregnancy rate of 50.4% (Bó et al., 2016). As most FTAI programs are applied to suckling beef cows in South America, the use of eCG at the time of removal of progesterone device improves the pregnancy rate outcome (Baruselli et al., 2004; Bó et al., 2013). The beneficial effect of eCG administered to a progesterone and estradiol-based protocol in anestrus beef cows were the increasing in: (1) ovulation rate, (2) ovulatory follicle diameter, (3) growth follicular rate and (4) area and serum progesterone concentration during subsequent early and mid-luteal phase (Baruselli et a., 2004; Núñez-Olivera et al., 2014). For practical recommendations, the ideal moment to initiate a FTAI program should be ~40–45 days after calving with the addition of eCG (400 UI) when BCS is low or a high percentage of animals present anestrus in suckled postpartum beef cows.

The recommended doses of eCG for beef heifers should be 300 UI if BCS is low and/or if anestrus rate is elevated in the lot.

GnRH-based treatment protocols that were developed for dairy cows are widely used in North America and Europe in beef cattle (Geary and Whittier, 2001; Day et al., 2012). The treatment consists of the administration of GnRH analogues (busereline acetate or gonadoreline acetate) and insertion of a progesterone device on Day 0 to induce ovulation of a dominant follicle (>10 mm) if there is one present, with emergence of a new follicular wave 1.5–2 days later. $PGF_2\alpha$ is given 7 days later to induce luteolysis and in beef cattle a second dose of GnRH is administered at the time of FTAI on Day 9 (54–66 h later) to synchronize ovulation (Day et al., 2012; Bó et al., 2016). Protocols based on GnRH and $PGF_2\alpha$ are generically named Co-Synch (Fig. 1.4). A recent modification of the traditional 7 day-Co-synch protocol, is a novel protocol (Fig. 1.4) that reduced the time of insertion of the progesterone device to 5 days instead of 7 days plus a double injection of $PGF_2\alpha$ 12 h apart (to ensure the luteolysis of immature CL or "accessory CL" with the application of the initial GnRH), and prolonged the proestrous period (FTAI 72 h after progesterone device removal) with a subsequent increased of circulating estrogen levels and higher progesterone concentrations in the subsequent luteal phase, named 5-day Co-Synch (Bridges et al., 2008; 2012; 2014). Bridges et al. (2008) compared a 7-day Co-Synch protocol plus progesterone device with FTAI at 60 h and a 5-day Co-Synch protocol plus progesterone device with FTAI 72 h in postpartum beef cows. Across experiments, 5-day Co-Synch increased FTAI pregnancy rate by 10.5% over the 7-day Co-synch protocol (70.4% [214/304] and 59.9% [187/312], respectively; P<0.05). Similar results were reported by Whittier et al. (2013), in a study carried out in Angus beef cows (n=1817), in which cows synchronized with the 5-day Co-Synch had higher FTAI pregnancy rate (58.1%) than those that received the 7-day Co-Synch (55.1%; P=0.04). The 5-day Co-synch protocol is available to synchronize beef heifers, achieving acceptable FTAI pregnancy rate (Perry et al., 2012). Omission of the initial GnRH and a single dose of $PGF_2\alpha$ would be advantageous to simplify the 5-day Co-Synch in beef heifers. However, results are contradictories indicating a negative effect by the omission of GnRH at Day 0 in beef heifers in one study (Kasimanikam et al., 2014), while non-effect was reported in pregnancy rate in yearling beef heifers in other (Cruppe et al., 2014). Nevertheless, either a single or double dose of $PGF_2\alpha$ resulted in similar FTAI pregnancy rate in both publications (Cruppe et al., 2014; Kasimanikam et al., 2014).

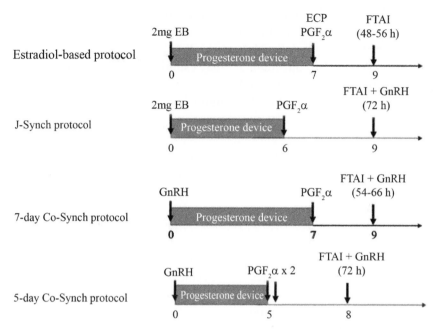

FIGURE 1.4 Common synchronizing programs for fixed-time AI in beef cattle. EB = estradiol benzoate; ECP = estradiol cypionate; $PGF_2\alpha$ = prostaglandin $F_2\alpha$; GnRH = gonadotropin releasing hormone; Progesterone device = intravaginal progesterone-releasing device; FTAI = fixed-time artificial insemination. Estradiol benzoate + progesterone treatments are used to regress follicles and induce a new follicular wave emergence few days later (3–5). With GnRH administration, if a dominant follicle greater than 10 mm is present on the ovaries, produces the ovulation and the emergence of a new follicular wave few days later (1.5–2). $PGF_2\alpha$ injection at device removal is used to induce luteolysis and collaborates together with ovulatory inducers (GnRH or ECP) to synchronize the ovulation of a dominant follicle. FTAI could be carried out at a predefined timing without the necessity of estrus detection.

A recent strategy proposed by our group, was to investigate for extending proestrus in an estradiol and progesterone-based estrous synchronization protocol in *Bos taurus* beef heifers which has been named J-Synch (de la Mata and Bó, 2012; Fig. 1.4). The treatment consists of the administration of 2 mg EB at the time of insertion of a progesterone device that is removed 6 days later. A single dose of $PGF_2\alpha$ is given at device removal, and animals receive GnRH at the time of FTAI, 72 h later (Day 9; de la Mata and Bó, 2012; de la Mata et al., 2018). In several studies (de la Mata and Bó, 2012, de la Mata et al., 2018; Ré et al., 2014; Núñez Olivera et al., 2016; Sanz et al., 2019) heifers submitted to J-Synch protocol had: lengthen duration of proestrus (period between progesterone source removal up to ovulation) that lasted 94–105 h (de la Mata and Bó, 2012; Ré et al., 2014; de la Mata et al., 2018), higher pregnancy rates in comparison with the conventional 7-day estradiol and progesterone-based protocol (de la Mata et al., 2018) or 5-day Co-Synch protocol (Sanz et al., 2019 in press) in FTAI. These improvements in heifers treated with J-Synch was related to an increased rate of growth of preovualtory follicle, greater progesterone concentrations during subsequent luteal phase and a differential uterine gene functionality expression that promoted a healthier milieu for embryo development (de la Mata et al., 2018).

In summary, from a practical point of view, practitioners and producers count with a vast knowledge in issues referred synchronizing ovulation for FTAI in beef cattle. The use of either GnRH-based or estradiol-based protocols with the insertion of progesterone release-device is an effective strategy to enhance reproductive beef heifers and postpartum anestrus beef cows, and pregnancy outcomes would achieve 50–60% (Bó et al., 2018a). A multiplicity of factors such female physiological status, nutrition, BCS, semen quality, synchronization treatment protocol, and the practitioner's experience will affect the success of the technique for maximizing the improved genetics in a herd.

1.4 USE OF SEXED-SORTED SEMEN IN BEEF CATTLE: UPDATE OF NEW TECHNOLOGIES

Sex ratio of resulting progeny through NS or trough FTAI programs is genetically controlled, and naturally the probability of male calf's births is higher than the female births. Field data from an Argentinian Angus stud that accumulates a total of 6713 calves birth registrations, informed 48.5% females calving and 51.5% males calving (personal communication). Sexed-semen sorted by flow cytometer/cell sorting technology is commercially available from many years ago with about 90% accuracy without unduly damage of sperm (Seidel, 2003). In the past, the use of sexed-sorted semen (XY Legacy method) in breeding programs had a compromised fertility because of sperm damage and fewer sperm concentration used per insemination dose (Seidel, 2013) and the recommendations were to apply HD and AI programs only in heifers. New methods have been developed in semen handling and processing before, during and after the sorting process. New machines have enhanced digital electronics with considerable automation, and these multiple changes have led to a new product called SexedULTRA (Vishwanath, 2015; Vishwanath and Moreno, 2018). Data of three years of experience in New Zealand using liquid-stored SexedULTRA semen (1 million total sex-sorted) into dairy cows (n=34,600) reported high pregnancy rates raising fertility to 65–67% (Vishwanath, 2015). Also, Vishwanath and Moreno (2018) reported an improvement of conception rates when Holstein heifers were inseminated in huge field trials of commercial herds in the United States and in Germany. The new SexdULTRA with 4 million sperm per dose achieved higher pregnancy rates when it was compared with the old XY Legacy technology, and results were comparable to those achieved by conventional non-sexed semen with 15 million sperm per dose (55.9% *vs.* 66.7% *vs.* 66.5%, for XY Legacy method, SexedULTRA 4 M and Conventional 15 M, respectively; P<0.01).

In beef cattle, various experiments have been reported (Table 1.2) comparing the field fertility of new technology SexedULTRA with 4 million sperm per dose in beef heifers and suckled beef cows (Thomas et al., 2017; Bó et al., 2018a,b; Crites et al., 2018; Silva et al., 2018; Thomas et al., 2019). Besides different synchronization protocols for FTAI have been used among publications, some practical considerations must be taken. In general, conventional non-sexed semen achieved higher significant pregnancy rates among studies (~10%) and fertility with SexedULTRA was improved when split-timing AI programs were applied using tail painting or patches on the top of the tail to detect rubbed off. In this way, delaying the time of AI closer to the time of ovulation or limiting the AI with SexedULTRA to those animals showing estrus would result in pregnancy rate AI between 40 and 50% or even higher. Also, bull intrinsic fertility was determinant to attain higher pregnancy rates (Thomas et al., 2017; Bó et al., 2018a). Even though, SexedULTRA pregnancy rates did not overcome conventional non-sexed semen in FTAI programs, average pregnancy rates of the major data of publications tend to approximate to 50%, confirming that this new technology is suitable for commercial purpose. Additionally, the potential usage of the sexed-sorted semen to generate productive animals aims to produce high-merit bulls or heifers from certain sire or dam combination or to produce crossbred high-quality carcass steers. These will maximize the utilization of sexed-sorted semen for genetic improvements in the beef cattle industry.

TABLE 1.2   Field Results of Fertility Comparing the Use of SexedULTRA Semen *vs.* Conventional (Non-Sexed) Semen in Beef Heifers and Beef Suckled Cows Synchronized with Different Protocols for Fixed-Time AI.

Protocol	Cat.	n	Sexed ULTRA (4 million)	Conven- tional (Non-sexed)	P-value	Author
14 d-CIDR	Heifers[a]	951	52.0%	60.0%	<0.05	Thomas et al., 2017
J-Synch+eCG	Heifers[a]	850	49.3%	58.3%	<0.05	Bó et al., 2018
7-d Co-Synch	Both[b]	394	49.2%	56.7%	>0.1	Crites et al., 2018
7-d E2+EB	Cows[c]	294	49.0%	52.4%	<0.01	Silva et al., 2018
7-d E2+ECP	Cows[c]	297	51.0%	68.2%	<0.01	Silva et al., 2018
J-Synch+eCG	Cows[c]	662	40.8%	65.8%	<0.05	Bó et al., 2019
7-d Co-Synch	Cows[c]	1,620	47.9%	64.6%	<0.01	Thomas et al., 2019

[a] Indicates beef heifers.
[b] Indicates suckled beef cows and beef heifers.
[c] Indicates suckled beef cows.

KEYWORDS

- **beef heifers and cows**
- **synchronization of the ovulation**
- **fixed-time artificial insemination**
- **natural breeding**
- **sex-sorted semen**

REFERENCES

Acuña, C. M.; Rojas Panelo, M.; Mendonça, C. The Use of Very High Serving Capacity Bulls to Achieve a High Early Pregnancy Rate in Suckling Beef Cows. *Taurus.* **2014,** 16, 20–24.

Anderson, K. J.; LeFever, D. G.; Brinks, J. S.; Odde, K. G. The Use of Reproductive Tract Scoring in Beef Heifers. *Agri Pract.* **1991,** *12,* 19–26.

Barth, A. Review: The Use of Bull Breeding Soundness Evaluation to Identify Subfertile and Infertile Bulls. *Animal* **2018,** *12,* pp. 158–164.

Baruselli, P. S.; Reis, E. L.; Marques, O. M.; Nasser, L. F.; Bó, G. A. The Use of Hormonal Treatments to Improve Reproductive Performance of Anestrous Beef Cattle in Tropical Climates. *Anim. Reprod. Sci.* **2004,** *82–83,* 479–486.

Baruselli, P. S.; Ferreira, R. M.; Sá Filho, M. F. and Bó. G. A. Review: Using artificial insemination v. natural service in beef herds. *Animal.* **2018**, *12*, pp 45–52.

Bó, G. A.; Cutaia, L.; Tríbulo, R. Hormonal Treatments for Fixed Time Artificial Insemination in Beef Cattle: Some Experiments in Argentina. *Taurus.* **2002**, *15*, 17–32.

Bó, G. A.; Cutaia L.; Peres, L. C.; Pincinato D.; Maraña, D.; Baruselli, O. S. Technologies for Fixed-Time Artificial Insemination and Their Influence on Reproductive Performance of Bos indicus Cattle. In *Reproduction in Domestic Ruminants VI.* Juenguel J. L., Murray J. F., Smith M. F. Eds., Nottingham University Press: Nottingham, UK, **2007**. pp 223–236.

Bó, G. A.; Baruselli, P. S.; Mapletoft, R. J. Synchronization Techniques to Increase the Utilization of Artificial Insemination in Beef and Dairy Cattle. *Anim Reprod.* **2013**, *10*, 137–142.

Bó, G. A.; de la Mata, J. J.; Baruselli, P. S.; Menchaca, A. Alternative Programs for Synchronizing and Resynchronizing Ovulation in Beef Cattle. *Theriogenology.* **2016**, *86*, 388–396.

Bó, G. A.; Hugenine, E.; de la Mata J. J.; Núñez-Olivera, R.; Baruselli, P. S.; Menchaca, A. Programs for Fixed-Time Artificial Insemination in South American Beef Cattle. *Anim Reprod.* **2018a**, *15*, 952–962.

Bó, G. A.; Huguenine, E. E.; de la Mata, J. J.; de Carneiro, R. L. R.; Menchaca, A. Pregnancy Rates in Suckled Beef Cows Synchronized with a Shortened Progesterone/Oestradiol-Based Protocol (J-synch) and Inseminated with Conventional or Sexed-Sorted Semen. *Reprod. Fert. Dev.* **2018b**, *31*, 129–129 (abstract 7).

Bridges, G. A.; Helser, L. A.; Grum, D. E.; Mussard, M. L.; Gasser, C. L.; and Day, M. L. Decreasing the Interval Between GnRH and PGF$_2\alpha$ from 7 to 5 Days and Lengthening Proestrus Increases Timed-AI Pregnancy Rates in Beef Cows. *Theriogenology.* **2008**, *69*, 843–851.

Bridges, G. A.; Mussard, M. L.; Pate, J. L.; Ott, T. L.; Hansen, T. R.; Day, M. L. Impact of Preovulatory Estradiol Concentrations on Conceptus Development and Uterine Gene Espression. *Anim. Reprod. Sci.* **2012**, 133, 16–26.

Bridges, G. A.; Mussard, M. L.; Hesler, L. A.; Day, M. L. Comparison of Follicular Dynamics and Hormone Concentrations Between the 7-Day and 5-Day CO-Synch + CIDR Program in Primiparous Beef Cows. *Theriogenology.* **2014**, *81*, 632–638.

Colazo, G. M.; Kastelic, J. P.; Mapletoft, R. J. Effects of Estradiol Cypionate (ECP) on Ovarian Follicular Dynamics, Synchrony of Ovulation, and Fertility in Cidr-Based, Fixed-Time AI Programs in Beef Heifers. *Theriogenology.* **2003**, *60*, 855–865.

Crites, B. R.; Vishwanath, R.; Arnett, A. M.; Bridges, P. J.; Burris, W. R.; McLeod, K. R.; Anderson, L. H. Conception Risk of Beef Cattle after Fixed-Time Artificial Insemination Using Either SexedUltra™ 4M Sex-Sorted Semen or Conventional Semen *Theriogenology.* **2018**, *118*, 126–129.

Crowe, M. A.; Diskin, M. G.; Williams, E. J. Parturition to Resumption of Ovarian Cyclicity: Comparative Aspects of Beef and Dairy Cows. *Animal.* **2014**, 8 (1), pp 40–53.

Cruppe, L. H.; Day, M. L.; Abreu, F. M.; Kruse, S.; Lake, S. L.; Biehl, M. V.; Cipriano, R. S.; Mussard, M. L.;Bridges, G. A. The Requirement of GnRH at the Beginning of the Five-Day CO-Synch + Controlled Internal Drug Release Protocol in Beef Heifers. *J. Anim. Sci.* **2014**, *92*, 4198–4203.

Day, M.L. State of the art of GnRH-based timed AI in beef cattle. *Anim. Reprod.* **2012**, *79*, 1–4.

de la Mata, J.J. y Bó, G.A. Sincronización de celos y ovulación utilizando un protocolo de benzoato de estradiol y GnRH en periodos reducidos de inserción de un dispositivo con progesterona en vaquillonas para carne. *Taurus.* **2012**, *55,* 17–23.

de la Mata, J. J.; Núñez-Olivera, R.; Cuadro, F.; Bosolasco, D.; de Brun, V.; Meikle, A.; Bó, G. A., Menchaca, A. Effects of Extending the Length of Pro-Oestrus in Ano Estradiol-and Progesterone-Based Oestrus Synchronisation Programo N Ovarian Function, Uterine Environment and Pregnancy Establishment in Beef Heifers. *Reprod. Fert. Dev.* **2018**, *30,* 1541–1552.

D'Occhio, M. J.; Baruselli, P. S.; Campanile, G. Influence of Nutrition, Body Condition, and Metabolic Status on Reproduction in Female Beef Cattle: A Review. *Theriogenology* **2019**, 125, 277–284.

Ferreira, R. M.; Conti, T. L.; Gonçalves, R. L.; Souto, L. A.; Sales, J. N. S.; Sá Filho, M. F.; Elliff, F. M.; Baruselli, P. S. Synchronization Treatments Previous to Natural Breeding Anticipate and Improve the Pregnancy Rate of Postpartum Primiparous Beef Cows. *Theriogenology* **2018**, 114, 206–211.

Geary, T. W. and Whittier, P. A. S. Effects of a timed insemination following synchronization of ovulation using the Ovsynch or CO-Synch protocol in beef cows. *The Professional Animal Scientist* **2001**, *14,* 217–220.

Gutierrez, K.; Kasimanickam, R.; Tibary, A.; Gay, J. M.; Kastelic, J. P.; Hall, J. B.; Whittier, W. D. Effect of Reproductive Tract Scoring on Reproductive Efficiency in Beef Heifers Bred by Timed Insemination and Natural Service Versus Only Natural Service. *Theriogenology* **2014**, *81,* 918–924.

Herd, D. B. and Sprott, L. R. Body Condition, Nutrition and Reproduction Of Beef Cows. Texas Agricultural Extension Service. Texas A & M Univ 1986; B-1526.

Hugenine, E.; Cledou, G.; Bó, G. A. and Callejas, S. Effect of Progesterone Intravaginal Device Combined with eCG upon Pregnancy Anestrous Cows During Breeding Season. *Taurus* **2017**, *76,* 28–31.

Kasimanickam, R. K.; Firth, P.; Schuenemann, G. M.; Whitlock, B. K.; Gay, J. M.; Moore, D. A.; Hall, J. B.; Whittier, W. D. Effect of the First GnRH and Two Doses of PGF$_2\alpha$ in a 5-day Progesterone-Based CO-Synch Protocol on Heifer Pregnancy. *Theriogenology.* **2014**, *81,* 797–804.

Lemos Motta, J. C.; Colli, M. H. A.; Penteado, L.; Bayeux, B. M.; Mingoti, R. D; Bó, G. A.; Lugo, L. C.; Rezende, R. G.; Baruselli, P. S. Pregnancy Rate to FTAI in Nelore and Crossbreed Heifers Submitted to J-Synch protocol (6 days). Proceedings of the 30th Annual of the Brazilian Embryo Technology Society (SBTE); Foz de Iguaçu, PR, Brasil, August 25th to 27th, and Meeting of the European Embryo Transfer Association (AETE); Barcelona, Spain, September 9th and 10th, **2016**. pp 401 (abstract).

Lucy, M. C.; Billings, H. J.; Butler, W. R.; Ehnis, L. R.; Fields, M. J.; Kesler, D. J.; Kinder, J. E.; Mattos, R. C.; Short, R. E.; Thatcher, W. W.; Wettemann, R. P.; Yelich, J. V.; and Hafs, H. D. Efficacy of an Intravaginal Progesterone Insert and an Injection of PGF$_2\alpha$ for Synchronizing Estrus and Shortening the Interval to Pregnancy in Postpartum Beef Cows, Peripubertal Beef Heifers and Dairy Heifers. *J. Anim. Sci.* **2001**, *79,* 982–995.

Meikle, A.; de Brun, V.; Carriquiry, M.; Soca, P.; Sosa, C.; de Lourdes Adrien, M.; Chilibroste, P.; Abecia, J. Influences of Nutrition and Metabolism on Reproduction of the Female Ruminant. *Anim. Reprod.* **2018**, *15,* 899–911.

Nebel, R. L. Detección de cello y momento de inseminación artificial. Memorias de las Sextas Jornadas Taurus de Reproducción Bovina 13 y 14 de septiembre de 2012, Ciudad Autónoma de Buenos Aires, Argentina. **2012**, pp. 16–23.

Núñez-Olivera, R.; de Castro, T.; Gracía-Pintos, C.; Bó, G.A.; Piaggio, J.; Menchaca, A. Ovulatory Response and Luteal Function After ecG Adminsitration at the End of a Progesterone and Estradiol' Based Treatment in Postpartum Anestrous Beef Cattle. *Anim. Reprod. Sci.* **2014**, *146*, 111–116.

Núñez-Olivera, R.; Bó, G. A.; Menchaca, A. 2016. Association Between Proestrus Length, Preovulatory Folicular Diameter, Estrus Behavior and Pregnancy Rate in Progesterone-Estradiol' based Treatment J-Synch for FTAI in Bos taurus Beef Heifers. 18th International Congress on Animal Reproduction (ICAR), June 26–30th, **2016**, Tours, France. pp 447–478 (Asbtract).

Pérez Wallace, S.; de la Mata, J. J.; de la Mata, C. A.; Cutaia, L. Effect of Intravaginal Progesterone Device or Intramuscular Injection of Progesterone on the Reproductive Performance in Lactating Aberdeen Angus Cows in Bull Breeding Soundness. Proceedings of the 3rd International Congress of the Sociedad Argentina de Tecnologías Embrionarias (SATE), June 2–3, **2016**, Universidad Católica Argentina, Ciudad Autónoma de Buenos Aires, Argentina. pp 150–151 (abstract).

Perry, G. A.; Grant, J. K.; Walker, J. A.; Bridges, G. A.; Kruse, S. G.; Bird, S.; Heaton, K.; Arias, R.; Lake, S. L. Comparison of Three CIDR Based Fixed-Time AI Protocols for Beef Heifers. *J. Anim. Sci.* **2012**, *90* (suppl. 3), 237 (abstract).

Perry, G. A. and Cushman, R. Effect of Age at Puberty/Conception Date on Cow Longevity. *Veterinary Clinics of North America: Food Animal Practice.***2013**, *29*, 579–590.

Pincinato, D.; Peres, L. C.; Lorentz, L.; Santana, G. S.; Machado, M. K.; Borges, A. J.; Lacerda, L. S.; Bó. G. A. Pregnancy Rates in Nelore Heifers Using a Shortened Estradiol/Progesterone-Based Protocol that Provides for a Lengthened Proestrus (J-Synch). *Anim Reprod.* **2018**, *15*, 350–350 (abstract).

Ré, M.; de la Mata, J. J.; and Bó, G. A. Synchronization of Ovulation in Dairy Heifers Using a Shortened Estradiol-Based Protocol That Provides for A Lengthened Proestrus. *Reprod. Fert. Dev.* **2014**, *26* (abstract 118).

Sanz, A.; Macmillan, K.; y Colazo, M. G. Revisión de los programas de sincronización ovárica basados en el uso de hormona liberadora de gonadotropinas y prostaglandina $F_2\alpha$ para novillas de leche y de carne. *ITEA-Inf. Tec. Econ. Agrar.* **2019**. *115*(4), 326–341.

Seidel Jr., G. E. Sexing Mammalian Sperm—Intertwining Of Commerce, Technology, And Biology. *Anim Reprod Sci.* **2003**, *79*, 145–156.

Seidel Jr., G. E. Application of Sex-selected Semen in Heifer Development and Breeding Programs. *Vet. Clin. North Am. Food. Anim. Pract.* **2013**, *29*, 619–625.

Short, R. E.; Bellows, R. A.; Staigmiller, R. B.; et al. Physiological Mechanisms Controlling Anestrus and Infertility in Postpartum Beef Cattle. *J. Anim. Sci.* **1990**, *68*, 799–816.

Silva, M. A. V.; Santos, C. S.; França, I. G.; Pereira, H. G.; Sá Filho, M. F.; Freitas, B. G.; Guerreiro, B. M.; Faquim, A.; Baruselli, P. S.; Torres-Júnior, J. R. S. Hormonal Strategy to Reduce Suckled Beef Cow Handling for Timed Artificial Insemination with Sex-Sorted Semen. *Theriogenology.* **2018**, *114*, 159–164.

Thomas, J. M.; Locke, J. W. C.; Vishwanath, R.; Hall, J. B.; Ellersieck, M. R.; Smith, M. F.; Paterson, D. J. Effective Use of SexedULTRA Sexed-Sorted Semen for Timed Artificial Insemination of Beef Heifers. *Theriogenology* **2017**, *98*, 88–93.

Thomas, J.M.; Locke, J.W.C.; Bonacker, R.C.; Knickmeyer, E.R.; Wilson. D.J.; Vishwanath, R.; Arnett, A. M.; Smith, M. F.; Patterson, D. J. Evaluation of SexedULTRA 4M™ Sex-Sorted Semen in Timed Artificial Insemination Programs for Mature Beef Cows. *Theriogenology* **2019,** *123,* 100–107.

Uslenghi, G.; Vater, A.; Rodríguez Aguilar, S.; Cabodevila, J.; Callejas, S. Effect of Estradiol Cypionate and GnRH Treatment on Plasma Estradiol-17 β Concentrations, Synchronization of Ovulation and on Pregnancy Rates in Suckled Beef Cows Treated with FTAI-Based Protocols. *Reprod. Domest. Anim.* **2016,** *51,* 693–699.

Vishwanath, R.. Sexed Sperm *vs.* Conventional Sperm- A Comparative Discussion. Proceedings, Applied Reproductive Strategies in Beef Cattle. August 17 & 18, **2015,** Davis, CA, USA. https://beefrepro.unl.edu/proceedings.html.

Vishwanath, R.; Moreno, J. F. Review: Semen Sexing—Current State of the Art with Emphasis on Bovine Species. Theory to Practice—International Bull Fertility Conference 27–30 May 2018, Westport, Ireland. *Animal.* **2018,** *12*(Supplement s1), 85–96.

Whitthier, W. D.; Currin, J. F.; Schramm, H.; Holland, S.; Kasimanickam R. Fertility in Angus Cross Beef Cows Following 5-day CO-Synch + CIDR or 7-day CO-Synch + CIDR estrus Synchronization and Timed Artificial Insemination. *Theriogenology* **2013,** *80,* 963–969.

CHAPTER 2

Ultrasonography in Bovine Gynecology

GIOVANNI GNEMMI[1,2*], JUAN CARLOS GARDÓN[2], and
CRISTINA MARABOLI[1]

[1]Bovinevet Internacional, Bovine Ultrasound Services and Herd
Management, Calle de la Mecanica, 9, Huesca, 22006, Huesca, Spain

[2]Department of Animal Medicine and Surgery, Faculty of Veterinary
and Experimental Sciences Catholic University of Valencia,
San Vincente Mártir, Spain

*Corresponding author. E-mail: giovanni.gnemmi@bovinevet.com

ABSTRACT

Ultrasound is an indispensable tool today for the reproductive management of cattle (dairy and beef). It is a collateral examination, which by itself cannot and does not pretend to be the answer to the reproductive problems of the farm. Ultrasound can reduce the margin of error encountered with the manual evaluation of the uterus and ovaries, a margin of error that is only partially attributable to individual capabilities.

This extraordinary technique allows for real-time responses in any environmental condition, as it is a flexible technique. It is a technique that is easily repeatable and allows many services to be produced on farms. Thanks to the introduction of ultrasound in the reproductive management of the herd, it is possible to safeguard both the concept of animal welfare and that of food safety. This is mainly due to the accurate and timely use of antibiotic and hormonal therapies, thanks to an extremely precise diagnosis, as only ultrasound can achieve.

2.1   INTRODUCTION

The need to use or not the ultrasound in bovine gynecology is being discussed all over the world. Although ultrasonography has been proposed as a collateral examination in bovine reproduction (Pierson et al., 1984a, b; Pierson et al., 1986; 1987) for about 30 years, about 40% of the veterinaries working in gynecology (Gnemmi et al., 2005), use this tool.

Why is this technique so hard to succeed in boring? Are there "scientific" reasons that do not recommend its use? Is it still possible to deal with bovine gynecology, without using this technique? What services should "offer" to customers? These are just some of the questions that are asked when we talk about ultrasonography applied to bovine reproductive management.

2.2   ULTRASONOGRAPHIC UNITS AND PRACTICAL RECOMMENDATIONS

2.2.1   ULTRASOUND UNITS

The ultrasound units can be divided into non-portable and portable models.

The non-portable units are tools of great bulk and weight (20–30 kg), which on the one hand guarantee an extraordinary image quality, on the other they are not usable easily in field conditions, but they can find their place by working in fixed positions, or in the research area.

The portable units, in turn, can be divided into portable and ultra-portable. The weight of these units it is between 3.0–12.0 kg. Higher weight instruments require a transport trolley and, normally, line current: both situations limit their use in the field.

In conditions of extensive breeding, where the animals are subjected to gynecological examination in fixed locations, these instruments still find their place of use. Even the power supply problem can be overcome brilliantly, using an inverter and then a 12-volt battery.

Today there are 3.0–5.0 kg portable units, with good portability and autonomy, being equipped with an internal battery (2.5–4 h of work). This is a new generation of instruments, which have all the qualities of non-portable units, also guaranteeing less weight and a smaller size. They have LCD screens, some even touch screens.

The ultra-portable units de facto have allowed the use of ultrasonography in filed condition. The weight of these machines ranges from 850 to 2000 g.

The first "ultra-portable" unit for farm animals, entered in Europe in the mid-90s (Gnemmi et al., 2005; 2006; 2011): it was a unit of 5500 g. There are many ultra-portable units available on the market today: the price ranges from € 3500 to € 12,000. They are all units with LCD screens, some are not equipped with a built-in screen, but they using cameras inserted in a device similar to a pair of glasses or use a portable screen (even wrist and fixed with a Wi-Fi connection). Some have the possibility of using different types of probes, while others, only mount a linear probe, sometimes sectoral, for endorectal use, multifrequency (5.0–10.0 MHz), intended for use in gynecology. All these instruments are powered by a battery, which offers a variable working autonomy (2.5–7.5 h). These are very practical, light and space-saving instruments that are well suited to every work situation (Fricke et al., 2005; Gnemmi, 2010).

2.2.2 CHOICE OF INSTRUMENT

When you need to buy an ultrasound machine, you need to do a business plan, which is to verify exactly the cost–benefit of the purchase. Based on this study may be possible to decide which ultrasound unit to buy. We need to analyze several points:

- Financial aspect. How much money I have available? Is it more convenient to rent the money at a bank, or use the money I have available? The instrument is normally amortized in 3–12 months, based on the number of ultrasonographic examinations performed by the professional. It has been calculated that it takes less than 3 h of work a month to amortize the instrument, within tax amortization times (7 years) (DesCoteaux et al., 1998; Filteau et al., 1998; Gnemmi 1999; 2001).
- Practical aspect. How many hours a day, a week, a month and a year do I intend to use the ultrasound unit? What kind of service can I offer already now? What kind of services can I offer for the next 3–6–12 months? Do I intend to carry out ultrasound scans only of the reproductive apparatus, or to carry out extra genital scans? Only in cattle or even in other species? (Gnemmi, 1999).
- Economical aspect. What is the fee per hour of ultrasound work and/or ultrasound examination carried out? What is the break-even and what is the pay-back of this investment?

The ultrasound scanners are fairly simple instruments, consisting of a screen, a probe and a keyboard.

The screen: The screens were originally cathode ray tube, now they are LCD screen: this choice has made it possible to lighten the ultrasound units considerably, at the same time guaranteeing a remarkable image quality. Working outdoors, especially in summer, you may encounter difficulties in seeing the image on the screen: this problem can be solved by resorting to an integrated system of cameras mounted on special glasses, or more simply can use small black cardboard cones, which applied on the screen allow you to limit the noise derived from the light, or may be possible to use various protection systems.

The keyboard: In some cases, it is extremely simple, while in others, it is comparable to a computer keyboard. In all the instruments there are commands, which allow to fix the image (and possibly to memorize it), to change the brightness of the screen and to improve the contrast in specific points.

The probes: In bovine gynecologic are used endo-rectal probes of 5.0–8.0 MHz, linear (straight or curved) or sectorial: the linear are substantially easier to use, especially for those who are beginners, the latter at the same frequency allow to work at a greater depth.

Microconvex probes are also available, both for endo-vaginal use and for endo-rectal use Increasing the frequency reduces the depth of action of the probe but increases the definition. In practice, the higher the emission frequency, the shorter the wavelength of the ultrasounds produced, so we will have a lower depth of action, but a better definition: a 7.5 MHz probe, allows to better highlight follicular structures even of 3–4 mm, at a depth of 4–5 cm, while a 5 MHz probe, will allow to highlight follicular structures of 7–8 mm, at a depth (greater) of 8–10 cm (Table 2.1).

2.3 ULTRASONOGRAPHY IN BOVINE REPRODUCTION

Many veterinarians and breeders, believe that ultrasonography in bovine reproduction, has a reason to be only for the early diagnosis of pregnancy. It is actually a very limited vision of the potential benefits that this technique can guarantee. The margin of error in the evaluation of ovarian structures (corpus luteum, follicle) of an excellent technician with palpation with over 30 years of experience in this sector and no less than 60,000 cows examined manually/year, is 35–45%, while the margin of error in the manual evaluation of physio-pathological pictures of the uterus, excluding the diagnosis of pregnancy, is 70–80% (Gnemmi, 1999; 2001). This error leads to a considerable economic loss, in terms of therapeutic costs, labor and above all in terms of open days!

TABLE 2.1 Characteristics and Indications of Probes of Different Frequencies in Bovine Gynecology (adapted from Ginther, 1998).

Probes frequency and characteristics	
5 MHz	**7.5 MHz**
It works between 0–12 cm deep, detecting follicular structures of 7–8 mm	It works between 0–7 cm deep, detecting follicular structures of 3–4 mm
Good resolution	Excellent resolution
Physiopathology of ovary and uterus	Physiopathology of ovary and uterus
Early diagnosis of nonpregnancy–pregnancy	Early diagnosis of nonpregnancy–pregnancy
Early diagnosis of suffering and embryonic death	Early diagnosis of suffering and embryonic death
Fetal sex diagnosis	Fetal sex diagnosis

The ultrasonographic, routine evaluation of the ovary and uterus, with the aim of evaluating the physio-pathological condition, represents one of the services that are ablest to increase the income of the farmer.

2.3.1 THE CORPUS LUTEUM AND THE FOLLICULAR DYNAMICS

The most important structures present on the ovary are the corpus luteum and the follicles. The corpus luteum can be compact or with a cavity (often there are also more cavities separated from each other, or communicating). The presence of the cavity does not affect its functionality, which in all respects is a normal corpus luteum, regularly producing progesterone. The cavity CL is not correlated to lower rates of conception, or to higher rates of embryonic and/or fetal death, moreover it does not influence in any way the length of the estrous cycle. The shape, the diameter, the number and the diameter of the cavity, do not absolutely influence the functionality of the corpus luteum cavity. This cavitary CL is excellent for starting a super ovulation, as well as for embryo transfer. It is therefore difficult to attempt to frame it in a single diagnostic criterion, as some Authors have tried to do (Chastant-Maillard, 2010). The cavity CL is present in large numbers in the first ten days of the estrous cycle (35–70%) (DesCoteaux et al., 2010), while we still have 30% of corpus luteum bodies at the end of the estrous cycle (DesCoteaux et al., 2010), Between the 10th–15th day of the ovarian cycle, 70% of the cavitary corpus lute, loses the cavity, which is replaced by new luteinic tissue (which appears more echogenic than the luteinic tissue that constituted the cavity CL wall), or following the collapse of the cavity, an echogenic scar remains, instead of the cavity itself. Not all researchers and not all ultrasonographers agree on lutein tissue, filling the cavity of the corpus luteum; some believe that it is only fibrin and red blood cells. A 30% of cavity corpus luteum maintains the cavity for the entire duration of the estrous cycle: in many cases, this CL cavitation at the end of the cycle, have a cavity (sometimes even of significant size), circumscribed by a thin hyper-echogenic bright line (Fig. 2.1).

In principle, we can therefore say, that in the presence of a CL with a cavity filled with echogenic tissue, or in the presence of a scar inside it, or even in the presence of a cavity circumscribed by a thin and brilliant hyper echogenic, we are in the second decade of the estrous cycle. It must be said that this indication should be taken as a general rule: in fact, it can happen to be in the presence of CL with the characteristics mentioned above, already after 4–6 days from ovulation.

Wanting to establish more precisely the age of the corpus luteum and therefore the estral window in which the cow is found, it is good to analyze the follicular map present on both ovaries, also analyzing the characteristics of the uterus.

The cavitary corpus luteum can also be a gravid corpus luteum: about 10% of pregnant bodies between 28 and 35 days of gestation are cavitary (Gnemmi et al., 2009)

The follicular dynamics is clearer today thanks to the ultrasonographic study, which allowed us to confirm Rajakoski's hypothesis (Rajakoski, 1960).

Ultrasonographically, with a 5.0–7.5 MHz rectal-probe and an ultra-portable unit, follicular structures can be detected starting from 3 mm in diameter. All follicular dynamics can be monitored: recruitment, deviation, ovulation of the last dominant follicle. It is possible to evaluate the diameter of the largest follicle present on the ovaries at that moment; this is of fundamental importance in defining the therapeutic strategy: in the presence of follicular structures with a diameter less than 8 mm, a possible therapy with GnRH must be postponed as with a $PGF_2\alpha$, regardless of the diameter of the corpus luteum. The ultrasound evaluation of the dominant follicle diameter allows us to predict with good approximation, when the cow will come in heat in two and three follicular waves.

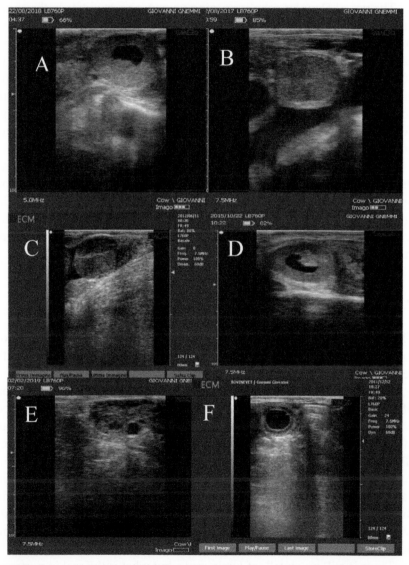

FIGURE 2.1 Ultrasonograms of different types of bovine CL: (A) Cavitary CL; (B) Compact CL; (C) ex Cavitary with scar; (D) CL with cavity partially full; (E) Hemorrhagic body; (F) CL with echoic ring.

The use of ultrasonography has also made it possible to optimize the results of the synchronization plans (synchronization of heat and ovulation), optimizing the detection of the corpus luteum and the dominant follicle, thus increasing the accuracy of the start of each synchronization plan.

The use of Doppler echo is opening up new opportunities in the study of physiology, but also of the pathology of the ovary and uterus (Gnemmi et al., 2013). There is a close correlation between the degree of vascularization of CL and the level of circulating progesterone (Herzog et al., 2007; Rauch et al., 2008). This makes it possible to make an accurate diagnosis of non-pregnancy already twenty days after insemination, but above all this technique can improve the accuracy of the ultrasound diagnosis, improving conception rates in synchronization plans and optimizing hormonal therapies: both for use therapeutic than for zootechnical use.

The application of ultrasonography in bovine reproduction has also improved the performance of estrous and ovulation synchronization programs. The use of ultrasonography to check for the presence of a CL at the end of the voluntary waiting period makes it possible to define which pre-synchronization strategy to use (Fricke et al., 2005; Gnemmi et al., 2011).

2.3.2   OVARIAN PATHOLOGIES.

The ultrasound examination of the ovary allows us to highlight pathological structures, which otherwise we would not be able to detect with rectal palpation (Fig. 2.2).

Ultrasonography allows us to establish the actual functional situation of the ovary: very often at the palpation the ovulatory anestrus is confused with anovulation (absence of persistent lutein structures for not less than 10 days). Thanks to ultrasonography, the concept of anaestrus is clearer (Peter et al. 2009; Gnemmi et al., 2010; 2012a, 2012b; Gnemmi, 2013). At the same time, we have seen that the accuracy of manual diagnosis in case of cystic degeneration of the ovary is very low (Farin et al., 1992) and that over 30% of follicular cysts (anestrus type III) are contemporaneous with a corpus luteum (Al-Dahash et al., 1977; Gnemmi et al., 2011) and therefore they are not functionally a problem.

There is still much talk of lutein cysts, but what is the real importance of these structures? How many of these alleged cysts are not actually a cavitary corpus luteum or a follicular cyst in the process of luteinization?

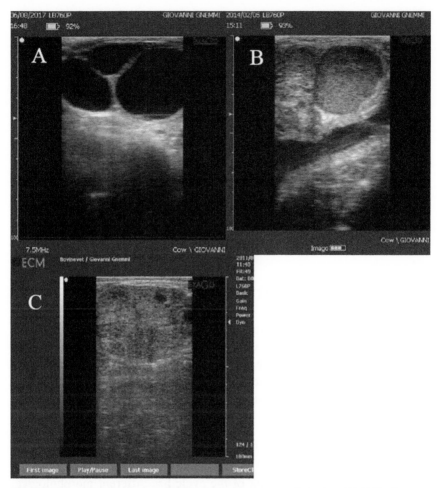

FIGURE 2.2 Ultrasonograms of different bovine ovary pathologies: (A) follicular cyst; (B) cyst of the ovary bag; (C) tumor of granulosa cells.

The differential diagnosis today is based on the thickness of the lutein wall: > 3 mm CL, <3 mm luteinic cyst. Other authors speak of an average thickness of the luteinic wall of 5 mm (3–10 mm) and of the presence of a cavity of not less than 30 mm (Chastant-Maillard, 2010; Hanzen et al., 2008): under field conditions this differential diagnosis is very difficult to make, even admitting that it has its own prognostic value.

Among the ovarian pathologies,, the abscesses and the hematomas of the ovarian bursa can be easily highlighted with the ultrasound examination and the ultrasound examination allow a diagnosis to be made (also establishing the degree of connectivity and calcification of the abscess) and especially a differential diagnosis with the corpus luteum.

The cyst of ovarian bursa is a pathology that does not seem to negatively affect the fertility of the cow. These are cystic formations of varying diameter (they can reach 10–15 cm in diameter), which form in the ovarian bursa and are clearly distinguished from the cystic degeneration of the ovary. Ultrasound diagnosis is relatively simple, but above all it allows a differential diagnosis with ovarian cysts.

Ovarian neoplasms (tumor of granulosa cells, lutein cell tumor), can be detected with an ultrasound examination, however the diagnosis must be confirmed with a biopsy.

The ovary dysplasia, considered by some to be a pre-tumor stage, by others a finding correlated with the advanced age of the animal.

2.3.3   ULTRASOUND UTERUS EVALUATION

The margin of error in the evaluation of the uterus (physio-pathological) of an excellent "palpator" with a very big experience it is 65–75% (Gnemmi, 1999; 2001), obviously the pregnancy diagnosis is not referred to. Both in terms of sensitivity and specificity, manual palpation of the uterus does not allow obtaining acceptable results.

2.3.3.1   PHYSIOLOGICAL UTERUS.

The uterus at different moment of the cycle has different morphological characteristics, determined by the hormonal setting. These characteristics can be evaluated on ultrasonography.

During oestrus, the endometrium appears thickened (edema) with low echogenicity and dotted with anechoic spots (blood vessels, edema), separated from the myometrium by the ticker vascular tunic, which in cross-section appears as an anechoic ring (Fig. 2.3 A). The uterine lumen is dilated and anechoic in the absence of endometritis. Numerous specular reflections ("good" artifact) characterize this moment of the cycle. The myometrium presents itself, contracted and more environmentally friendly.

During the meta-estrus, the uterine characteristics change: in the immediate meta-estrus, the ultrasound the uterus will be very similar to the estrous uterus, but as you move away from ovulation (36 hs), lowering the level of estrogen, the thickness is reduced of the endometrium, of the uterine lumen (specular reflexes are also reduced) and of the vascular tunica, while the thickness of the myometrium increases.

During the di-estrus, there are some differences between the beginning, the intermediate phase and the end (5th –15th day in a two-wave cows). On the 10th day of the cycle, approximately in correspondence with the atresia of the first dominant follicle (bovine with two waves), the thickness and the ultrasonographic characteristics of endometrium and myometrium are very similar, separated by a very thin vascular habit (anechoic), in absence of a uterine lumen (unless an endometritis persists). This picture is typical of a hormonal profile characterized by progesterone.

In pro-estrus, the thickness of the endometrium begins to increase, just as its echogenicity gradually decreases; increases the diameter of the uterine lumen, increases the thickness of the vascular tunic, decreases the thickness of the myometrium and with it also increases its echogenicity.

Establishing the moment of the cycle, due to the ultrasound characteristics of the uterus, is not possible: this evaluation should always be carried out considering the follicular map of both ovaries. In the case of cows with two growth waves, this assessment is rapid and precise. Attention to cases of co-dominance (presence of more than one dominant follicle in the same wave) and/or persistent dominant follicles, which can make the picture equivocal.

2.3.3.2   *NO PREGNANCY DIAGNOSIS.*

Most of the veterinarians and technicians who use the ultrasound machine in the clinic, limit their use to the early diagnosis of pregnancy only. This is a very limited view.

More than the early examination of pregnancy, it is important to be able to carry out the early examination of non-pregnancy: these are the cows, the ones that have the greatest impact on the economic losses, increasing the open days.

A certain diagnosis of pregnancy is based on the presence of one or more corpus luteum on one or both ovaries, on the presence of fluid in the uterus, but above all on the presence of one or more embryos.

The mere presence of a corpus luteum (or more than one) and liquid in the uterus, allows only to make a diagnosis of suspicion of pregnancy.

The emergence of the embryo is theoretically possible even very early (19th day). It is much easier to detect the embryo at 25th day of gestation (width 3–5 mm and length about 8 mm). This is obviously a relative ease: in less than 50% of cases, the embryo can be detected ultrasonographically in a very early stage of gestation (24th–25th day), without having to manipulate the uterus. (Ginther, 1998; Gnemmi et al., 2005; Fricke et al., 2005). The manipulation of the uterus always involves a release of $PGF_2\alpha$, responsible for an increase in late embryonic death. The sensitivity of the embryo to PGF is greater the younger the embryo. Therefore, if the diagnosis of non-pregnancy/pregnancy should be started at twenty-five days post-insemination, do not manipulate the uterus. At twenty-eight days of gestation, the diagnosis of non-pregnancy/pregnancy is easier, faster and more accurate; the doubtful cows are few and it is easier to make the diagnosis of twin pregnancy. Furthermore, the non-pregnant cows that have cycled have a CL of 6–8 days, that is very easy to highlight unlike a hemorrhagic CL (Gnemmi et al., 2005).

When to start making the diagnosis of non-pregnancy/pregnancy? The choice must be made based on the rate of detection of the heat of the farm, based on the use of re-synchronization systems and on the frequency of gynecological visits (Gnemmi et al., 2015).

In farms where gynecology is carried out weekly, to start the no-pregnancy/pregnancy exam before 30–32, don't reduce the days open, in particularly using a Resynch program (Resynch25).

Where gynecological examinations take place every fifteen days, especially if the heat detection is low ($\leq$ 40%), there may be a need to anticipate the diagnosis at 25–26 days, stressing the fact that the number of doubtful cows increases, that it is more difficult to make the diagnosis of twinning and that it is more difficult to highlight the embryo and therefore evaluate its vitality (Gnemmi et al., 2008).

2.3.3.3   EMBRYO VIABILITY

During the diagnosis of pregnancy, one should not limit oneself to this, but it is useful and appropriate to evaluate the quality of the pregnancy itself. Embryo death (Fig. 2.3 B) is an important problem in the gynecological management of cattle breeding, from dairy, but also from meat. This is not an abstract problem or even a random one, heavily affecting corporate balance sheets (Vasconcelos et al., 1997; Fricke et al., 2005; Gnemmi et al., 2011a, b; 2013a, b, c). The criteria for evaluating the quality of pregnancy are different:

- Heart rate
- Echogenicity of amniotic and/or allantoic fluid
- Separation of the corion-allantoic membrane
- Edema of the endometrium
- Integrity of the amniotic membrane
- Absence of the embryo
- Size of the embryo

Certainly, at a very early stage (27–28 days) the most immediate assessment is the observation of the heartbeat, which appears ultrasonographically as a rapid succession of echogenic points (Fig. 2.3 C). Normally, at this age the heartbeat has a frequency between 120–130 beats per minute (Ginther, 1998; DesCoteaux et al., 2010). Timing beats in field conditions is difficult, but normally it can be said that, if the heart rate is so slow that it can be counted easily, there is a state of embryonic suffering, whereas when the speed of the beat is so rapid as to make counting difficult to impossible, the embryo's state of health is regular.

2.3.3.4   FETAL SEXING

Fetal sexing is a useful service in every business environment. It should not be thought that this is a technique intended only for elite of breeders, who produce genetics. The reasons for extending fetal sexing to all types of businesses are different:

- The value of sexed female or male pregnancies increases.
- It is possible to carry out contracts for male pregnancies.
- Culling decision improves surprisingly.
- It is possible to improve the management of delivery assistance in the heifers.
- It is possible to improve the calving management (beef races).
- It is possible to improve the management of the nursery: spaces and work.
- It is possible to improve the efficiency of the breeding plan.

The sexing is performed by determining the position of the genital tubercle (TG): in the male it will be retro umbilical (Fig. 2.3 D), in the female under the tail (Fig. 2.3 E). TG is ultrasonographically presented as a double bright echogenic structure, in the male as in the female. In the male the TG becomes tri-lobed from seventy days for the appearance of the corpus cavernosum of the penis. After the 70th day of gestation, the breasts and the scrotum can be detected (Ginther, 1998; Gnemmi et al., 2008). Migration of the genital tubercle begins at day 45 and ends in the female at 52–53 days, in the male at 55 days. Therefore, it is not advisable to perform fetal sexing before the 55th day (Ginther, 1998; Fricke et al., 2005; Gnemmi et al., 2005; 2008; 2015). From the 55th to the 60th day, the skill and experience of the technician are decisive: between 60–90 days it is simple: between 90–110 days the technician's experience is decisive, while from 110 to 130 days it depends from the position that the fetus is assuming (Gnemmi et al., 2005; 2008; 2015). A good technician has an accuracy of 99.99%.

2.3.3.5   TWIN PREGNANCY DIAGNOSIS

Twinning is certainly an emerging "pathology" in high production dairy cattle breeding. The twin rate has doubled in just over fifteen years: if the twins are looking for us, the twins will be found! (Gnemmi, 2006; Gnemmi et al., 2006, 2008).

The 99% of twin pregnancies are heterozygous (two corpora lutea on the same ovary or distributed on both ovaries; two males or two females, or one male and one female), 1% are monozygotic (a corpus luteum, two females, or two males) (Ginther, 1998; Fricke et al., 2005; Gnemmi, 2006; Gnemmi et al., 2006; 2008).

The rate of late embryonic death, in the case of twins is about 30% higher than in single pregnancies, similarly the abortion rate is greater. Ultrasound diagnosis is necessary, given the low accuracy of manual diagnosis (Fig. 2.3 F). Once the diagnosis is made, these cows will have to be constantly monitored (do no less than four confirmations of pregnancy during gestation), furthermore it will have to be brought up to ten days earlier (the delivery will be anticipated by ten days) and assistance must always be given to the birth. Possibly these animals should receive a suitable food supplement during the dry period, to reduce the predisposition towards puerperal pathologies (placenta retention, metritis, ketosis, LDA/RDA,) (Gnemmi, 2006; Gnemmi et al., 2006; 2008).

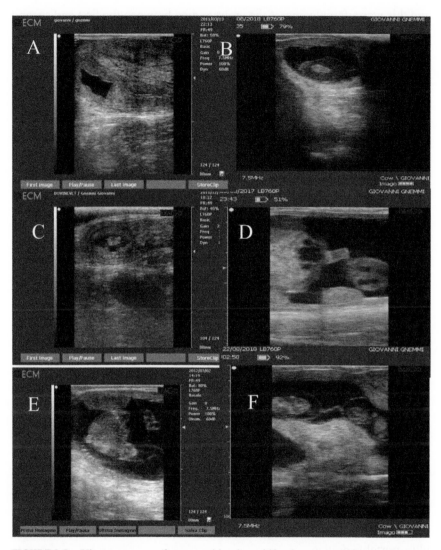

FIGURE 2.3 Ultrasonograms of non–gravid and gravid bovine uterus: (A) uterus in estrus; (B) embryo death; (C) pregnancy 28 days; (D) male pregnancy; (E) female pregnancy; (F) twin pregnancy.

Make twin pregnancies! In the case of male and female pregnancy, the female must be considered at high risk of Free Martinism. This pathology is always suspected even when only one embryo was present in the sexing and this was a female one: if the embryo died between the first and second pregnancy diagnosis was a male and if it died after the 30th day of gestation, the possibility that the female fetus is not a Free Martin is very few.

2.3.3.6 PATHOLOGICAL UTERUS.

Ultrasonography is not the best diagnostic method for the diagnosis of metritis (puerperal or septical) in the early postpartum days. After the 10th day, the introduction of this technique for monitoring the uterus is decisive, given the very low accuracy of the manual examination. From the 20th postpartum day, it is possible to ultrasonologically diagnose clinical endometritis (purulent, muco-purulent, pyometra, mucometra) and sub-clinical endometritis and endometrial fibrosis (DesCoteaux et al., 2010; Gnemmi et al., 2010a,b).

Both purulent and muco-purulent endometritis is easily identifiable thanks to the ultrasound examination, working with a linear probe with a frequency of 5.0–7.5 MhZ. The uterine content will have a variable echogenicity based on the concentration of PMN (> or <50%). The uterine content always looks like a "snow storm" (Fig. 2.4 A and B). The content will be more eco-friendly when the PMN concentration is ≥ 50%, while it will be hypo-echogenic when the PMN concentration is <50% (Gnemmi et al., 2010a).

The presence of pyometra is worth the considerations just made for clinical endometritis. The pyometra in most cases is characterized by the presence of one or two persistent CLs (Gnemmi et al., 2010a)

In the presence of mucometra, the uterine content will be anechoic, often with small hypo-echogenic points. There is always one more than one persistent CL. Pay attention to the differential diagnosis with a gestation (Gnemmi et al., 2010a). These diagnoses are also possible with an ultra-portable device.

The ultrasonographic diagnosis of sub-clinical endometritis can be carried out with extreme accuracy: endometrial thickness > 8 mm, uterine content > 3 mm are general guidelines, which however make the diagnosis not very sensitive (Fig. 2.4 C and D). Sensitivity increases greatly by verifying the presence of artifacts (shadows or specular reflections) that can guide the diagnosis, as well as the verification of the follicular map (Gnemmi et al., 2010b).

The ultrasonographic examination of the uterus also allows us to highlight pathological structures of the uterine wall: abscesses (Fig. 2.4 F), hematomas, cysts (Fig. 2.4 E).

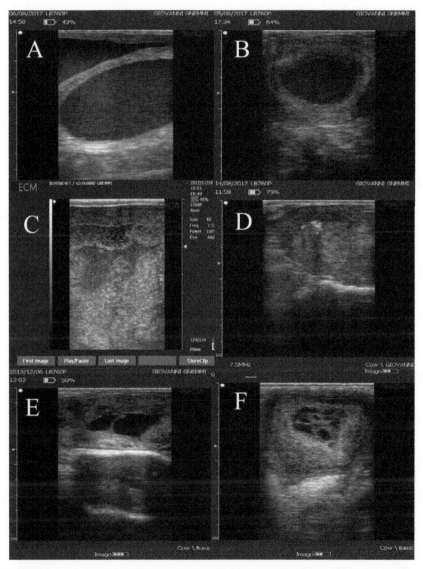

FIGURE 2.4 Pathologies of bovine uterus: (A) purulent endometritis; (B) muco–purulent endometritis; (C) clinical metritis; (D) subclinical endometritis; (E) uterus cyst; (F) abscess of the uterus.

KEYWORDS

- ultrasound units
- reproductive evaluation
- follicular dynamics
- ovarian pathologies
- pregnancy diagnosis
- uterus pathologies
- herd management

REFERENCES

AlDahash, S. Y. A.; David, J. S. E. Anatomical Features of Cystic Ovaries in Cattle Found During an Abattoir Survey. *Vet Rec.* **1977**, *101*, 320–324.

Chastant-Maillard, S. Importanza dell'ecografia delle cisti ovariche. *Summa Anno.* **2010**, *5–8*, 38–44.

DesCoteaux, L.; Fetrow, J. Does it Pay to Use an Ultrasound Machine for Early Pregnancy Diagnosis in Dairy Cows?, Proceedings of the 31th Annual Convention AABP. Spokene, 1998. Sep 24–28.

Des Coteaux, L.; Gnemmi, G.; Colloton, J. Ultrasonography of the Bovine Female Genital Tract. *Vet Clin North Am Food Anim Pract.* **2009**, *25*, 733–752.

DesCoteaux, L.; Colloton, J.; Gnemmi, G. *Practical Atlas of Ruminant and Camelid Reproductive Ultrasonography.* Ed.; Wiley-BlackWell: New York, **2010**; Chapter 4; pp 35–62.

Farin, P. W.; Youngquist, R. S.; Parfet, J. R.; Garverick, H. A. Diagnosis of Luteal and Follicular Ovarian Cysts by Palpation per Rectum and Linear-Array Ultrasonography in Dairy Cows. *J. Amer. Vet. Med. Assoc.* **1992**, *200*, 1085–1089.

Filteau, V.; DesCoteaux, L. Predictive Values of Early Pregnancy Diagnosis by Ultrasonography in Dairy Cattle, Proceedings of the 31th Annual Convention AABP. Spokene 1998. Sep. 24–28.

Fricke, P. M, Lamb, G. C. Potential Applications and Pitfalls of Reproductive Ultrasonography in Bovine Practice. *Vet Clin Anim.* **2005**, *21*, 419–436.

Ginther, O. J. *Ultrasonic Imaging and Animal Reproduction: Cattle. Book 3.* Equiservices Publishing, Cross Plains, WI. **1998**; p 304.

Gnemmi, G. Ultrasonografia ginecologica in buiatria: valutazioni economiche nell'allevamento del bovino da latte. *Summa Veterinaria.* **1999**, *8*, 59–62.

Gnemmi, G. Analisi economica dell'uso dell'ecografia ginecologica buiatrica. *Summa Veterinaria.* **2001**, *6*, 61–64.

Gnemmi, G. 2001. Degenerazione cistica dell'ovaio nel bovino da latte. *Summa Veterinaria Animali da Reddito.* **2001**, *18–1*, 35–40.

Gnemmi, G. Diagnosi ecografica di sessaggio fetale. *Summa Veterinaria Animali da Reddito.* **2005,** *22—1,* 5–8.

Gnemmi, G. Gestacion Doble: Patología Emergente en Tambos de Alta Producción. *Taurus Argentina.* **2006,** *8–32,* 24–35.

Gnemmi, G. Improving Bovine Fertility: Look Again at Ultrasonography. *Ir. Vet. J.* **2007,** *60–7,* 435–438.

Gnemmi, G. Practical Uses for Transrectal Ultrasonography in Reproductive Management of Cattle. Proceedings XXVI WBC Santiago de Chile, November 14–18, 2010.

Gnemmi, G. Anestrusus in bovine reproduction: diagnosis and therapy. *Lecznica Poland.* **2013,** *4,* 42–45.

Gnemmi, G.; Maraboli, C. Gestazione Gemellare. *Summa Veterinaria Animali da Reddito.* **2006,** *1–6,* 17–22.

Gnemmi, G.; Maraboli, C. Diagnosi ultrasonografica precoce di gravidanza. *Summa Veterinaria.* **2008,** *3,* 1–6.

Gnemmi, G.; Maraboli, C. Il sessaggio fetale. *Summa Veterinaria.* **2008,** 2, 3–6.

Gnemmi, G.; Maraboli, C. 2008. La gravidanza gemellare. *Summa Veterinaria.* **2008,** *6,* 43–48.

Gnemmi, G.; Maraboli, C. Ultrasonografia e corpus luteum: applicazioni cliniche. *Summa Veterinaria Animali da Reddito.* **2009,** *4–5,* 9–16.

Gnemmi, G.; Maraboli, C. Anaestro nel bovino da latte ad alta produzione: diagnosi eterapia. *Summa Veterinaria Animali da Reddito.* **2010,** *5–1,* 7–12.

Gnemmi, G.; Maraboli, C. Diagnosi ultrasonografica delle patologie uterine nella bovina. *Summa Veterinaria.* **2010,** *2,* 7–14.

Gnemmi, G.; Maraboli, C. Endometrite subclinica nel bovino da latte. *Summa Veterinaria.* **2010,** *6,* 38–42.

Gnemmi, G.; Maraboli, C. Inseminazione a tempo fisso: ultime novità in tema di sincronizzazione dell'ovulazione. *Summa Veterinaria Animali da Reddito.* **2011,** *5,* 1–6.

Gnemmi, G.; Maraboli, C. OCD: nuovi approcci. *Summa Veterinaria Animali da Reddito.* **2011,** *6–9,* 9–16.

Gnemmi G.; Maraboli C. Morte embrionale. Diagnosi ecografica Parte I. *Summa Veterinaria Animali da Reddito.* **2011a,** *6–6,* 7–12.

Gnemmi, G.; Maraboli, C. Morte embrionale. Diagnosi ecografica Parte II. *Summa Veterinaria Animali da Reddito.* **2011b,** *6–7,* 37–41.

Gnemmi, G.; Maraboli, C. Il corpo luteo & la diagnosi precoce di gestazione/non gestazione. *Summa Veterinaria Animali da Reddito.* **2012,** *7,* 56–62.

Gnemmi, G.; Maraboli, C. L'anaestro nella bovina: diagnosi e terapia. *Rivista di Medicina Veterinaria.* **2012a,** *46–1,* 21–26.

Gnemmi C.; Maraboli C. L'anaestro nella bovina: fisiopatologia di un evento multifattoriale. *Rivista di Medicina Veterinaria.* **2012b,** *46–1,* 17–20.

Gnemmi, G.; Maraboli, C. Eco color Doppler in riproduzione bovina. Parte I: Fisica del Color Doppler. *Summa Veterinaria Animali da Reddito.* **2013,** *8–2,* 43–46.

Gnemmi, G.; Maraboli, C. Diagnosi precoce di morte embrionale tardiva. *Summa Veterinaria Animali da Reddito.* **2013a,** *8–4,* 52–61.

Gnemmi, G.; Maraboli, C. Diagnosi ecografica di morte embrionale. Parte I. *Summa Veterinaria Animali da Reddito.* **2013b,** *8–4,* 62–67.

Gnemmi, G.; Maraboli, C. Diagnosi ecografica di morte embrionale. Parte II. *Summa Veterinartia Animali da Reddito.* **2013c,** *8–4,* 68–72. 40 Biotechnologies Applied to Animal Reproduction

Gnemmi, G.; Maraboli, C. Il sessaggio fetale. *Summa Veterinaria Animali da Reddito.* **2015,** *10–1,* 1–9.

Gnemmi, G.; Marboli C.; Colloton J. Ultrasonografia in ginecologia buiatrica. *Summa Veterinaria Animali da Reddito.* **2006,** *9,* 11–16.

Gnemmi, G.; Ferrari, E.; Maraboli, C. La re–sincronizzazione nel bovino da latte e da carne. *Summa Veterinaria Animali da Reddito.* **2015,** *10–3,* 1–9.

Hanzen, C. H.; Bascon, F.; Theron, L.; Lopez-Gatius, F. Les kystes ovariens dans l'espèce bovine. Partie I. Définitions, symptômes et diagnostic. *Ann. Med.Vet.* **2008,** *152,* 17–34.

Herzog, K.; Bollwein, H. Application of Doppler Ultrasonography in Cattle Reproduction. *Reprod. Dom. Anim.* **2007,** *42–2,* 51–58.

Peter, A. T.; Vos, P. L.; Ambrose, D. J. Postpartum Anestrus in Dairy Cattle. *Theriogenology.* **2009,** *71,* 1333–1342.

Pierson, R. A., Ginther, O. J. 1984. Ultrasonography for the Detection of Pregnancy and Study of Embryonic Development in Heifers. *Theriogenology.* **1984a,** *22,* 225–233.

Pierson, R. A.; Ginther, O. J. Ultrasonography of the Bovine Ovary. *Theriogenology.* **1984b,** *21,* 495–504.

Pierson, R. A.; Ginther, O. J. Ovarian Follicular Population During Early Pregnancy in Heifer. *Theriogenology.* **1986,**,*26,* 649–659.

Pierson, R. A.; Ginther, O. J. Ultrasonographic Appearance of the Bovine Uterus During the Estrus Cycle. *J. Amer. Vet. Med. Assoc.* **1987,** *190,* 995–1001.

Rajakoski, E. The Ovarian Follicular System in Sexually Mature Heifers with Special Reference to Seasonal, Cyclical and Left-Right Variation. *Acta Endocrinolol.* **1960,** *34,* 7–68.

Rauch, A. L; Krüger, A.; Miyamoto, H.; Bollowein, H. Colour Doppler Sonography of Cystic Ovarian Follicles in Cows. *J. Reprod. Develop.* **2008,** *54–6,* 447–453.

Vasconcelos, J. L. M; Silcox, R. W; Lacerda, J. A. et al. Pregnancy Rate, Pregnancy Loss, and Response to Heat Stress After AI at 2 Different Times from Ovulation in Dairy Cows [abstract]. *Biol. Reprod.* **1997,** *56–1,* 140.

CHAPTER 3

Ultrasonography of the Bovine Reproductive System: Ultrasound Management of the Male Reproductive System

GIOVANNI GNEMMI[1,2*], JUAN CARLOS GARDÓN[2], and
CRISTINA MARABOLI[1]

[1]Bovinevet Internacional, Bovine Ultrasound Services and Herd Management, Spain

[2]Department of Animal Medicine and Surgery, Faculty of Veterinary and Experimental Sciences, Catholic University of Valencia, San Vincente Mártir, Spain

*Corresponding author. E-mail: giovanni.gnemmi@bovinevet.com

ABSTRACT

The natural service is still extremely widespread today and, in the breeding of beef cattle, it is the most important form of insemination. Functional evaluation of the reproductive efficiency of the bull is as important as that of the cows, in fact, it is even more important considering that a bull awaits several females. Being able to have a procedure that allows evaluating the reproductive potential of the bull is fundamental, both for bulls used in the herd and for bulls destined, for their genetic merit, to the production of seminal material for artificial insemination. Ultrasound has not yet been officially introduced in the breeding soundness evaluation; however, it has been used extensively for over 20 years to complement the clinical evaluation of the bull. It becomes a fundamental tool whenever there is teratospermia, low semen concentration, leukospermia or pyospermia, oligospermia or azospermia, little vitality after thawing, presence of testicular pain for no apparent reason, or when we have anatomical modifications of the bull's reproductive system. It is a simple technique, repeatable in any environmental condition and requires very basic ultrasound instrumentation.

3.1   INTRODUCTION

Reproductive management represents one of the fundamental critical points in the intensive or extensive breeding of beef or dairy cattle (Pursley, 2007; Gnemmi and Lefebvre, 2010). Infertility continues to be the main cause of involuntary elimination in cattle breeding (Santos, 2013). There is much talk, and with reason, of the infertility associated with female factor: repeating cow syndrome in the USA costs between 1 and 2 billion dollars per year (Pursley, 2007). Unfortunately, very little is said about the importance (determinant) of the bull in this aspect, whether it is used for semen production or in natural service. The main limiting factor in modern reproductive management is undoubtedly the low efficiency in the detection of oestrus (Gnemmi, 2007; 2013), which is why in dairy herds natural service is often used, which is a common resource in bovine and bubaline beef herds, at least after the first IA (FTAI). The reproductive efficiency of the bull is important for the herds, because of the economic consequences in case of failures (increase in open days); also, in the case of bulls used for semen production, a constant reproductive efficiency is essential in order to guarantee, on the one hand, good or optimal conception rates, and on the other hand, for the recovery of the economic investment in the reproducer, which is undoubtedly important.

The choice of a breeder is first made on the basis of genealogical (genomic and genetic) and morphological criteria. The morphology is undoubtedly a very considered aspect; attention is paid to the general clinical state, its libido, its ability to mount a female. In some cases, there is also a qualitative–quantitative evaluation of the semen. Sometimes, the bull is subjected to a general clinical examination and a particular examination of the reproductive apparatus: inspection, palpation, superficial, and deep palpation of the testicles, with the aim of evaluating their elasticity. A complete clinical examination is carried out, without resorting to complementary examinations, except (sometimes) for the spermogram.

However, the cost of a reproducer is usually very important, if it is bought as a bull of the year. Although andrological examination (Breeding Soundness Evaluation; BSE) has been used for several years, there are still few establishments that have incorporated ultrasonography (Kastelic and Brito, 2012).

It is difficult to understand reasons for this malpractice, especially in view of the fact that often not even the best clinical examination, carried out by the best professional, makes it possible to highlight the location of a possible lesion, neither the extent of it nor, much less, to issue a prognosis. Ultrasonography has been used for 15 years in the evaluation of the bull's reproductive system, with the same equipment used for gynecological diagnosis (Ginther, 1995; Gnemmi, 2007; Gnemmi and Lefebvre, 2009, 2010). With this article, authors want to show how to incorporate the ultrasound technique in the BSE, demonstrating its ability to adapt to any environment.

3.2 BREEDING SOUNDNESS EVALUATION

The BSE is not a fertility test, but a systematic clinical approach to identify bulls with low reproductive potential (Gnemmi and Lefebvre, 2009). It includes clinical examination of the bull, semen collection, and evaluation (Kastelic and Thundathil, 2008; Gnemmi and Lefebvre, 2009; 2010; Kastelic and Brito, 2012). This test is designed to evaluate the fertility of a bull before it is destined for reproduction (or semen production), but it is also used to establish the cause or causes of infertility of a bull already in production (Gnemmi and Lefebvre, 2010).

Generally, it can be said that the BSE traditionally includes three general evaluations:

1. Determination of the scrotal circumference
2. Inspection and palpation (superficial and deep) of external and internal genitalia
3. Evaluation of seminal quality

In more recent years, it has been proposed to incorporate ultrasonography into BSE (Gnemmi, 2007; Gnemmi and Lefebvre, 2009, 2010; Kastelic and Brito, 2012), as well as biochemical tests, such as the determination of adiponectin (Kasimanickam et al., 2013).

3.2.1   ULTRASONOGRAPHY AND ANDROLOGICAL EXAMINATION

The ultrasound examination is a complementary test that is incorporated into the BSE and should always follow the clinical examination. It is a mistake to do ultrasound of the testicle and/or vesicular glands without first having done a complete clinical examination. It is a minimally invasive examination, especially in comparison with a biopsy, the result of which was especially questioned by the risk of production of anti-sperm antibodies, which may be a consequence of this examination. Recently, however, emphasis has again been placed on biopsy (Chapwanya et al., 2008). It is economically advantageous and allows us to obtain a photograph of the bull's reproductive system in real time, but especially, it is not an invasive examination (Ginther, 1995; Gnemm 2007; Gnemmi and Lefebvre, 2009, 2010; Kastelic and Brito, 2012). The ultrasound examination is necessary because with the clinical examination it is often not possible to identify the type of lesion present, its location/extension and above all it does not allow a prognosis to be made (Gnemmi, 2007; Gnemmi and Lefebvre, 2009, 2010). As in the case of semen evaluation, it is not always possible to determine the location of the lesion (Gnemmi 2007; Gnemmi and Lefebvre, 2009, 2010). It is a safe, minimally invasive and non-traumatic technique, unlike biopsy (Roberts, 1986; MacGowan et al., 2002; Goovaerts et al., 2006).

Ultrasound examination is considered necessary whenever there is a poor semen quality such as (Rault and Gèrard, 2006; Gnemmi, 2007; Gnemmi and Lefebvre, 2010):

1. Presence of abnormal spermatozoa
2. Low sperm concentration
3. Low viability after thawing
4. Presence of piospermias and/or azoospermia, or if it's discovered (Gnemmi, 2007; Gnemmi and Lefebvre, 2010)
5. Presence of testicular inflammation or presence of abnormal testes in form and/or size
6. Presence of pain for no clear reason

The ultrasound examination should be a routine examination, both in semen production centers and in the case of bulls used for natural service. This examination should be performed whenever there have been quali–quantitative alterations to the straws produced, or as a preventive measure, 2–4 weeks before the bull begins the mounting period (Gnemmi, 2007; Gnemmi and Lefebvre, 2010).

3.2.1.1 PREPARATION OF THE BULL

It is essential to work ensuring both the respect of the animals and the safety of the operator. Thus, regardless of the age, size and temperament of the bull, ultrasonography must be carried out under appropriate conditions, which guarantee the possibility of an optimal ultrasonographic examination, without risk and without the possibility of the bull being injured.

In order to do this, we must ensure the following paragraphs:

1. First evaluate the animal's attitude before approaching it.
2. The examination must be carried out in a favorable environmental condition. Away from noise, avoiding sudden noises. Speaking only when necessary and always in a moderate tone.
3. Place the animal in the operating box: check that both the operator and the bull are in a safe condition. It is important that the box is adequate to the size and strength of the animal. Inspect the box before entering the bull, carefully checking that there are no protruding points that could be dangerous to the safety of the bull itself (Fig. 3.1).
4. Before approaching the bull, allow the animal a few minutes to adapt to the new situation.
5. Warn the bull of its presence. Talk to the bull in a low tone, patting it on the head, neck, withers, chest, and rump.
6. Evaluate the bull's reaction to palpation. If the bull shows excessive aggressiveness, light sedation may be used.
7. To sedate a bull, xylazine (0.02 mg/kg) or diazepam (0.05 mg/kg) can be used. In the case of very nervous animals and/or in the case of some breeds or fighting bulls, the recommended doses can also be increased by 50–100%.
8. Before resorting to sedation, in an attempt to calm the bull, ejaculation can be stimulated. After mounting the bull tends to be more relaxed, calm, and easier to handle, and also the testicles will be more pendulum. Ejaculation prior to ultrasonographic examination will discharge the ampulla from the vas deferens and vesicular glands. However, it should be remembered that electroejaculation

increases the temperature of the skin of the scrotum covering the tail of the epididymis, and therefore alters the infrared scrotal thermogram (i.e. the evaluation of the surface temperature of the scrotum), and it is not known how it affects the ultrasound image (MacGowan et al., 2002).

9. Proceed to palpation of the testicles, head and tail of epididymis, and spermatic cord. This palpation serves to alert the bull of our presence, at the same time as allowing the particular clinical examination.

10. In case of hyperkeratosis and/or scleroderma, present especially in winter in old bulls, before the ultrasound examination it is good to degrease the surface of the skin of the area to be scanned (testicle and spermatic cord) with alcohol.

11. Before applying the gel, it is good to wet the surface of the seat to be examined with water at 35–38°C, in order to soften the surface, which allows a better adhesion of the ultrasound gel.

12. It is possible to make the ultrasound examination without using the gel, but with alcohol. In winter, especially in old bulls with very thick scrotum skin and keratosis, this is not a good alternative. In the summer, especially when working at high temperatures (>25–27 °C), the alcohol evaporates very quickly.

13. In summer, the gel should be kept refrigerated to avoid an excessive decrease in density.

14. If the gel is kept refrigerated, or in winter, when it is kept at room temperature, before applying it to the surface you wish to examine, check that it is not too cold. The gel also has a softening action on the skin and prevents air from remaining between the hairs of the scrotum, which makes ultrasound examination impossible.

3.2.1.2   EQUIPMENT

Ultrasound of the bull's reproductive system is performed with the same equipment used in bovine gynecological diagnosis. An ultra-portable, portable, or non-portable ultrasound machine with a linear transducer of 5.0–7.5 MHz (Gnemmi, 2007; Gnemmi and Lefebvre, 2010). Sectoral transducers are not normally used because their spherical surface is poorly adapted to the surface of the testicles. In addition to the 5.0–7.5 MHz linear transducer, an 8–11 MHz probe (T-Line), normally used in tendons and ligaments in equine clinics, can be used. This probe allows a more accurate evaluation of small lesions (Gnemmi 2007; Gnemmi and Lefebvre, 2010).

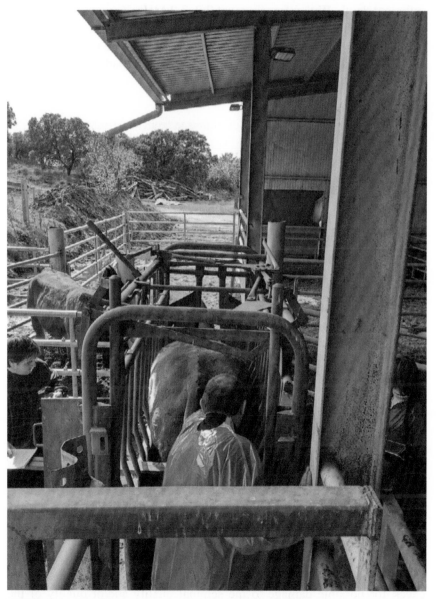

FIGURE 3.1 Operating box or squeeze chute, the necessary facility for working with bulls.

Even the linear or convex probe 2.0–5.0 MHz is very useful, allowing a simultaneous evaluation of the testicular parenchyma of both testicles in pubescent bulls. The 5.0 MHz probe is no longer able to guarantee sufficient depth. With a frequency of 2.0–3.0 MHz, it is possible to determine the total depth of the two, even in the testicles of a large adult bull. The ultrasound is performed by direct apposition of the transducer, after the application of ultrasound gel. The use of silicone pads is not necessary (Fig. 3.2).

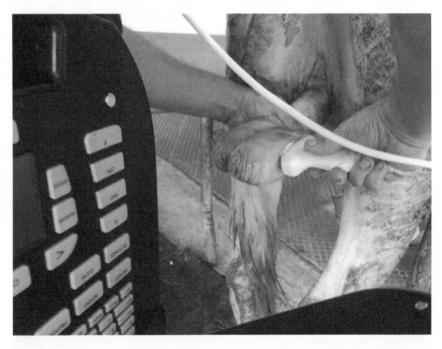

FIGURE 3.2   Ultrasound testicle examination: In sagittal view location of the probe is parallel to the long axis of the testicle. Also, it allows the evaluation of the parenchyma of both testicles.

3.2.1.3   ULTRASOUND TECHNIQUE

The ultrasound examination is an absolutely risk-free examination. To check for possible damage to the seminal quality and/or quality of the testicular parenchyma, a young beef bull was subjected to an ultrasound of the testicles, using a 5 MHz linear transducer, prior to semen extraction twice a week, for about 10 weeks (Coulter and Bailey, 1988).

A spermatogenesis cycle lasts about 70 days. The bull's testicles subjected to ultrasound evaluation were examined after this period, evaluating weight and morphology and also taking into account the amount of sperm present in the epididymis and semen production in general, including any anomaly (Coulter and Bailey, 1988). In this case, it was not possible to demonstrate any effect on semen quality.

The ultrasound examination is carried out by placing it on the posterior or lateral side of the bull. In the case of very nervous bulls, it is advisable to maintain an elevated hind limb (Gnemmi, 2007; Gnemmi and Lefebvre, 2010). It is advisable to carry out the examination in the dark, especially if working with LCD screens. It is possible to protect the screen of the ultrasound by the light, by means of a canvas or an umbrella, creating a shadow or resorting to the special cylinders that are applied to the screen. There is also the possibility of using cameras mounted on special glasses or handheld screens, or ultralight screens, connected through Bluetooth to the ultrasound unit.

3.2.1.3.1   External Genitalia

3.2.1.3.1.1   Testicles

First, a comparative evaluation of the two testicles should be carried out, taking the total depth. This measure, although not yet coded, may be an alternative to scrotal circumference. Unlike the latter, it is more faithful to reality, because it allows the testicular parenchyma to be measured specifically. The scrotal circumference may not reflect reality, for example, in the case of hydro-pio-haematocele (Gabor et al., 1996). After the comparative study of the two testicles, we examine each testicle separately. The right hand holds the left testicle, pushing it down, while the thumb and index finger of the same hand push the right testicle up (Gnemmi, 2007; Gnemmi and Lefebvre, 2010). Then, with the left hand, the right testicle is taken, making the same movements that we have just mentioned. We generate longitudinal and transversal cuts or sections. In the longitudinal section, the main axis of the ultrasound probe is parallel to the major axis of the testicle. In the cross-section, the main axis of the probe is perpendicular to the major axis of the testicle (Gnemmi, 2007; Gnemmi and Lefebvre, 2010).

In the longitudinal section it's evaluated:

1. Testicular parenchyma
2. Mediastinum
3. Length of testicle
4. Width of testicle
5. Albugineous tunic
6. Vaginal Tunic
7. Epididymis (head and tail)

In the cross-section, it's evaluated:

1. Testicular parenchyma
2. Mediastinum
3. Width of testicle
4. Albugineous tunic
5. Vaginal Tunic
6. Epididymis (head and tail)

3.2.1.3.1.2   Epididymis

It is possible to evaluate the head and tail of the epididymis. In the longitudinal section, but only in young bulls (with small testicles), it is possible to jointly evaluate the head and tail of the epididymis. In adult bulls, the head or tail can be evaluated, with both longitudinal and transverse sections.

3.2.1.3.1.3   Spermatic Cord

The spermatic cord grows to 14 months of age (Kastelic and Thundathil, 2008). The spermatic cord is circumscribed by the vaginal tunic (visceral and parietal lamina lamina); inside is the pampiniform plexus, formed by the two testicular veins and the tortuous testicular artery. The two testicular veins communicate with each other and form an extraordinary tangle of vessels near the artery. The vas deferens also form a part of the spermatic cord. Outside the vaginal tunic is the crematorium muscle. The spermatic cord is always evaluated with a posterior approach, in the transversal sections or with a longitudinal section.

3.2.1.3.1.4 Penis

The penis is boarded laterally. It is evaluated mainly in the cross-section. Before carrying out the ultrasound examination of the penis, you should shave the area with electric razor blade No. 40 and apply plenty of gel. The probe is moved perpendicular to the main axis of the cranio-caudal penis to verify the presence of any swelling (hematoma, abscess) (Gnemmi, 2007; Gnemmi and Lefebvre, 2010).

3.2.1.3.2 Internal Genitalia

3.2.1.3.2.1 Ampoules

The approach is posterior. After the fecal matter is evacuated from the rectum, the catheter is inserted trying to create a good contact with the rectal area. First, a longitudinal section, right and left, and then a cross-section (Gnemmi, 2007; Gnemmi and Lefebvre, 2010).

3.2.1.3.2.2 Vesicular Glands

The approach is posterior. After the fecal matter is evacuated from the rectum, the catheter is inserted trying to create a good contact with the rectal area. First a longitudinal section, right and left, and then a cross-section, sliding the probe in a cranio-caudal direction (Gnemmi, 2007; Gnemmi and Lefebvre, 2010).

3.2.1.3.2.3 Bulb-Urethral Glands

The approach is posterior. After the fecal matter is evacuated from the rectum, the catheter is inserted trying to create a good contact with the rectal area. Given the very caudal location of the bulbo-urethral glands, the probe is inserted into the rectum the length of the hand (Gnemmi, 2007; Gnemmi and Lefebvre, 2010).

3.2.1.3.2.4 Prostate

The approach is posterior. Both the body and the disseminated portion of the prostate can be seen. After the fecal matter is evacuated from the rectum, the catheter is inserted trying to create a good contact with the rectal area. First, a longitudinal, right, and left section is performed, and then a cross-section, sliding the cranial-caudal probe (Gnemmi, 2007; Gnemmi and Lefebvre, 2010).

3.2.1.3.2.5   Urethra

The approach is posterior. After the fecal matter is evacuated from the rectum, the catheter is inserted trying to create a good contact with the rectal area. First a longitudinal section, right and left, and then a cross-section, sliding the craniocaudally probe (Gnemmi, 2007; Gnemmi and Lefebvre, 2010).

3.2.1.4   ULTRASOUND ANATOMY

3.2.1.4.1   External Genitalia

3.2.1.4.1.1   Testicles

The normal testicle has a moderate, homogeneous echogenicity, very similar to the echogenicity of the corpus luteum. The echogenicity of the testicles increases with sexual maturity as a consequence of an increase in the density of the testicles (Kastelic and Brito, 2012).

The echogenicity of the rete testis increases between 20 and 40 weeks of life. This period is characterized by a greater growth capacity of the seminiferous tubules (Evans et al., 1996; Gnemmi, 2007; Gnemmi and Lefebvre, 2010). In breeds of *Bos taurus* for meat production (Angus, Charolais, Hereford and their crosses), the greatest increase in echogenicity is between 20 and 46 weeks of age (Kastelic and Brito, 2012). In crosses *Bos taurus* x *Bos indicus*, the increase in testicular density is delayed, compared to bulls *Bos taurus*. The maximum testicular intensity develops between 49 and 62 weeks of age (Brito et al., 2004). These changes in testicular density occur simultaneously with histological changes in the pre-pubertal testicles and indicate the differentiation of Sertoli cells, the formation of the blood–testis *barrier* (BTB), the increase in the diameter of seminiferous tubules, the increase in the volume of testicular parenchyma occupied by seminiferous tubules, and also a rapid growth of all germ cells and the onset of spermatogenesis (Brito et al., 2012; Kastelic and Brito, 2012). It has been shown that in *Bos indicus* and *Bos Taurus* individuals and their crosses older than 18 months, the density of the testicular parenchyma does not change. This leads us to believe that the composition of the testicular parenchyma remains almost constant after puberty (Brito et al., 2003; Kastelic and Brito, 2012); the sensitivity–specificity of ultrasound evaluation of testicular density to evaluate sexual precocity (early *vs.* late), puberty (no puber *vs.* puber), and sexual maturity (not good seminal quality *vs.* good seminal quality) is not statistically superior to the determination of scrotal circumference (Brito et al., 2004, 2012; Kastelic and Brito, 2012). The possibility of individual variations in testicular density, easy to find, especially in young bulls near puberty, should also not be underestimated. These individual variations make it difficult to define a cut-off point for density (Brito et al., 2012; Kastelic and Brito, 2012). The presence of echogenic (white) or hypo-echogenic/anechogenic foci is generally related to testicular parenchymal pathologies. With a transversal section, in the central part of the testicles, the mediastinum (2–4 mm) can be seen as an echogenic star (white). Similarly, in a longitudinal section (Fig. 3.3), the rete testis can be seen as a thin echogenic band (Gnemmi, 2007; Gnemmi and Lefebvre, 2009, 2010). The parietal and visceral vaginal tunic are thin and hyper-echogenic, separated by a thin echogenic line (2 mm). The space between the two layers increases in the case of hydropium or hematocele. Under the vaginal tunic, the albuginea tunic is seen as a thin echogenic line (Gnemmi, 2007; Gnemmi and Lefebvre, 2009, 2010).

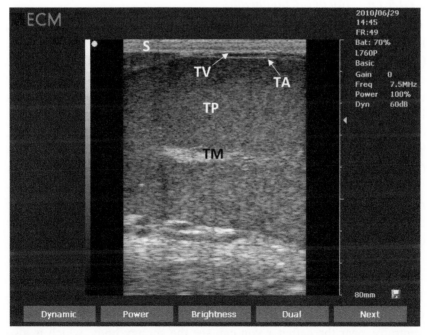

FIGURE 3.3 Ultrasonographyc appearance of testicular image in longitudinal section. S: scrotal skin; TA: tunica albuginea; TV: tunica vaginalis; TP: testicular parenchyma; TM: testicular mediastinum.

3.2.1.4.1.2   Head of Epididymis

The head of the epididymis is near the dorsal part of the testicle, under the pampiniform plexus (Gnemmi, 2007; Gnemmi and Lefebvre, 2009, 2010). Ultrasound examination to reveal the head of the epididymis is not always easy. Oblique sections are usually used. The head of the epididymis is clearly more echogenic than the testicular parenchyma and contrasts well with the anechogenicity of the vessels belonging to the pampiniform plexus.

3.2.1.4.1.3   Body of the Epididymis

The body of the epididymis, if there is no pathological dilation (sperm cysts), is not easily visible. The body of the epididymis runs along the medial side of each testicle (Gnemmi, 2007; Gnemmi and Lefebvre, 2009, 2010; Kastelic and Brito, 2012). In the longitudinal section, there is a small anechogenic conduit, whose walls are weakly echogenic.

3.2.1.4.1.4   Tail of the Epididymis

The tail of the epididymis is the most accessible part of the epididymis, located in the ventral part of the testicle with the typical conical shape (Gnemmi, 2007; Gnemmi and Lefebvre, 2009, 2010). The tail of the epididymis is visualized ultrasonographically by means of oblique transversal cuts. A small linear probe (TLine) produces excellent images thanks to the reduced contact surface of the probe itself. The tail of the epididymis seems less echogenic than the testicular parenchyma, but above all less homogeneous. It differs very well from the testicles (Fig. 3.4).

In the spermatic cord, the presence of the pampiniform plexus is dominant, characterized by tortuous anechogenic ducts. Only through the use of color Doppler, it is possible to distinguish the arterial branches of the dense network of venous anastomosis, forming a part of the plexus.

3.2.1.4.1.5   Penis

The albugineous tunic surrounds the penis and looks echogenic. Inside you can see the cavernous body hypoechogenic and homogeneous. Ventrally, near the catheter you can see the spongy body, which is also hypoechogenic, inside which you can see the urethra, as a virtual anechogenic space.

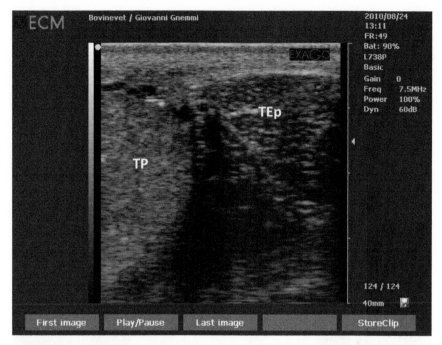

FIGURE 3.4 Epididymis evaluation: To evaluate the tail of the epididymis, each testicle is pushed toward the bottom of the scrotum. TP: testicular parenchyma; Tep: tail of epididymis. Spermatic cord.

3.2.1.4.2 Internal Genitalia

3.2.1.4.2.1 Ampoule

The two ampoules deferens are located cranially and dorsally with respect to the bladder neck (anechogenic). They are the most cranial glands of the entire glandular system. They have a tubular shape and are, on average, 10–12 cm long and 1.5 cm wide. In cross-section, they appear as two small hypoechogenic structures with an anechogenic light (Gnemmi and Lefebvre, 2009, 2010).

3.2.1.4.2.2 Vesicular Glands

Located near each of the corresponding vas blisters, they branch out near the bladder neck. They have an oblong shape and under physiological conditions the size is proportional to the age of the animal.

In general, we can say that the vesicular glands have a size in relation to the age of the bull (Table 3.1). Echographically, they have the same echogenicity of a compact corpus luteum being of moderate echogenicity and physiologically homogeneous (Gnemmi, 2007; Gnemmi and Lefebvre, 2009; 2010) (Fig. 3.5).

TABLE 3.1 Size of the Vesicular Glands, According to the Age of the Bull (Buczinski, 2008).

Age	Length	Thick	Width
1 year	7.0–9.0 cm	1.5–2.0 cm	1.5–2.5 cm
5 year	10–15 cm	2.0–4.0 cm	3.0–7.0 cm

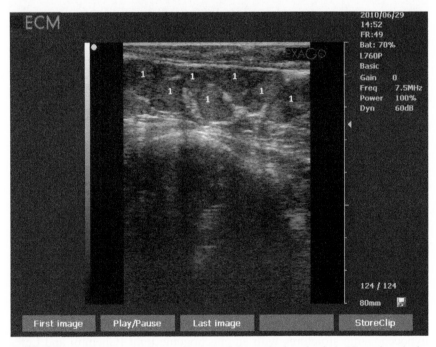

FIGURE 3.5　Ultrasonographic evaluation of the vesicular gland. 1: Normal vesicular gland lobes.

3.2.1.4.2.3　Bulbourethral Glands

They are the most caudally located glands of the entire glandular system. They are not detectable by rectal palpation, as they are covered by the bulbous spongy muscle (Gnemmi and Lefebvre, 2009, 2010). Although they are not easily identifiable by ultrasound, they have an ovoid or fusiform shape with an average diameter of 2 cm. Echographically, they appear hypoechogenic in comparison with m. bulb-spongiosum.

3.2.1.4.2.4 Prostate

The prostate is divided anatomically into two parts: the body and the disseminated part. The body is located in correspondence with the bladder neck, measures approximately 3.4 × 1.5 cm; the disseminated part is approximately 12 cm long and cannot be detected by palpation (Gnemmi and Lefebvre, 2010). The prostate, especially the disseminated part, is detectable in the longitudinal and transverse section during evaluation of the pelvic urethra. The prostate disseminated in the longitudinal section appears as a hypoechogenic band between the dorsal and ventral muscle of the urethra, which tends to be echogenic (darker) (Gnemmi and Lefebvre, 2009).

3.2.1.4.2.5 Urethra

The pelvic urethra extends between the bladder neck and a horizontal line corresponding to the ischial tuberosities. It has a length of about 20 cm and a diameter of about 3 cm (Gnemmi and Lefebvre, 2009). It is detectable both longitudinally and transversally. In this last section (Fig. 3.6), the C-shaped urethral muscle is observed, and tends to be echogenic (darker), with the thicker part ventrally placed (Gnemmi and Lefebvre, 2010).

3.2.1.5 ULTRASOUND OF PATHOLOGIES

3.2.1.5.1 External Genitalia

3.2.1.5.1.1 Testicles

The testicular parenchyma may be affected by inflammatory, degenerative, and neoplastic processes. However, it can also present cysts and torsion (Gnemmi, 2007; Gnemmi and Lefebvre, 2009, 2010). In some cases, the scrotum may also be involved in a pathological process: accumulation of fluid (hydro, hemato, or pio-cele) or inguinal hernia. Hydrocele is an accumulation of fluid between the parietal and visceral layers of the tunica albuginea. The virtual space (2 mm), which normally separates the two sheets, widens and becomes more evident (anechogenic space). Hydrocele is usually the result of torsion of the spermatic cord, but may be associated with testicular neoplasms, orchitis, or cardiac or renal pathologies (Gnemmi and Lefebvre, 2010).

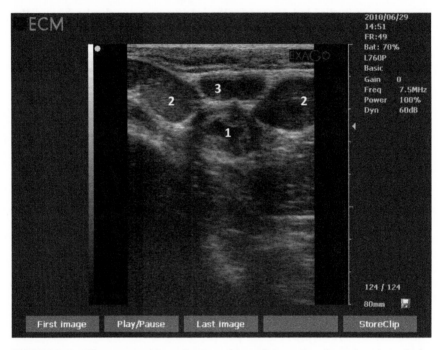

FIGURE 3.6   Ultrasonographic evaluation of the pelvic urethra. 1: urethra, 2: vesicular glands (right and left), and 3: ampulla of the deferent (right and left).

Hematocele is an accumulation of blood between the leaves of the vaginal tunic. To the ultrasound initially it appears anechogenic, with diverse echogenic points (red blood cells). At an advanced stage, hyperechogenicity will appear. The cause may be testicular trauma or torsion of the testicles. In the case of bacterial contamination of unhydrocele or hematocele, a piocele may develop, which echographically resembles a snowstorm: an anechoic background with a series of echogenic points (Gnemmi, 2007; Gnemmi and Lefebvre, 2009, 2010).

3.2.1.5.1.2 Orchitis

In acute forms, the testicle shows an increase in volume and appears warm to the touch. Echographically, the testicular parenchyma loses its usual homogeneity and tends to appear echogenic. In the case of chronic inflammation, areas of parenchyma can be seen, completely replaced by a bright hyperechogenic thickening (fibrosis, calcification), below which evident artifacts, such as shadow cones (shadows) (Gnemmi, 2007; Gnemmi and Lefebvre, 2009, 2010).

3.2.1.5.1.3 Hematoma

Hematomas usually have a traumatic base and are just below the surface. Their size is variable due to the trauma that created them. Echographically, they are observed hypoehcogenic (dark) in comparison with the testicular parenchyma that surrounds them. Their presence is always accompanied by pain.

3.2.1.5.1.4 Fibrosis

Fibrosis is observed as an echogenic thickening, hyperechogenic more or less large, more or less widespread, by virtue of which, if the acoustic density is high, the cone of shadow (shadow) can be seen (Fig. 3.7). Often, especially in bulls, it can highlight an echogenic thickening, hyperechogenic, without the company of shadows. In the absence of these artifacts, it is difficult to correlate densification to poor semen quality (Gnemmi, 2007; Gnemmi and Lefebvre, 2009, 2010).

In the presence of fibrosis, there is always poor quality (azoospermia)—quantity of semen. A recent study of these areas of "fibrosis" (Barth and Oko, 1989) has allowed us to bring to light, especially in prepubertal bulls (5–6 months) with "fibrosis", with a tendency to grow in number and extension, in the same animals when they reach 12–14 months of age. The cause of these lesions is not known; it is assumed that they may be related to respiratory syncytial virus (BRSV) infections (Barth and Oko, 1989). Histological examination of these lesions showed fibrous tissue between the seminiferous tubules, with a reduction in the number of germ cells. Some tubules were absolutely devoid of germ cells and Sertoli; however, they were always devoid of inflammatory cells. No abnormalities in sperm morphology have been observed in mild or moderate cases of testicular fibrosis (Barth and Oko, 1989; Kastelic and Brito, 2012).

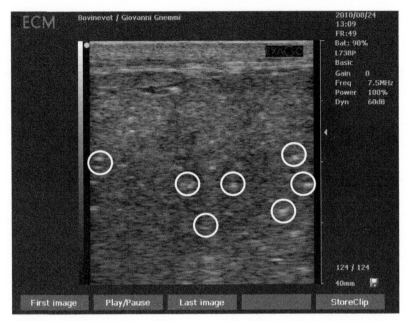

FIGURE 3.7   Ultrasonagraphic appearance of a testicular image in longitudinal section with fibrosis (white circles).

3.2.1.5.1.5   Hypoplasia

It can be uni- or bilateral. In any case, bulls with hypoplasia, even unilateral should never be used for breeding. The testicles are smaller in volume and less consistent to the touch. Echographically, the testicular parenchyma tends to be anechogenic (dark), although the mediastinum appears poorly echogenic and is often difficult to see (Fig. 3.8).

3.2.1.5.1.6   Abscess

The abscess capsule appears echogenic more or less bright. Inside you can see pus in the form of a snowstorm, but only at an early stage. Then appears the interior of the echogenic abscess, hyper-echogenic (if replaced by a connective tissue-calcification) and heterogeneous (Gnemmi and Lefebvre, 2009, 2010).

3.2.1.5.1.7   Neoplasia

It is possible to find interstitial cell tumors, Sertoli cell tumors, and seminomas. The swelling is not always visible or palpable from the outside. Echographically, it is seen that the testicular parenchyma loses its homogeneity and hypoechogenic, echogenic, hyperechogenic areas are seen, often alternating with liquid (anechoic), limited by an echogenic capsule, sometimes several millimeters thick. The diagnosis of type cannot be done by ultrasound, but histologically (biopsy) (Gnemmi and Lefebvre, 2009, 2010).

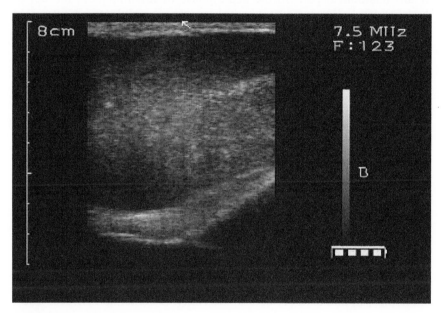

FIGURE 3.8 Testicle hypoplasia.

3.2.1.5.1.8 Cyst

Within the testicular parenchyma it is possible to see small cysts, ultrasonographically anechogenic. They are not related to subfertility or infertility: the quality and quantity of semen are generally not affected. Testicular cysts should not be confused with dilation of the central vein of the testicles: differential diagnosis requires color Doppler.

3.2.1.5.1.9 Epididymal Head

The most frequent pathology of the head of the epididymis are abscesses. Its capsule may be a few millimeters thick, echogenic, while the content is heterogeneous: there may be hyperechogenic areas (calcification), along with hypoechogenic areas. Cysts of the head of the epididymis with hypoechogenic areas within the tissue have also been reported (Matuszewka and Sysa, 2002).

3.2.1.5.1.10   Epididymal Tail

Inflammation of the tail of the epididymis is the most common pathology of this anatomical part. In the acute phase of inflammation, the tail of the epididymis increases in size and becomes painful on palpation and ecohgenic. When the process becomes chronic, the tail of the epididymis is very heterogeneous and hypoechogenic, probably due to the presence of edema. You can also see some hyperechogenic zones (Gnemmi and Lefebvre, 2009, 2010).

3.2.1.5.1.11   Spermatic Cord

It is possible to find inflammation, torsion of the spermatic cord in various degrees, varicocele, which can be considered the most frequent pathology in this anatomical location (Gnemmi, 2007; Gnemmi and Lefebvre, 2009, 2010). The varicocele is a consequence of a malfunction of the valvular system of the two sperm veins; the veins dilate, then the ultrasound, you will see an anecogenic tortuosity more or less dilated. Mild varicocele is physiological in old bulls. The varicocele, if it does not reach a high degree, is not related to infertility. The diagnosis of varicocele is confirmed with Doppler color. The torsion of the spermatic cord is paraphysiological in the old bull and is not related to infertility. If the torsion exceeds 180°, clinical symptoms appear: dilation of the ventral spermatic cord at torsion, with an increase in testicular volume (hydrocele), increase or decrease of the echogenicity of the testicles (Gnemmi, 2007; Gnemmi and Lefebvre 2009, 2010). It is possible to find hyperplasia of the lymphatic tissue of the spermatic cord (BLV): the hyperplastic gland induces compression of the pampiniform plexus, it could also induce the formation of hydrocele. Hyperplastic lymphatic tissue looks hypoechogenic (Gnemmi and Lefebvre, 2009).

3.2.1.5.1.12   Penis

The pathological forms of ultrasound interest at this anatomical location are abscesses and hematomas. Abscesses are usually located between the foreskin and scrotum and usually develop as a complication of a hematoma. The hyperechoic capsule of the abscess, which circumscribes a heterogeneous area, containing hyperechogenic, echogenic and anechogenic subareas, can be seen ultrasonographically. However, the ultrasound aspect of the penile abscess changes over time: the older the abscess, the greater its echogenicity (Gnemmi and Lefebvre, 2009, 2010). The hematoma of the penis is normally formed by the rupture of the dorsal surface of the tunica albuginea, with blood coming out of the *corpus cavernosum*. Therefore, the greater the rupture of the albugineous tunic, the larger the hematoma that forms. Often, the hematoma of the penis is accompanied by a prolapse of the foreskin, which is in fact the reason, in many cases, why the bull is checked. Echographically, the hematoma of the penis is presented as a multilobular mass with heterogeneous ehcogenicity, covered by an echogenic capsule (Gnemmi and Lefebvre, 2010).

3.2.1.5.2   Internal Genitalia

3.2.1.5.2.1   Ampoule
Pathologies are not usually described in this location.

3.2.1.5.2.2   Vesicular Glands
Inflammation of the vesicular gland is the most common pathology affecting this anatomical site; however, with a low frequency (9%) (Bagshaw and Ladds, 1974; Gnemmi and Lefebvre, 2009, 2010). Acute forms are characterized by glandular hypertrophy, palpation pain, and sometimes localized pelvic peritonitis (Gnemmi, 2007; Gnemmi and Lefebvre, 2009, 2010). The gland is ultrasonographically enlarged and hypoechogenic. In case of abscess, it is possible to see an echogenic capsule, which circumscribes a more or less extended area, such as a snowstorm. In the case of unilateral inflammation, the comparison of the two glands makes diagnosis easier (Gnemmi, 2007; Gnemmi and Lefebvre, 2009, 2010). In the case of acute infection and abscess formation, leukocytosis is always present, even piospermia. In chronic inflammation, the gland is slightly enlarged, and fibrosis may occur, making it ultrasound more echogenic and bright compared to normal contralateral. Hypertrophy of the vesicular gland should always be considered as a pathology in the young animal, whereas it is a paraphysiological condition in old bulls.

3.2.1.5.2.3   Bulb-Urethral Glands

Pathologies are not usually described in this location.

3.2.1.5.2.4   Prostate

Pathologies are not usually described in this location.

3.2.1.5.2.5   Urethra

Normally the pelvic urethra cannot be seen ultrasonographically, but it appears as a virtual space. A dilation of the urethra, which appears in longitudinal section as an anechogenic channel, may be the consequence of urethral obstruction/stenosis, urethritis, or urolithiasis (Gnemmi and Lefebvre, 2009, 2010).

3.3   CONCLUSIONS

Some authors have shown that a small testicular degeneration cannot be diagnosed with an ultrasound examination, since the ultrasound aspect of the testicle does not change (Sidibe et al., 1992; Brito et al., 2003; Arteaga et al., 2005). But we must also ask ourselves if these same microscopic lesions were/are always correlated with quantitative changes in semen. The ultrasound density of the testicles was statistically correlated with the production of semen (Brito et al., 2012; Kastelic and Brito, 2012), but not with the volume of the ejaculate, much less with the concentration of sperm or the total amount of sperm in the ejaculate (Gabor et al., 1996; Brito et al., 2012). In some studies, it has been impossible to demonstrate the correlation between the density of the ultrasound of the testicles and the quality of the semen (Gabor et al., 1998; Brito et al., 2003; Kastelic and Brito, 2012). In these studies, however, they have tried to demonstrate a correlation between semen quality and testicular density, determined on the same day as the ultrasound, when we know that spermatogenesis lasts about 70 days. Therefore, the ultrasound density of the testicle must be related to the quality of semen that will be produced 60–70 days after the ultrasound (Barth and Oko, 1989; Brito et al., 2004; Arteaga et al., 2005; Kastelic and Brito, 2012). Practically, the ultrasound density of the testicle has a predictive value, rather than giving a snapshot of the situation at the time of determination. Ultrasound examination of the bull's reproductive system requires statistical validation to standardize the technique. Despite of this, it is a test that must be included in a BSE. It is a convenient, minimally invasive test, capable of determining the source of a problem and its severity, also offering the possibility of providing a prognosis. Ultrasound examination, together with scrotal thermography, is surely the most interesting technique that the clinician currently has available to make a diagnosis under field conditions.

KEYWORDS

- **bull**
- **breeding soudness evaluation**
- **ultrasound**
- **andrological examination**
- **reproductive pathologies**

REFERENCES

Arteaga, A. A.; Barth, A. D.; Brito, L. F. Relationship Between Semen Quality And Pixel-Intensity Of Testicular Ultrasonograms After Scrotal Insulation In Beef Bulls. *Theriogenology* **2005,** *64*, 408–415.

Bagshaw, P. A.; Ladds, P. W. A Study Of The Accessory Sex Glands Of Bulls In Abattoirs In Northern Australia. *Austral. Vet. J.* **1974,** *50*, 489–495.

Barth, A. D.; Oko, R. J. *Abnormal Morphology of Bovine Spermatozoa*; Iowa State University Press: Ames, 1989; pp 23–24.

Brito, L. F.; Barth, A. D.; Wilde, R. E.; Kastelic, J. P. Testicular Ultrasonogram Pixel Intensity During Sexual Development And Its Relationship With Semen Quality, Sperm Production, And Quantitative Testicular Histology In Beef Bulls. *Theriogenology* **2012,** *78*(1), 69–76.

Brito, L. F.; Silva, A. E.; Barbosa, R. T.; Unanian, M. M.; Kastelic, J. P. Effects Of Scrotal Insulation On Sperm Production, Semen Quality, And Testicular Echotexture In Bos Indicus And Bos Indicus X Bos Taurus Bulls. *Anim. Reprod. Sci.* **2003,** *79*, 1–15.

Brito, L. F.; Silva, A. E. D. F; Unanian, M. M.; Dode, M. A. N.; Barbosa, R. T.; Kastelic, J. P. Sexual Development In Early And Late Maturing Bos Indicus And Bos Indicus X Bos Taurus Crossbred Bulls In Brazil. *Theriogenology* **2004,** *62*, 1198–1217.

Chapwanya, A.; Callanan, J.; Larkin, H.; Keenan, L.; Vaughan, L. Breeding Soundness Evaluation Of Bulls By Semen Analysis, Testicular Fine Needle Aspiration Cytology And Transscrotal Ultrasonography. *Ir. Vet. J.* **2008,** *61*, 315–318.

Coulter, G. H.; Bailey, D. R. Effects Of Ultrasonography On The Bovine Testis And Semen Quality. *Theriogenology* **1988**, *30*, 743–749.

Evans, A. O. C.; Pierson, R. A.; Garcia, A.; McDougall, L. M.; Hrudka, F.; Rawling, F. Changes In Circulating Hormone Concentration, Testes Histology And Testis Ultrasonography During Sexual Maturation In Beef Bulls. *Theriogenology* **1996**, *46*, 345–357.

Gabor, G.; Szasz, F.; Sasser, G.; Bozo, S.; Völgyi, J.; Barany, I. In *Using Digitized Video Method For The Measuring Of Testes Sizes And Prediction The Testis Volume In Bulls*, Proceedings of the 13th ICAR Congress, Sydney, July 30, **1996**.

Gabor, G.; Sasser, R. G.; Kastelic, J. P.; Mezes, M.; Falkay, G.; Bozo, S.; VCsik, J.; Barany, I.; Hidas, A.; Szasz Jr., F.; Boros, G. Computer Analysis Of Video And Ultrasonographic Images For Evaluation Of Bull Testes. *Theriogenology* **1998**, *50*, 223–228.

Ginther, O. J. *Ultrasonic Imaging and Animal Reproduction: Cattle. Book 3*. Equiservices Publishing: Cross Plains, WI, USA, **1995**.

Gnemmi, G. Fisiopatologia delle ovaie e del ciclo. Gestione clinica della riproduzione bovina, a cura di G. Sali. *Le Point Veterinaire Italie* **2013**, *5*, 89–118.

Gnemmi, G. Place de l'echographie du taureau en pratique. *Le Point Veterinaire* **2007**, *275*, 40–45.

Gnemmi, G.; Lefebvre, R.C. Bull Anatomy and Ultrasonography of the Reproductive Tract. In *Practical Atlas of Ruminant and Camelid Reproductive Ultrasonography*; DesCoteaux, L., Colloton, J., Gnemmi, G., Eds.; Wiley-Blackwell: New York, **2010**, 9, pp 143–162.

Gnemmi, G.; Lefebvre, R. C. Ultrasound Imaging Of The Bull Reproductive Tract: An Important Field Of Expertice For Veterinarians. *Vet. Clin. Food. Anim.* **2009**, *25*, 767–779.

Gnemmi, G.; Maraboli, C.; Perkins, J. Rilevazione del calore nella bovina: nuovi approcci ad un vecchio problema. *Summa Animali da Reddito* **2007**, *5*, 37–43.

Goovaerts, I. G. F.; Hoflack, G. G.; Van Soom, A.; Dewulf, J.; Nichi, M.; de Kruif, A.; Bols, P. E. J. Evaluation Of Epididymal Semen Quality Using The Hamilton-Thorne Analyzer Indicates Variation Between The Two Caudal Epididymides Of The Same Bull. *Theriogenology* **2006**, *66*, 323–330.

Kasimanickam, V. R.; Kasimanickam, R. K.; Kastelic, J. P.; Stevenson, J. S. Associations Of Adiponectin And Fertility Estimates In Holstein Bulls. *Theriogenology* **2013**, *79*(5), 766–777.

Kastelic, J. P.; Thundathil, J. Breeding Soundness Evaluation And Semen Analysis For Predicting Bull Fertility. *Reprod. Domest. Anim.* **2008**, *43*(2), 368–373.

Kastelic, J. P.; Brito, L. F. C. Ultrasonography For Monitoring Reproductive Function In The Bull. *Reprod. Dom. Anim.* **2012**, *47*(3), 45–51.

MacGowan, M. R.; Bertran, J. D.; Fordyce, G.; Fitzpatrick, L. A.; Miller, R. G.; Jayawardhana, G. A.; Doogan, V. J.; De Faveri, J.; Holroyd, R. G. Bull Selection And Use In Northern Australia 1. Physical Traits. *Anim. Reprod. Sci.* **2002**, *71*, 25–37.

Matuszewka, M.; Sysa, P. S. Epididymal Cysts In European Bison. *J. Wildl. Dis.* **2002**, *38*, 637–640.

Pursley, J. R. In Practical OvSynch® Programs, Proceedings of the 40th Annual Convention of the American Association of Bovine Practitioners, Vancuver, British Columbia, Canada, Sep 20–22, **2007**.

Rault, P.; Gèrard, O. Examen èchographique génital du taureau. *Point Veterinaire*. **2006**, *37*, 32–39.

Roberts, S. J. Infertility in Male Animals (Andrology): Diagnosis of Sterility and Infertility in the Male and avaluation of Breeding Soundness. In *Veterinary Obstetrics and Genital Disease–Theriogenology*; Roberts, S. J., Ed.; Edwards Brothers, Inc.: Michigan, USA, **1986;** pp 856–870.

Santos, J. E. P. Animal Health and Reproduction. Dairy Cattle Reproduction Conference, Indianapolis IN, **2013.**

Sidibe, M.; Franco, L.A.; Fredriksson, G.; Madej, M.; Malmgren, L. Effects On Testosterone, LH And Cortisol Concentrations, And On Testicular Ultrasonographic Appearance Of Induced Testicular Degeneration In Bulls. *Acta Vet. Scand.* **1992,** *33*, 191–196.

CHAPTER 4

Postpartum Management in Dairy Cows

GIOVANNI GNEMMI[1,2*], JUAN CARLOS GARDÓN[2], and
CRISTINA MARABOLI[1]

[1]Bovinevet Internacional, Bovine Ultrasound Services & Herd
Management, Spain

[2]Department of Animal Medicine and Surgery, Faculty of Veterinary
and Experimental Sciences Catholic University of Valencia,
San Vincente Mártir, Spain

*Corresponding author. E-mail: giovanni.gnemmi@bovinevet.com

ABSTRACT

Modern cattle health management is basically based on prevention. This approach finds its natural justification in the fact that today it is necessary to guarantee the health of the consumer (through a proper and measured use of medicaments, in particular antibiotics and chemotherapy) and animal welfare. The economic aspect should not be underestimated: 70–75% of the cost of a disease depends on the lack of production. It, therefore, becomes natural to focus all health management on the prevention of pathologies. In the transition phase almost 70% of all cattle diseases are concentrated, therefore limiting the occurrence of diseases in this delicate period to a minimum is of fundamental importance. Equally important is the early diagnosis of sick cows, but above all the rapid identification of cows at risk. Electronic devices capable of creating a daily attention list of cows at risk of infirmity are available today. However, these systems can be completed or replaced by a careful observation of post-calving cows, integrating this clinical evaluation with collateral tests, which will allow determining which animals are at risk, also allowing them to establish a risk order.

4.1   INTRODUCTION

The transition period is a critical time for dairy cattle (Overton and Fetrow, 2008). Didactically, this period is identified during the 2–3 weeks prior to delivery and the 2–3 weeks after delivery (Block, 2010). However, we must face this "period" with some flexibility, especially today, that nutritional management strategies, which until yesterday were considered "indisputable," are questioned (dry off and close up). For this reason, the transition period could be started 30 days before the delivery and we could end it with the end of the voluntary waiting time, or with the first artificial insemination (AI).

During the transition period, the cow suffers from physiological changes (Goff et al., 1997; Drackley et al., 1999; Overton and Fetrow, 2008). The cow is preparing for calving and milk production, events that, especially for future primiparous heifers, they represent a true physiological "cyclone" (LeBlanc, 2013, 2014).

We know that during the first part of the transition, ecological and zootechnical environment conditions must be created such as the cancellation or, at least, the drastic reduction of stress factors. In this way, the dry matter intake can be maintained high; in the primiparous, never should fall below 10–11 kg; while that in the cow, it should always be higher than 11–12 kg (Gnemmi et al., 2018).

Especially during the first part of lactation, the nutrients deviate greatly toward the udder. The metabolism of glucose is altered and, as a consequence of the resulting hypoglycemia, the mobilization of fat and protein reserves begins (LeBlanc, 2013, 2014). The cow loses weight and cows that cannot compensate for these imposing transitions can develop puerperal diseases, that is, retention of fetal membranes, puerperal metritis, ketosis, abomasal displacement, etc. (LeBlanc, 2013, 2014).

This situation can affect to a different extent, even 30–50% of the cows (LeBlanc, 2010). The cows that develop pathologies during the transition period are often compromised their productive/reproductive capacity. Therefore, it is essential that the environmental and zootechnical management be such that it reduces or cancels the risk of diseases in the pre- and postpartum. In addition to this, we must try to identify the problem cows as soon as possible.

The productive and reproductive performance of the cow and herd is related to the incidence of different transition pathologies, but also, and probably above all, to the ability to identify problem animals very early.

In this regard, it is essential to observe the cattle, trying to identify the sick cows in each moment (Hulsen, 2003).

4.2 THE METHOD

Every postpartum pathology more or less compromises the animal's productive and reproductive performance. If we take for example two pathologies of the uterus such as the retention of fetal membranes and metritis, analyzing the cost, we can see that the higher cost item refers not to veterinary costs and/or to the costs for medicalization, but to the failure production (Gnemmi et al., 2016) (Table 4.1).

In other studies, it has been seen that the cost of drugs is between 16 and 28% due to the use of an ampicillin or a third-generation cephalosporin, respectively. The cost of elimination (different because of parity, production, and Days in Milk (DIM) at the time of cow's elimination) would affect between 22 and 26%, whereas the reduction in reproductive performance would affect the order of 28–33% (Overton and Fetrow, 2008).

Evaluating the cost of puerperal pathologies is a very complex analysis; the four main cost chapters must be taken into consideration, which in turn can be divided into 18 sub-chapters, of which veterinary expenses, labor costs, the cost for medicalization, the cost of eliminating contaminated milk from medicaments, and the lack of production are 5 of 18 items.

However, to look at it, it is clear that when a cow gets sick, the farmer starts to lose money. This is especially related to the greater predisposition of the bovine to develop, even in the postpartum, more than one puerperal pathology. Due to the lack of production determined by the sanitary conditions in which the cow is found, its state of health is compromised by the greater risk that this animal develops other puerperal pathologies. For all this, prevention on the one hand and the early identification of problem cows take on fundamental importance.

The goal is not to have and/or drastically reduce the number of sick cows during the transition period. This means focusing attention on four fundamental points of the management program (Gnemmi et al., 2019):

- Nutritional management
- Environmental management (ecological and zootechnical environment) and cow comfort

TABLE 4.1   Impact of Different Cost Items on the Complex RFM-Metritis and Endometritis.

Disease	Day open cost (+ 30 dd)	>AI cost	<Risk culling	Total cost	% Vet cost	% Drug	% Milk elim.	<Milk prod.	% Labor cost
RMF	180 €	88 €	85 €	1.439€	6.9%	10.9%	0.5%	86.0%	2.6%
Metritis	180 €	88 €	85 €	1.469€	8.8%	10.5%	6.4%	80.4%	2.7%
Endometritis	180 €	88 €	85 €	1.445€	8.3%	4.4%	7.6%	88.8%	3.2%

Reprinted with permission from Gnemmi et al., 2016.

- Handling drying period
- Prevention of pathologies (metabolic diseases, hypocalcemia, infection, etc.)

We must be able to identify sick cows and especially subclinical cows as soon as possible. A cow with retained placenta and/or metritis is not necessarily a sick cow. More than 50% of the cows with retention of the fetal membranes do not develop fever, which means they undergo spontaneous healing (Gilbert, 2008) and 55–70% of the cows with metritis have a spontaneous recovery (Santos et al., 2014) without where to resort to therapy, especially to antibiotic therapy. The ability to manage postpartum, that is, limiting the use of antibiotics only to the cows that really need it, has direct and indirect positive effects on the economic balance of the herd, but also on the welfare of the herd and consumer health.

Today, there are electronic detection systems, a kind of artificial intelligence, that allow the monitoring of several biological parameters. These systems can be applied as ear tags or as necklaces (www.scrdairy. com, 2019). They not only allow the identification of cows close to heat and/or in heat, or with disorders of the reproductive sphere (cystic degeneration of the ovaries), but also allow detecting body temperature, hours of rumination, resting hours, and the hours that the cow spends eating/drinking (www.scrdairy.com, 2019). These systems detect the state of the animal every hour, sending all the information to a server, which collects and classifies all this data. In practice, it is possible to verify in real time the state (physiological or pathological, or close to the pathology) of the bovine.

These systems are no longer the future, but the present and, undoubtedly, in the coming years, will become crucial in the raising of livestock, especially in those farms that want to address the problem of reducing the drug (antibiotics and hormones), to through the reduction of sick cows in the transition period.

It is possible to monitor the herd in the postpartum period and identify the problems of the cows, even without the help of these technological supports. It is necessary to "only" observe the herd, very carefully, observing everything that seems to be nonphysiological. The observation is important; however, it is very useful to be able to recognize and remember the problem of the cow (Table 4.2).

Observe the cows to understand what they are telling us. We often do not understand what cows manifest, only because instead of observing we limit ourselves to look superficially without knowing how to grasp fundamental nuances.

TABLE 4.2 Postpartum Pathologies Acronyms.

RFM	RP
Uterus Prolapse	UP
Dystocia	DS
Hypocalcemia	HCa
Puerperal Metritis	MT
Ketosis	K
Mastitis	MS
Lameness	LA

We must be able to observe or be educated in observation. It is necessary to observe minutely and without prejudice (Hulsen, 2003).

What am I seeing? Why is it happening? What does it mean? Is it an individual problem or does it concern more cows? Which cows are interested in: all cows or just the lactating heifers? These are some of the questions that an attentive observer, walking in the postpartum group every morning, must ask themselves. It is necessary to observe the cow completely, without leaving out the details. It is necessary to observe the cow, but also the ecological and zootechnical environment in which the cow is found. In practice, a precise evaluation of the cow is made both individually and collectively, without neglecting to observe the environment in which the cow lives, trying to understand the degree of adaptation and satisfaction of the cow and the group toward the ecological environment (light, climate, ventilation, cooling, flooring, berths, lanes, cleaning, etc.) and zootechnical environment (nutrition, quality of human management, etc.) in which the cow lives.

In this sense, an excellent strategy is to "write" in cows, between the iliac tuberosity and the ischial tuberosity, indicating with an acronym, the pathology that has affected the cow (Fig. 4.1).

On farms where the rectal temperature is detected daily in the first 10 days after calving, a row is applied every day, so that there are five rows on the right and five rows on the left at the end of the temperature monitoring. If the measured temperature is higher than 39.5°C, the line on the rump is made in a different color, so that the person looking at the cow, even if he/

she does not detect her number, can determine from how many days she delivered and, if so, when a thermal increase is determined (Fig. 4.2).

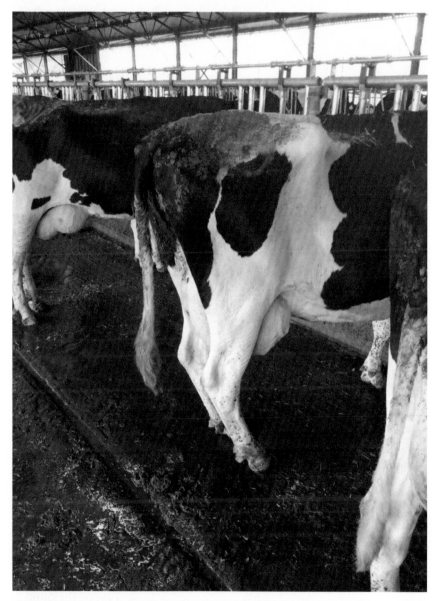

FIGURE 4.1   Acronym indicating pathology of affected cow.

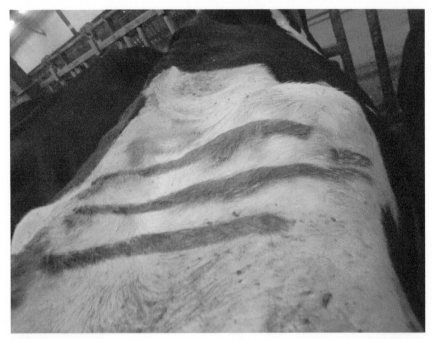

FIGURE 4.2   Cow with high temperature; line on the rump is made in a different color.

4.3   MONITORING

The first problem that needs to be addressed is which animals focus our attention.

All animals after parturition must be kept under control; however, this does not mean that all cows must be visited daily. In small and medium herds (<100 cows in milk), daily monitoring of each animal may be feasible, but one wonders what the benefit of a daily visit of each postpartum bovine might be.

There are many farms where all the cows of the group 0–10 DIM are subjected to an intravaginal visit every 48 h (to verify the presence and type of vaginal discharge) and to a daily rectal exploration to verify the uterine involution. Why carry out a manual exploration of the vagina, being able to produce a precise and punctual diagnosis without resorting to invasive methods? Let's not forget that, especially in the primiparous, there may be postpartum vaginal lacerations: also, for this reason, manual exploration of the vaginal vestibule, if possible, should be avoided. All postpartum animals should be monitored daily, but only sick or suffering animals should be visited. How to detect these animals early?

Through observation and daily monitoring of the group 0–10 DIM, it is possible to control the health status of the herd in the immediate postpartum.

We have already seen that there is the possibility of controlling the rectal temperature. In addition, it may be possible to control Body Condition Score (BCS), the ketosis test (Beta Hydroxy Butyrate [BHB]) level in blood or milk, rumen fill scoring, locomotion scoring, mobility scoring, edema scoring, fecal scoring, metritis scoring, etc. Most of these evaluations can be done mainly by observing the cows (Table 4.3).

TABLE 4.3   Bovine Monitoring Procedures.

Time	Production	RS	LS	MS	AS	RF	BHB	FS	VD	ES	VL	T
Every 24 h	X	X	X	X	X	X			X			X
Every 48 h								X				X
Every 72 h										X		X
Every 120 h							X				X	

AS, abdominal shape; ES, edema score; FS, Fecal score; LS, locomotion score; MS, mobility score; RF, respiratory frequency; RS, Rumen score; T, temperature; VD, vaginal discharge; VL, vaginal laceration.

Before doing one or all of the different tests that we have discussed, it is necessary to verify the production of each postpartum cow. A healthy cow progressively increases milk production, from the first days of lactation. A cow that does not produce milk and/or falls is a cow that must be observed in a special way: there is always a problem at the base of this situation. All herd management software can be configured so that cows that do not rise to milk and/or that decrease milk production by 6–8%, compared to the last milking, are brought to attention by the system. The clinician should check these animals immediately.

Attention: controlling them does not necessarily mean visiting them. First, verify that these animals are interested in the food and their score in the rumen.

4.3.1   MILK PRODUCTION

A healthy cow, immediately after the delivery, begins to eat and then increases its milk production progressively. A cow that does not increase milk production, or that decreases milk production by 6–8% compared to the last milking must be subjected to an accurate clinical examination as soon as possible.

Every morning, before anything else, the person in charge of the postpartum, must verify the production of all the animals of this group, selecting those animals that have not increased or decreased production compared to the last milking. These animals must be visited as soon as possible.

4.3.2   FRONTAL OBSERVATION

The frontal observation of the cows must be carried out carefully and with great discretion. The cows must not be harassed but must be observed without causing stress. We must observe the cows of this group, trying to understand the hierarchies; but above all, it is fundamental to understand if each cow is well in the group, or if there are reasons for stress and/or tension.

It must be observed if the cow can easily access the food, if she can access the water easily, and if there are comfortable bunks where the cow can rest. It is also necessary to observe the location of the postpartum group with respect to the rest of the farm.

4.3.2.1   INTERESTS IN FOOD

Observe the herd as it behaves in front of the food and observe the interest in the food of each individual cow. Do the animals eat regularly? Are there cows that are choosy? Are there cows that disturb the other cows that want to eat? How much food do they grow on average each morning in this group? Does the unloading of food occur regularly? Is the mixture well made? Do cows have an appetite? If cows refuse food, is it because they are not hungry (why?) or, because the mixture has problems (smell)?

4.3.2.2   POSITION, MOVEMENT, AND TEMPERATURE OF THE EARS

A healthy cow is attentive to everything that surrounds it. The ears are an excellent indicator of the state of the cow's sensory. A healthy cow has straight ears and moves whenever something catches the cow's interest. Low ears are an indicator of a cow's malaise. Cold ears are an indication that cows have fever: normally cold ears are an indication of a drop in skin temperature of at least 3°C, which roughly corresponds to an increase in the internal temperature of 1°C.

4.3.2.3   HORNY SHINE, TEARING (KIND OF TEARING)

A healthy cow has bright corneas. The eyes follow with attention everything that happens near the cow. A sick cow has opaque corneas and a half-closed eye. The presence of excessive tearing can be an indication of an ocular pathology. It is always necessary to verify if the tears are single or bilateral. It is also necessary to verify what type of tearing is involved: serous, mucopurulent, or purulent.

4.3.2.4   MUZZLE

The cow is an animal that cares very much for its personal hygiene!

A healthy cow constantly cleans the muzzle, which will be clean and moist. In a sick cow, the muzzle will be dirty and dry. Also, pay attention to the presence of nasal leaks: are they unilateral or bilateral? Are they serous, mucus-purulent, or purulent? Are they odorless or stinky?

All these signs point the clinician toward a diagnosis of high or low airway pathologies.

4.3.2.5   PRESENCE OF COUGH AND TYPE OF COUGH

The presence of cough, the frequency of cough, and the type of cough (dry and oily) help the clinician to suspect a pathology of the respiratory system, but also allow hypotheses to be made about the site of the pathology (upper or lower respiratory tract).

4.3.3   POSTERIOR OBSERVATION

The subsequent observation of the cows in the group 0–10 DIM allows completing the clinical evaluation initiated with the frontal examination. At the end of this observation, it will be decided if it is necessary to submit the cow to a complete clinical visit.

4.3.3.1   RUMEN FILL SCORING

One element that determines the health of the cow in transition and not only in transition is its ability to ingest dry matter. In principle, we can say that a cow that eats is not suffering and that the greater the ingestion of dry matter, the less the risk of becoming sick.

An excellent indicator of the health of the cow is the Rumen Fill Score or Rumen Score. A healthy rumen is an indication of a healthy cow; therefore, the rumen score is indirectly an indicator of the cow's health status. Obviously, when evaluating the efficiency of rationing also in the postpartum, the analysis must not be limited to the rumen score, but other parameters must also be evaluated (palatability of the ration, homogeneity of the ration, possibility of the animals to choose, amount of food advanced, type of advanced food, etc.). However, for the technician who must evaluate the postpartum group on a daily basis, the evaluation of the rumen score is a precise and rapid indicator. It provides very useful indications related to the quantity of food ingested and on the speed of food transit in the last hours, which in turn are mainly related to the characteristics of the forage, its structure, and the relationship between the different nutrients (Hulsen, 2003).

The filling of the rumen depends on the amount of dry matter ingested, the composition of the ration, the digestive capacity of the rumen, and the speed of rumen transit. Rumen Fill Scoring is used to monitor ingestion disorders and is based on a 5-point score: score 1, the cow has not eaten anything in the last 24 h and score 5, the cow is eating regularly. For simplicity, a score of 3 is proposed, where score 1 is a cow that does not eat at least 24 h (skin fold from hook bone falls vertically, so hollow shape looks rectangular), score 3 that of a cow that eats regularly and so enough.

4.3.3.2 UDDER OBSERVATION PERCENTAGE OF EDEMA SCORE

Pay attention to the size, shape, symmetry, presence of swellings (position, number, size, and consistency), color, smell (inguinal sores, intra-mammary sores), and presence of edema. Observe the teats (shape, size, direction, and presence of lesion); check if the cow loses milk spontaneously.

The Edema Score is an important indirect indicator of the nutritional and environmental management of the cow in the first part of the transition period. The edema of the udder can be associated with a genetic predisposition, but much more to an excess of sodium and/or potassium in the close-up ration, to very long dry period (> 70 days), to rations with low content of magnesium or protein, to poor drainage lymphatic caused by little space available for movement (overcrowding).

4.3.3.3 LOCOMOTION SCORE AND MOBILITY SCORE

The locomotion scoring makes it possible to make precise assessments of foot health, establishing whether and which feet and hooves does a disease possibly affect. The scoring used is 1–5, where 1 corresponds to a healthy cow, 3 to a slight lameness, and 5 to a severely lame cow. Sometimes, the locomotion scoring is ≥ 3, although there is no lameness; this can occur in case of gastro-enteric diseases (foreign body syndrome, abomasal volvulus, enteritis, etc.), abdominal diseases (peritonitis), or diseases of the reproductive system (puerperal metritis and vaginal lacerations). For this reason, in all cases of doubt, or when we want to ascertain a diagnostic suspicion, mobility scoring should also be carried out. This is a score ranging 0–4, where 0 corresponds to a cow with good or excellent mobility, being able to walk with a uniform load rhythm on all four feet, with a flat back; whereas score 3 corresponds to a cow unable to keep up with the healthy herd and an uneven load on a limb that is immediately identifiable or which cams with shortened strides and an arched back (www.dairy.ahdb.org.uk).

4.3.3.4 SHAPE OF ABDOMEN

In healthy cows, observation of the abdominal form from the right side allows a pear profile to be detected. The presence of an apple profile is an indication of an abdominal pathology (peritonitis) or gastrointestinal (bloating rumen, abomasum dilatation, abomasal volvulus, intestinal volvulus, etc.).

4.3.3.5   TYPE AND FREQUENCY OF BREATHING

The observation from the left side of the type and frequency of breathing allows to establish if there are signs of a respiratory pathology that involves the upper or lower respiratory tract, or if there is only an increase in respiratory frequency associated with heat stress.

4.3.3.6   OBSERVATION OF FECES

Faces are the expression of the cow's digestive efficiency. It is necessary to evaluate the consistency, color, smell, quantity, and quality of the undigested material contained therein. Also, the "noise" that the fecal material makes falling on the ground, once expelled by the rectum, gives us precise indications.

The characteristics of the feces can also be determined by observing the ventral part of the tail and the tuft of the tail: the cows with diarrhea and/or who have had recent episodes of diarrhea have their tail smeared.

It is possible to carry out a fecal scoring: the score goes from 1 to 5. A score 1 corresponds to a cow with glossy, creamy, homogeneous stools, within which undigested parts are not visible or palpable. The score 5 corresponds to a cow with opaque stools, not homogeneous, inside which there is a lot of undigested food (Hulsen, 2003).

4.3.3.7   VAGINAL DISCHARGE

Almost all cows immediately after delivery suffer from bacterial uterine contamination (Sheldon et al., 2011). However, only a part of them develops puerperal metritis, or gets sick. Most cows with postpartum uterine inflammation undergo spontaneous recovery. However, it is essential to identify the animals that fall ill with puerperal metritis early. Observation of vaginal discharge, their quantity, consistency, color, and odor are useful to identify these animals. All cows with vaginal discharge, very liquid, red-brown putrid, must be observed with great attention (Sheldon et al., 2006).

4.3.3.8   OBSERVATION OF THE VAGINA

In the case of vaginal and/or cervix-vaginal lacerations, the cow may present a locomotion scoring > 3, without lameness. A vaginal or cervix-vaginal laceration is usually painful and can compromise the health of the cow, which reduces up to suspending the feed intake, predisposing the cow to other puerperal pathologies (ketosis, Left Displacement Abomasum (LDA), etc.). In the presence of a locomotion score ≥ 3, in the absence of lameness, always check for vaginal lacerations by opening the vulva.

4.3.3.9   RECTAL TEMPERATURE

Rectal temperature is an excellent indicator of the health of the cow. Usually, a cow with an acute puerperal metritis has a rectal temperature > 39.5°C. However, the presence of fever is not indicative of a uterine pathology or in another place: 48% of the cows manifest a thermal rise > 39.5°C at least once in the first 10 days postpartum, without having any pathology of the reproductive system, or elsewhere (Wagner et al., 2007). Rectal temperature detection can be an excellent strategy to impose a work strategy based on animal observation: in the 10–15 s necessary to detect rectal temperature with a digital thermometer, a good observer can verify:

1. Locomotion Scoring
2. Mobility Scoring
3. Rumen Fill Scoring
4. Presence of vaginal discharge and their analysis (color, odor, and consistency)
5. Status of the udder (edema, swelling, symmetry, color, odor, loss of milk, shape and size of the teats, etc.)
6. Shape of the abdomen
7. Frequency and type of breathing

Rectal temperature detection is therefore not the end, but the means by which to train the dairy workers in charge of postpartum cows to observe. In stables where the staff is attentive and well trained, it is possible to avoid taking rectal temperatures to all the animals in the first 10 DIM, limiting this detection only to the cows that actually need it. Normally, a cow of the postpartum group, which increases its production, which eats regularly, does not require rectal temperature measurement.

4.4 CODE DEFINITION

At the end of the frontal and posterior observation, the clinician obtained a series of information. This information, together with the data related to the production of the cow, will allow the professional to establish whether to present the bovine to a clinical examination (Gnemmi et al., 2019).

In big, very big farms, it is possible to code each cow: a color is associated to each cow and, depending on the given color, the cow must be visited immediately, monitored in the next 12 h or monitored in the next 24 h. This is a system that allows the coding of cows due to the severity of each case (Gnemmi et al., 2019).

The clinical examination of the bovine will include other tests, such as BHB, the diagnosis of the abomasal displacement, the rumen function evaluation, and others diagnostic tests. Some time may also be required for complementary tests such as ultrasound (Table 4.4).

TABLE 4.4 Definition of Codes According to the Clinical Characteristics Identified

	Red code	Orange code	Yellow code
T°C	≥ 40°C	39.5–40.0°C	38.5–39.5°C
LC	4–5	4	3
MS	3	2	1
RS	1	2	3
MT	Liquid, red-brawn, fetid	Dense, red-pink	Dense, white-yellow or pink, any smell
P	< 8–10%	=	= or a little increased

LC, locomotion score; P, production; MS, mobility score; MT, type, color, and smell of the vaginal discharge; RS, Rumen score; T, temperature.

4.5 CLINICAL VISIT

The clinical visit must be carried out as a personal qualifier and according to the classical scheme (Rosenberger, 1979), or through an accurate anamnestic collection, a general objective examination, and a special physical examination of the apparatus that have been affected by the disease. Not all postpartum cows must be visited daily; only sick cows or those suspected of having a quiescent disease must undergo a clinical examination.

The tools that the professional must equip themselves with are few, but essential:

1. Stethoscope
2. Digital thermometer
3. BHB and blood glucose equipment
4. Gloves for rectal exploration
5. Short latex or nitrile gloves
6. Chalk to write on the cows
7. Palm-computer or smart phone or notebook to record cow data
8. 2.5 cc syringes with 18G° needles

The clinical examination serves to confirm the diagnostic suspicion. The cows in red code will have to be visited immediately; cows in orange code will be monitored for 12 h before the eventual clinical visit; the cows in yellow code will be monitored for 24 h before the eventual clinical visit.

KEYWORDS

- **dairy cow**
- **post partum pathologies**
- **uterine pathologies**
- **diagnosis**
- **monitoring procedure**
- **transition management**
- **herd prevention**

REFERENCES

Block, E. Transition Cow Research: What Makes Sense Today? The High Plains Dairy Conference **2010,** Amarillo Texas. 75–98.

Dairy Cow Monitoring and Herd Management Solutions, Precision Dairy Farm Technology | SCR Dairy. http://www.scrdairy.com (accessed March 23, 2019).

Drackley, J. K. Biology of Dairy Cows during the Transition Period: The Final Frontier? *J. Dairy Sci.* **1999,** *82,* 2259–2273.

Gilbert, R. Postpartum Uterine Health and Disease. Dairy Cattle Reproductive Council Convention. Omaha, Nebraska. **2008**. 29–38.

Gnemmi, G.; Maraboli, C. Impatto del Metaboilismo Sull'insorgenza di Infezioni Uterine nel Postpartum. *Summa Veterinaria Animali da Reddito.* **2018**, *9*, 1–5.

Gnemmi, G.; Maraboli, C. From Calving to 1st AI: Rational Management of the Post-Partum. *Proc. Int. Con. Bovine Reprod. Med.* March 11–12th **2019**. Faculty of Veterinary and Experimental Sciences Catholic University of Valencia, San Vincente Mártir, Valencia, Spain.

Gnemmi, G.; Morini, G.; Calvo, A.; Maraboli, C. Complesso Ritenzione Placenta-Metrite-Endometrite: Valutazione Economica. *Rivista di Medina Veterinaria.* **2016**, *54–1*, 15–25.

Goff, J. P.; and Horst, R. L. Physiological Changes at Parturition and Their Relationship to Metabolic Disorders. *J. Dairy Sci.* **1997**, *80*, 1260–1268.

Hulsen, J. *Koesignalen.* Ed.; Vetvice, The Netherlands, **2003**.

LeBlanc, S. J. Monitoring Metabolic Health of Dairy Cattle in the Transition Period. *J. Reprod. Dev.* **2010**, *56*, 29–35.

LeBlanc, S. J. Inflammation, Metritis and Reproduction. Dairy Cattle Reproduction Conference Indianapolis IN, **2013**, 89–97.

LeBlanc, S. J. Reproductive Tract Inflammatory Disease in Postpartum Dairy Cows. 2014. BSAS Annual Meeting, Westport, May **2014**.

Overton, M.; Fetrow, J. Economics of Postpartum Uterine Health. DCRC **2008**, Omaha Nebraska, 39–43.

Rosenberger, G. *L'esame clinico del bovino.* Ed.; Essegivi, Bologna, **1993**; 548.

Santos, J. E. Enfermedades Uterinas en la vaca Lechera: Un Tema Controvertido. *Proc. XIX Cong. Inte. ANEMBE de Med. Bovina.* June 25–27, **2014**.

Sheldon, M. Mechanism of Infection and Immunity in the Bovine Female Genital Tract Post-Partum. *Proc. Dairy Sympos.* August 13, **2011**. Hilton Milwaukee City Center. Milwaukee, Wisconsin.

Sheldon, I. M.; Lewis, G. S.; LeBlanc, S.; Gilbert, R. O. Defining Postpartum Uterine Disease in Cattle. *Theriogenology.* **2006**, *65*, 1516–1530.

Wagner, S. A.; Schimeck, D. E.; Chend, F. C. Body Temperature and White Blood Cell Count in Postpartum Dairy Cows. *Bovine Pract.* **2007**, *42*, 18–26.

CHAPTER 5

Reproductive Efficiency in Dairy Cows: Change in Trends!

ANA HERAS-MOLINA[1], JOSÉ LUIS PESANTEZ PACHECO[1,2] and SUSANA ASTIZ[1*]

[1]Department of Animal Reproduction, INIA, Avda Pta. de Hierro s/n, 28040 Madrid, Spain

[2]School of Veterinary Medicine and Zootechnics, Faculty of Agricultural Sciences, University of Cuenca, Avda. Doce de Octubre, Cuenca, Ecuador

*Corresponding author. E-mail: astiz.susana@inia.es

ABSTRACT

Dairy cattle industry has gone through a series of changes during the last decades to improve competitiveness. However, this has correlated to a detriment in reproductive parameters. Efforts in improving and understanding this situation have meant in practice changes in many fields. Milestones have been: (1) a deeper study and understanding of the estrus cycle of the cow, with the development of synchronization and resynchronization protocols more and more detailed and with improving fertility results after insemination; (2) better insight of how cow's parity affects reproduction; (3) the consideration of the length of the voluntary waiting period as an essential decision in order to maintain an optimal reproductive efficiency in farms; (4) the understanding of the process and relevance of the pregnancy loss during the early fetal phase; (5) improvement in estrus detection rates through novel technologies. These advances in technology have resulted also in earlier and more precise pregnancy diagnoses.

But reproduction control alone is not enough. Nutrition, genetics, and welfare have a deep effect on reproductive performance. A better understanding of the energy during the production cycle and its effects have been pivotal in the improvement of dairy cattle fertility in high-yielding animals. In recent years, fertility has been added as a trait to be taken into account in selection programs, since they are fundamental for maintaining farm's profitability. Animal welfare, with growing importance in animal production, has been focused on an increase of published studies, studying the effect of stress (social, environmental) on reproduction, helping to give strategies to minimize it or even to void it.

All in all, changes in veterinary advice in farms have been accomplished by this better understanding of the dairy production systems, transforming the trend of reproductive efficiency up to figures even better than the historically 50% fertility after artificial insemination.

5.1   INTRODUCTION

In the last decades, there has been a major change in dairy cattle industry. In order to be more competitive, this sector has developed into an economy of scale, looking for high production, higher profitability of the investments, and reducing the production costs (European Commission, 2013). This can be seen in the changes suffered by herd size and milk yield. By 1950, the herd size was on average of 6.5 dairy cows per farm (Stevenson and Britt, 2017), but since then it has increased exponentially. In the European Union (EU) average herd size has increase from 24 lactating animals in 1997 in the EU-15 (van Arendonk and Liinamo, 2003) to 55 in 2010 (European Commission, 2013). In the United States, the number of lactating cows per herd is even larger, being on average of 180 in 2015 (NMPF Centennial Booklet, 2016). Not only the number of animals has risen, but also the average milk production per cow, incrementing the annual yield from 5000 kg/cow (van Arendonk and Liinamo, 2003; NMPF, 2016) to 7000 kg/cow in EU from 1997 to 2010 (EU Dairy Farms 2010 Report, 2013) (Fig. 5.1).

These two factors imply a total transformation of the management of the herd at different levels, being especially important in bigger farms, since individual cows that produce more milk are usually found in them (Lucy, 2001). For example, during the early half of the 20th century, most of the dairy cattle grazed pastures, being housed in tie-stalls or stanchion barns (Fig. 5.2) only during winters (Stevenson and Britt, 2017). However, nowadays the more common installations are freestalls (Fig. 5.3) and dry-lot systems (NAHMS, 2009), although in recent years loose-housing methods with compost or straw bedding are increasingly being used (Barberg et al., 2007). These new ways of keeping the cattle mean a drastic modification in the herd nutrition and feeding systems (NAHMS, 2009). Other change can be seen in the number of cows managed by a single dairy worker (Stevenson and Britt, 2017). The greater number of animals under the control of a worker is extremely important in different factors in the farm. For instance, the volume of milk managed by each person is larger (Stevenson and Britt, 2017), as it is the number of cows milked per minute per operator (Progressive Dairy Operators, 2016). Related to the reproductive management, these new farm situations affect it at various levels. For example, it limits drastically the capacity to observe estrus, which has stimulated the study of different strategies to make easier and more efficient the estrus detection (Palmer et al., 2010), or even that makes unnecessary estrus detection to be able to inseminate the cows by the implementation of timed artificial insemination (TAI) (Stevenson, 2016). Another factor affected by the changes in dairy cattle industry is the increased numbers of calves per worker. Some studies reported increases in calf mortality risk according to herd size (Gulliksen et al., 2009; Mellado et al., 2014; Seppä-Lassila et al., 2016), which could be caused by the increase care in management of fewer and more valuable animals in smaller farms (Seppä-Lassila et al., 2016).

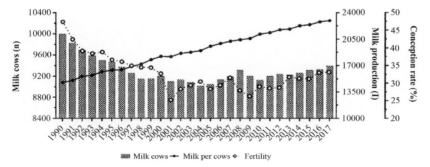

FIGURE 5.1 Evolution of number of milk cows, milk per cows and fertility from 1990 to 2017. Data combined coming from López-Gatius et al., 2002; Norman et al., 2009; Huang et al., 2009; Feijoo et al., 2018, USDA, 2019.

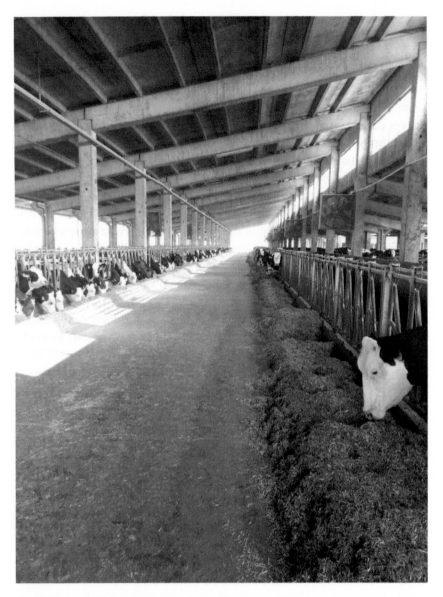

FIGURE 5.2   A dairy cattle herd in a typical barn, nowadays.

All in all, there has been a shift in the way we understand dairy cattle medicine. As veterinarians, we find ourselves as health professionals with no patients, not even with just a group of patients. As in other species, like swine or poultry, we are dealing with a very complex system, that includes the cow itself, the herd, the farm staff, the livestock facilities, etc. (Astiz et al., 2018a). We are no longer working in the traditional individual medicine, but in production medicine, also called "herd health medicine" (Van der Leek, 2015).

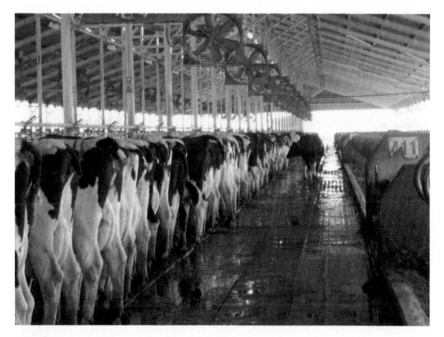

FIGURE 5.3   A dairy cattle herd in a typical stall, nowadays.

The development of the dairy cattle industry has driven to modifications in its productivity, not always leading to an optimal situation, especially regarding the reproductive efficiency of our herds. The trend in the increase of milk production has been concomitant with a decrease in fertility, since in some systems cows with the greatest milk yields have the highest incidence of infertility (Lucy, 2001). The first service conception rate has declined from approximately 65% in 1951 (Butler, 1998) to 40% in 1996 (Lucy, 2001), with an average of 1.5–2.5 artificial insemination (AIs) per conception being necessary (van Arendonk and Liinamo, 2003). The decline of fertility when AI is used can also be found, that could be up to 30% in the case of TAI (Pursley et al., 1997a,b; Schmitt et al., 1996). The reproductive physiology of dairy cattle has evolved over the past 50 years to cope with the high milk production, which could explain some (but not all) of the reproductive problems that have been common in the industry until 2000 (Lucy, 2001). It is important to highlight that, even though benefits of improving reproduction are obvious, specific causes of poor reproductive performance are hard to identify and resolve (Stevenson, 2016).

However, in the last decade has occurred a great increase of approximately 5% in daughter pregnancy, even though the milk yield is still boosting (Stevenson, 2016). What has happened? Is this change random? Is it the consequence of one certain factor or of several strategies and circumstances?

In this chapter, the authors try to briefly review, resume and explain this change in tendency of the reproductive efficiency of our high yielding dairy cow, assuming its health (we will not cover specific health issues, but the reproductive difficulties when dealing with healthy dairy adult cows). In this transformation, it has been vital the effort of a variety of professionals that includes advisors, scientists, practitioners, farmers, etc. With their work, it has been possible to understand the high producing dairy cow in its different aspects: reproductive physiology, immunology, health, welfare, herd medicine, and genetic selection (Astiz et al., 2018a.; Weigel, 2006). Thanks to this deeper knowledge, we can conclude that the decrease in fertility was not only caused by the increasing milk yield, but by many other factors as well (Lucy, 2001; Stevenson, 2016). It is impossible to improve reproduction with unhealthy and not well-being animals, so it is important to take care of feeding, care, management, facilities, etc. (Astiz et al., 2018b). Being aware of and optimizing all of them have caused the recent change in reproduction traits.

Therefore, factors affecting the healthy dairy cattle reproduction will be explained, as well as the different strategies used nowadays to keep reproductive efficiency at a satisfactory level at farms. These factors will be organized in four major categories: reproductive management, nutrition, genetics and welfare, especially focusing on the first one.

5.2   REPRODUCTIVE ISSUES

Several factors have had an important impact in the improvement of cattle reproduction. During the last decades, major advances have been made that have permitted the understanding of the underlying processes of reproductive physiology in dairy cows and heifers. These advances provide the basic technology that has been transferred to modern dairy farms (Thatcher, 2017). Also, the better understanding of the animals has made possible the improvement of dairy cattle management in order to improve fertility and production, in general. These factors, related to reproductive management are: synchronization and resynchronization protocols for TAI, parity, estrus detection, and voluntary waiting period (VWP). We will not cover the issues of the male and of the reproductive biotechnologies (embryo transfer and *in vitro* embryo production), which are also relevant for the actual global fertility in our farms, but out of our scope.

5.2.1 SYNCHRONIZATION AND RESYNCHRONIZATION PROTOCOLS FOR TAI

The knowledge of the endocrine events behind reproduction allowed the development of synchronization and controlled breeding programs. Firstly, these programs were focused on the synchronization of the estrus (with programs that allows the shortening of the time until a group of females should show estrus and the grouping of these cows), using either progesterone in the late 1940s and early 1950s (Ulberg, et al., 1951), progestins in the 1960s (Hansel, 1961) and prostaglandins in the 1970s (Cooper et al., 1976) first only to induce estrus for first AI services after observed estrus and later for inducing estrus in nonpregnant cows (Britt et al., 1981) but with a palpable corpus luteum (CL) (Plunkett et al., 1984). Once the progestin products for synchronization became available, management of the dairy cattle changed, being introduced the concept of clustering cows according to calving dates for group management (Britt et al., 1972). It was also discovered that a double injection of prostaglandin 14 days apart in cows, so that the cow will be responsive at least at the second injection and comes into estrus shortly afterwards, induce the grouping of estrus within the 4–10 days after the second hormone administration (Cooper et al., 1976; Squires, 2010). This system and its variations have been used since a long time and even now are currently implemented in bovine farms. The grouping schemes used in that period are prototypes for what is done today to cluster cows for TAI (Stevenson and Britt, 2017). Since the 1970s, several newly discovered hormones and delivered technologies were introduced not only for the control of estrus cycle, but also the ovulation in domestic animals (Stevenson and Britt,

2017). Reproductive management in dairy farms has markedly evolved in the last 20 years, especially because of the continuous development of synchronization programs that allows TAI. Early research on control of follicle development and CL span has as a goal to develop systems that synchronize follicle growth, luteolysis, and ovulation at a predictable time in which the TAI could be performed maintaining fertility at a satisfactory level (Thatcher et al., 1996). The studies focused on the control of the follicular wave with gonadotropin-releasing hormone (GnRH) (Macmillan and Thatcher, 1991) made possible the creation of the Ovsynch protocol in 1995 (Pursley et al., 1995). Today, the Ovsynch protocol and its variations are the most common TAI programs used for reproductive management of dairy cattle worldwide (Bisinotto et al., 2014). The most commonly used protocols will be briefly explained hereunder.

5.2.1.1   OVSYNCH AND COSYNCH

The original Ovsynch protocol (or 7-day Ovsynch) is considered as the basic ovulation synchronization TAI program (Stevenson, 2016). It consists on a GnRH injection on the day 0 of the protocol, followed by a prostaglandin $F_2\alpha$ ($PGF_2\alpha$) on day 7, another GnRH injection on day 9 and the TAI on day 10, 16 hours after the GnRH administration. The GnRH administrations induce a luteinizing hormone surge to cause ovulation of a dominant follicle when present, and the $PGF_2\alpha$ lyse the CL that is formed (Pursley et al., 1995). Even though it did not result in better pregnancy rates than cows inseminated after detected estrus (38 *vs.* 39%) and the results were even worse for heifers (35 *vs.* 74%, Ovsynch and detected estrus, respectively; Pursley et al., 1997), we have to think that, when compared to the results after inseminations when estrus observation was near 0%, the progress was huge.

One of the first variations of the Ovsynch was the Cosynch. The objective of this modification was not to increase fertility, but to reduce management of the cows, being the only difference with Ovsynch that TAI is done together with the final GnRH injection (Schmitt et al., 1996; Colazo and Ambrose, 2011). In fact, Cosynch induces a decrease in fertility of about 7% when compared to Ovsynch (Borchardt et al., 2018), but it has been demonstrated to be efficient in many productive systems (Sanz et al., 2019). In Figure 5.4, differences between both protocols can be seen.

Another variant of the Ovsynch protocol is the administration of estradiol cypionate on day 8 but maintaining the GnRH and the PGF$_2\alpha$ and being the TAI performed on day 10. However, the overall results were very similar between the two protocols (Pancarci et al., 2002), and it is worthy to remember, that the pharmaceutical estradiol forms are forbidden in animal production in Europe.

5.2.1.2 PROGRAMS INCLUDING PROGESTERONE

In the beginning of the investigation of estrus protocols, the usefulness of progestins were investigated (Hansel, 1961). Afterwards, different studies confirmed that the utilization of a progesterone intravaginal device such as CIDR, PRID, etc. within the Ovsynch protocol, between the first GnRH and the PGF$_2\alpha$ injection could improve the percentage of pregnant cows at day 60 after AI (34.2 *vs.* 29.6%) (Bisinotto et al., 2015), mainly for cows with scarce Body Condition Scores, with and without a CL at the beginning of the synchronization protocol. Cows benefitting the most from supplemental progesterone are those that are anovular or not in diestrus at the onset of the TAI program, confirming the therapeutical effect of the supplemented progesterone. This dissimilarity could be explained by the difference in amount of progesterone released by CL during diestrus and a single progesterone insert (Stevenson, 2016). The utilization of these devices has been studied in both 7-day and 5-day Ovsynch/Cosynch protocols (Fig. 5.4), with controversial results, that could depend on the initial percentage of noncycling cows. Some authors (Colazo and Ambrose, 2011; Wilson et al., 2010) did not find differences between both, but Bridges et al. (2008) reported an improvement of pregnancy rate when using CIDR for 5 days instead of 7 (60 *vs.* 70%). Thus, pregnancy rate could be more related to the programming of an adequate TAI taking into account the proestrus rather than the time of CIDR removal (Wilson et al., 2010).

Other hormones that have been studied in order to improve fertility after the implementation of Ovsynch protocol and its variants in dairy cattle are equine and human chorionic gonadotropin, eCG or hCG in addition to progestins. Studies where a dose of eCG is administered on the day of CIDR removal, has shown an improvement of fertility, especially in animals with detrimental nutrition status (Macmillan and Burke, 1996). On the other hand, utilization of hCG is effective in reducing the incidence of short return intervals (Schmitt et al., 1996), since the effectiveness of this

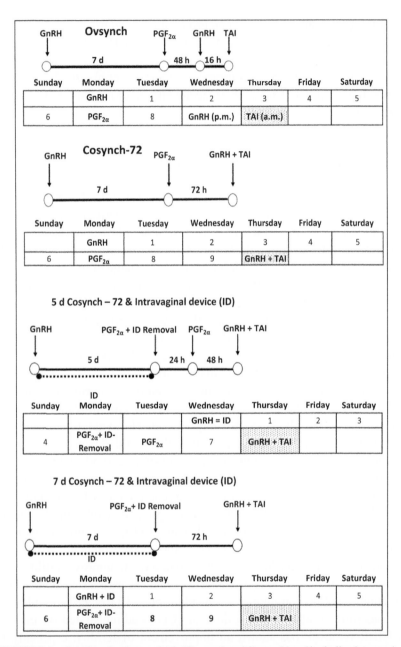

FIGURE 5.4 Synchronization methods (Ovsynch and Cosynch) and including intravaginal progesterone devices. GnRH, gonadotropin releasing hormone; PGF, prostaglandin $F_2\alpha$; TAI, timed artificial insemination.

hormone inducing the ovulation of the dominant follicle is similar to that observed after GnRH administration (Schmitt et al., 1996), but with a direct effect on the ovary and with a longer half-life (De Rensis et al., 2010).

5.2.1.3   PRESYNCHRONIZATION PROTOCOLS FOR FIRST TAIS

5.2.1.3.1   *Presynchronization Prostaglandin $F_2\alpha$ Programs*

Early studies after the original Ovsynch publication in 1995 indicated that pregnancy outcomes were better when beginning the TAI program on days 5 through 12 of the estrus cycle (i.e., during diestrus), with greater ovulatory responses to GnRH administration and fertility (Vasconcelos et al., 1999). A recent study confirms that the definitive factor is the amount of progesterone observed at the initial GnRH injection, that has to be moderate at this time point (coinciding with early diestrus-5 to 8th day of the cycle) to maximize probability of pregnancy after TAI (Carvalho et al., 2018). In order to get a greater proportion of cows in this cycle days at the beginning of the Ovsynch protocol, the injection of two PGF$_2\alpha$ 14 days apart (the old estrus induction program of prostaglandin-prostaglandin), was suggested.

In the first description of the so denominated "Presynch protocol" (PS), the Ovsynch protocol was started 12 days apart from the last PGF$_2\alpha$ of the presynchronization with prostaglandins (Moreira et al., 2000). However, some modifications focused on the days between the Presynch and the Ovsynch protocols have been made changing the interval from 10 to 14 days, always with the two PGF$_2\alpha$ injections administered 14 days apart, but the onset of the Ovsynch program was 14, 11, or 10 days, respectively (Fig. 5.5) (Stevenson and Britt, 2017). Among these programs, improved pregnancy outcomes were reported in cows after a Presynch-11 than a Presynch-14 (percentage of cows pregnant at 60 days 36.4 *vs.* 30.2%, respectively) (Galvão et al., 2007), since more cows were at the ideal stage of the cycle after this treatment (Stevenson, 2016). On average, the pregnancy risk using a Presynch + Ovsynch protocol was clearly superior to the one obtained using Ovsynch alone (46.5 *vs.* 35.4%, respectively; Stevenson, 2016).

Another benefit of Presynch programs is the possibility of inseminating cows after observed estrus that show heat before the beginning of the Ovsynch protocol, strategy that increased pregnancy rate when compared to a system with 100% of cows timed inseminated (Macmillan et al., 2017).

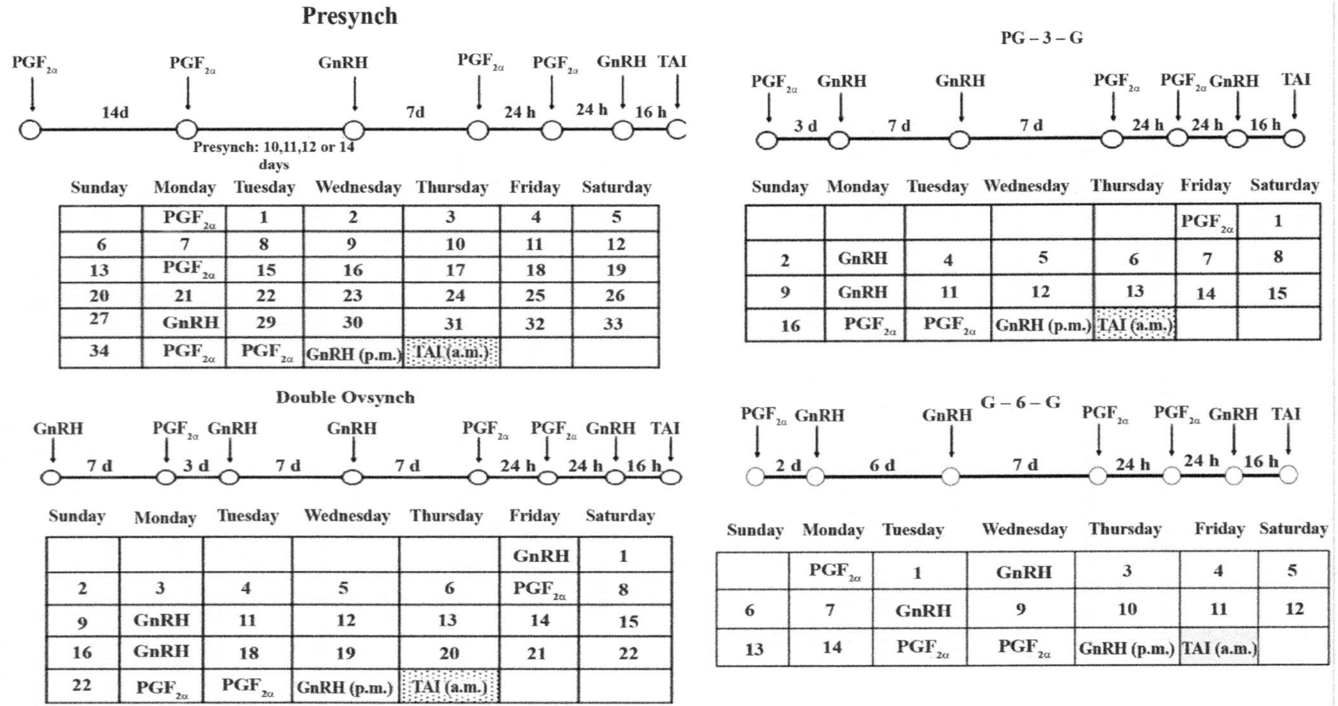

Presynch

Sunday	Monday	Tuesday	Wednesday	Thursday	Friday	Saturday
	$PGF_{2\alpha}$	1	2	3	4	5
6	7	8	9	10	11	12
13	$PGF_{2\alpha}$	15	16	17	18	19
20	21	22	23	24	25	26
27	GnRH	29	30	31	32	33
34	$PGF_{2\alpha}$	$PGF_{2\alpha}$	GnRH (p.m.)	TAI (a.m.)		

PG – 3 – G

Sunday	Monday	Tuesday	Wednesday	Thursday	Friday	Saturday
					$PGF_{2\alpha}$	1
2	GnRH	4	5	6	7	8
9	GnRH	11	12	13	14	15
16	$PGF_{2\alpha}$	$PGF_{2\alpha}$	GnRH (p.m.)	TAI (a.m.)		

Double Ovsynch

Sunday	Monday	Tuesday	Wednesday	Thursday	Friday	Saturday
					GnRH	1
2	3	4	5	6	$PGF_{2\alpha}$	8
9	GnRH	11	12	13	14	15
16	GnRH	18	19	20	21	22
22	$PGF_{2\alpha}$	$PGF_{2\alpha}$	GnRH (p.m.)	TAI (a.m.)		

G – 6 – G

Sunday	Monday	Tuesday	Wednesday	Thursday	Friday	Saturday
	$PGF_{2\alpha}$	1	GnRH	3	4	5
6	7	GnRH	9	10	11	12
13	14	$PGF_{2\alpha}$	$PGF_{2\alpha}$	GnRH (p.m.)	TAI (a.m.)	

FIGURE 5.5 Presynchronization protocols with two PGF before GnRH and TAI. GnRH, gonadotropin releasing hormone; PGF, prostaglandin $F_2\alpha$; TAI, Timed Artificial Insemination.

5.2.1.3.2 Presynchronization GnRH Programs

The major limitation of Ovsynch alone and Presynch $PGF_2\alpha$ programs is that they are unable to improve fertility in anovular cows (Bisinotto et al., 2014). Including GnRH administration in addition to injections of $PGF_2\alpha$ increases the odds for pregnancy by 1.65 times for this kind of animals (Bisinotto et al., 2014). Thus, different protocols were designed, such as Double Ovsynch (DO), PG-3-G and G6G (Stevenson, 2016).

The DO uses an Ovsynch protocol in order to induce cyclicity in anovular dairy cows before the use of a breeding Ovsynch protocol (Souza et al., 2008). Different studies have reported better fertility with this program in comparison with $PGF_2\alpha$ synchronization programs (Souza et al., 2008; Herlihy et al., 2012) (46.3 *vs.* 38.2% P/AI in DO and PS, respectively). This difference was especially important in primiparous cows (52.5 *vs.* 42.3%, DO *vs.* PS), probably due to the higher incidence of anovular cows with primiparous cows (Herlihy et al., 2012).

The PG-3-G consist on injecting $PGF_2\alpha$ 3 days before injection of the first GnRH of the Ovsynch (Peters and Pursley, 2002; Stevenson et al., 2012). In the literature, better P/AI was found with this protocol than with Presynch-10 (35 *vs.* 41.2%, respectively) (Stevenson and Pulley, 2012). However, it is a protocol not commonly implemented by the farmers, perhaps due to the difficulty to fix the program into a schedule with weekends free for the farm workers.

In the G6G program, cows are treated with a dose of $PGF_2\alpha$ and two days later, with GnRH, being this injection of GnRH administered 6 days before the Ovsynch protocol, since the 6 days interval increased the percentage of cows that ovulated in response to first GnRH of Ovsynch as well as the number of cows synchronized. With this method, improvement of fertility was obtained when compared with the Ovsynch program (Bello et al., 2006). This program achieves high conception rates at first TAI ranging from 37% (Astiz and Fargas, 2013) to 57% (Yousuf et al., 2016). However, when compared with other presynchronization GnRH programs such as DO, results show that DO is better for primiparous cows (44.3 *vs.* 36.3%, DO *vs.* G6G), but G6G tended to be better for multiparous in some studies (31.4 *vs.* 34.8%) (Astiz and Fargas, 2013).

Improved pregnancy outcomes of GnRH-Presynch programs may be done in herds with an elevated percentage of anovulatory cows when submitted to the TAI programs before first AI service (Stevenson, 2016).

This is a consequence of the association of all these programs with greater ovulation response to the first GnRH injection of Ovsynch (Vasconcelos et al., 1999; Bello et al., 2006; Chebel et al., 2006), greater number of cows with a functional CL (Galvão and Santos, 2010; Stevenson et al., 2012), more number of CL per cow at the first GnRH of Ovsynch (Stevenson et al., 2012) and greater ovulatory response to both GnRH injections of Ovsynch (Rutigliano et al., 2008; Galvão and Santos, 2010), and more appropriate serum progesterone levels at each key moment during synchronization (Carvalho et al., 2018).

As we can see, all these variations of the protocols for first AI after calving have been developed during this last century (Fig. 5.5), and have been rapidly implemented in commercial farms, so that their input to the improvement of the global fertility is clear.

5.2.1.4 RESYNCHRONIZATION PROGRAMS

Even with the programs mentioned above, conception at the first TAI after parturition can fail in 50% of the cases, at best (López-Helguera et al., 2012; Lopes et al., 2013). In order to increase efficiency on reproduction in the farms, it is important to detect as soon as possible those animals that are not pregnant (Fricke, 2002). In farms observing estrus, it is estimated that 40–60% of nonpregnant cows are detected on the next 23 days on average (Chebel and Ribeiro, 2016), but if a nonpregnancy diagnosis (NPD) has to be performed, this can be made as early as 26–28 days, being extremely important the interval to pregnancy diagnosis. Nowadays, ultrasound scanners have become portable and kits to measure pregnancy-associated glycoproteins (PAGS) have become cheaper and makeable at a farm, which means an improvement of dairy cattle reproductive strategies when used adequately and combined with other methods (Patron-Collantes et al., 2017). These are factors also responsible for the general advancement of the global fertility in dairy cows: the earlier and more exactly the NPD is made, the higher becomes the pregnancy rate of the herds. The refinement of these technologies together with the development of resynchronization programs has improved notably the reproductive efficiency after second AIs. However, we should not forget the required training time for the experts responsible for this exploration; when no sufficient, an enhanced pregnancy rate loss may be related to (Patron et al., 2017).

At first, the resynchronization programs consisted on the injection of $PGF_2\alpha$ to nonpregnant cows when a palpable CL was found upon nonpregnant diagnosis. Cows were either inseminated upon detected estrus or by appointment at 72 and 96 h after the hormone injection (Plunkett et al., 1984). However, when inseminations only occurred after detected estrus, failing to follow up on noninseminated cows resulted in longer AI-AI intervals, which affected overall fertility in farms, reducing pregnancy rates directly (Stevenson and Britt, 2017). For this reason, once the TAI programs were developed, studies were conducted using these programs initiated in nonpregnant cows starting a Resynch-Ovsynch/Cosynch program on the day of NPD (Stevenson and Britt, 2017). This program is the most commonly used one for resynchronization, with an average pregnancy risk of 29% (Stevenson, 2016), when detection of estrus is not applied and cows are only inseminated after a TAI program.

Recently, it has been demonstrated, that reducing the time between the first GnRH and the $PGF_2\alpha$ injections from 7 to 5 days would enhance fertility, since the embryo quality could be related inversely to length of follicle dominance (Santos et al., 2010). Shorter programs are an ideal solution for resynchronization protocols (Fig. 5.5). However, a limitation to manipulate the length of follicle dominance when GnRH is used is the fact that CLs are refractory to $PGF_2\alpha$ during the first 5 days of estrus cycle (Tsai and Wiltbank, 1998). In order to cope with this problem, two $PGF_2\alpha$ injections are administered at days 5 and 6, obtaining better pregnancy per AI (P/AI) results (39.3 *vs.* 33.9% for 5-day and 7-day Ovsynch protocol) (Santos et al., 2010). Anyway, it is now known that a double prostaglandin administered 24 h apart before the last GnRH administration (and AI) assures the correct luteolysis almost to a 95% of synchronized cows, independently of the length of the protocol. Therefore, it is advised to apply two doses of $PGF_2\alpha$, even when implementing 7 days Ovsynch protocols (Fig. 5.5) (Carvalho et al., 2018).

After the development of the shorter protocols, 5-day Ovsynch/ Cosynch and its variations have been used, and average fertility increased up to 45.3% (Patron et al., 2018; Colazo and Ambrose, 2015).

As we can see, the development of these resynchronization strategies has also notably improved the conception rates after second and later inseminations in the last 18 years.

It is important to keep in mind that the evaluation of the efficiency of any protocol program cannot be based exclusively on the fertility after the TAI, but on the global reproductive efficiency (pregnancy rate of the whole herd). Moreover, the economic efficiency has also to be evaluated. Therefore, some shorter programs with a lower fertility could be more efficient than other longer protocols with higher fertility. This has to be evaluated at each farm, specifically for resynchronization protocols using other programs such as G6G, originally designed for first inseminations because it takes 18 days to be implemented, but that also leads to optimal results, with an average of 38% of conception rates for second and more TAI (Patron et al., 2018).

Another very relevant factor when inseminating the second or higher time, is the time when cows are diagnosed for nonpregnancy or interval between AI-NPD, which must be the shortest in order to intensify efficiency. Thus, resynchronization protocols can include a presynchronization with GnRH or chorionic gonadotropin (hCG) administration 5-7 days even before knowing if the cows are pregnant. These methods increase pregnancy risk in 4–5% when compared with the Ovsynch resynchronization protocol (29 *vs.* 33.5%) (Stevenson, 2016).

Other option is to introduce intravaginal devices, which increase pregnancy risk when used with a 5-day Ovsynch program, as seen by Bissinotto et al. (2010) (51.3 *vs.* 43.1%, for cows with and without CIDR treatment, respectively).

Nevertheless, the best solution would be to adjust resynchronization to the individual ovarian status of each cow at NPD as demonstrated recently. In this case, animals with a CL ≥ 15 mm and a follicle ≥ 10 mm at NPD would receive $PGF_2\alpha$, $PGF_2\alpha$ 24 h later, GnRH 32 h later, and TAI 16–18 h later; NPD without a CL ≥ 15 mm or a follicle ≥ 10 mm would receive GnRH plus CIDR, $PGF_2\alpha$, and CIDR removal 7 days later, $PGF_2\alpha$ 24 h later, GnRH 32 h later, and TAI 16–18 h later. Although this new system didn't enhance conception rate when compared with classical 7-days Ovsynch (Ovsynch = 31.0% *vs.* new systems = 33.9%), it did reduce time to pregnancy because of reduction of the TAI-TAI interval in cows with a CL at NPD and greater conception rate in cows with no CL at NPD (Wijma et al., 2017). Moreover, we can see that the improvement of ultrasonography and its use on the study of ovarian cycle has permitted the utilization of this method in order to achieve globally better results in farms.

In general, AI-AI interval is reduced when increasing estrus detection, but it is important to adapt this to the efficiency of estrus detection and the fertility of the inseminations done after the observed estrus in each farm. All in all, the combination of both strategies, resynchronization for TAI and AI after estrus detection seems to be the most profitable strategy (Galvão et al., 2013; Denis-Robichaud et al., 2018), depending the optimal percentage of cows submitted to each protocol on the farms idiosyncrasies (Astiz et al., 2018b).

Many dairy herds have incorporated fertility TAI programs into a complete reproductive management program. For instance, Carvalho et al. (2018) implemented an aggressive reproductive management system for first and Resynch TAIs in high yielding herds. Firstly, all cows were submitted for first TAI between 76 and 82 DIM after a Double Protocol (Souza et al., 2008) with the addition of a second $PGF_2\alpha$ treatment 24 h after the first one. For Resynch TAI, all animals were treated with GnRH 25 days after TAI. Ultrasound was used for pregnancy diagnosis, and afterwards nonpregnant cows were classified as having or lacking a CL >10 mm in diameter. Those that have this CL size go on with an Ovsynch/Cosynch-56 protocol by the injection of a $PGF_2\alpha$ treatment 32 days after TAI, whereas those animals lacking a CL restart an Ovsynch/Cosynch-56 protocol that includes a second $PGF_2\alpha$ treatment 24 h after the first (Carvalho et al., 2015), including a P4 device. With this protocol, huge improvement of fertility was obtained being the conception risk averaged 50%. This protocol and similar ones are being used in different herds, which drastically improve their reproduction results.

Therefore, we have managed to change the situation of facing a steady, with time, declining fertility in line in our farms into a situation where we have achieved average fertility rates even greater than the historically limit of 50% after AI, and annual average pregnancy rates of more than 35% in our high producing dairy herds.

5.2.2   NUMBER OF CALVINGS: "PARITY"

The fact of having enhanced average rates of conception and pregnancy in our dairy farms is not only due to mastering the synchronization protocols and the improvement of individual fertility after AI. We have also learned to consider different characteristics of our cows that were not relevant for us before. One example of this is the parity of the cow.

Parity plays a very important role in reproductive management, since the reproductive physiology is different in multiparous and primiparous cows (Astiz et al., 2018b), which was not clear for professionals during the last century. Nowadays, we know that primiparous cows have been reported to have better fertility, since they have, in general, less reproductive problems or anovulation (Erb and Grohn, 1988; Gröhn and Rajala-Schultz, 2000). However, this idea is controversial because other studies reported a better fertility of multiparous cows and a higher incidence of anovular cows (De Kruif, 1978; Stevenson and Call, 1988).

The differences between primiparous and multiparous cows fertility could be explained by differences in endocrine parameters like IGF1, related with the delay of ovulation (Beam and Butler, 1999). However, more research is necessary, since some studies indicate a higher concentration in multiparous cows (Meikle et al., 2004), whereas other researchers have opposite results (Taylor et al., 2003).

Due to these endocrine divergences, it is known that the synchronization protocols are not as effective in both groups, and currently the parity of the cows must be considered in any reproductive study, because of its relevance when deciding the best protocol for the farm. For example, primiparous cows shows higher conception rates (> 10 points in conception rate) after first insemination when inseminated with the DO protocol (Souza et al., 2008; Astiz and Fargas, 2013), which can be explained by the fact that this protocol works better in anovulatory cows (and in some herds primiparous cows show an enhanced proportion of anovulation) (Souza et al., 2008; Herlihy et al., 2012) or because this protocol leads to intermediate progesterone values in a greater proportion of cows than the Presynch-Ovsynch protocol after TAI (Herlihy et al., 2012). On the other hand, multiparous cows inseminated after a G6G protocol have slightly better results than primiparous, because it leads to higher ovulation rates, higher rates of CL formation in anovular cows and, therefore, higher concentration of progesterone (Astiz and Fargas, 2013).

Therefore, currently we can find some reproductive management systems designed specifically for certain parity order of the cows, optimizing in this way their reproductive results, which also contributes to the general enhancement of the reproductive efficiency in the dairy cattle sector.

Parity also shows a strong interaction when trying to find the optimal VWP, as we will review later on this chapter. In brief, the VWP is the interval after calving until we decide to inseminate the cows. In a recent work (Stangaferro et al., 2018), extending the VWP from 60 to 88 days delayed time to pregnancy during lactation (20 days approximately) and increased the risk of leaving the herd for multiparous cows (hazard ratio = 1.21). This shift in time to pregnancy combined with the herd elimination policy resulted in longer lactations (22 days) and greater milk income for primiparous but not for multiparous in the VWP88 group. Under variable conditions, the longer VWP treatment increased cash flow for primiparous, but reduced it for multiparous. Therefore, the decision regarding the length of the VWP has to consider the parity of the cows.

5.2.3 ESTRUS DETECTION

Even though timed AI is a highly viable option to produce pregnancies in dairy cows, the implementation of an accurate and efficient estrus detection system is vital in farms (Stevenson and Britt, 2017).

Cows express a number of behavioral changes during estrus, like an increase in chin resting, anogenital licking and sniffing, aggressive interaction, mounting other cows and modifications in feed intake, and rumination time (Helmer and Britt, 1985; Kerbrat and Disenhaus, 2004; Stevenson and Britt, 2017). Other changes during estrus have been studied, such as vaginal cytology and pH, electrical resistance of vaginal mucus and genital tissues, body temperature, pulse and heart rates, blood flow, pheromones, blood metabolites and hormones, and milk yield (Stevenson and Britt, 2017).

Traditionally, visual monitoring of these signs of estrus has been used. In order to be efficient using this method, observation of cows should occur at least 30 min twice daily (once in the morning and the other in the late afternoon-early evening) (Stevenson and Britt, 2017). Although laborious and time consuming, the optimal estrus observation system is considered to be 20 min, 5 times per day (Diskin and Sreenan, 2000). However, the expression and hence detection of standing estrus is affected by different factors; in Holstein is assumed that only 58% of the cows expresses estrus (Roelofs et al., 2005). Factors are the number of animals in estrus simultaneously, lameness, housing type, and the surface underfoot (Hurnik et al., 1975; Sood and Nanda, 2006) (cows are likely to express estrus behavior more often and for longer duration on earthen surfaces rather than on dry grooved concrete surfaces (Britt et al., 1986), which is a common floor in dairy cattle farms (Somers, 2004). This change in the housing of the animals together with the increased herd size, has made that visual observation of individual cows is not practical in modern farms, resulting in large rates of unobserved estrus and remarkable economic losses (Reith and Hoy, 2018). Detection efficiency has often been below 50% in dairy herds (Van Vliet and Van Eerdenburg, 1996), which means a decrease of fertility in the farm, as well as higher culling rate, even though about 90% of the factors for low detection rates are attributable to management (Reith and Hoy, 2018).

In the 1970s, various devices were developed in order to facilitate visual estrus detection. Some examples are the simple use of tail-painting, video tapes (more useful in research than in farm), detectors on the cows (being the most used device of this type the KaMaR Heatmount Detector) or the chain ball mating device. With these two methods, an improvement of 15–53% on estrus visualization was obtained. Other changes such as vaginal measurements, hormone detection, or milk yield were studied, but were found less practical that visual detection (Foote, 1975). In the 1990s, mounting pressure-sensitive sensors to the rump of the cow that are activated herdmate were developed (Stevenson et al., 1996). They are highly efficient and accurate because they are associated with specific sexual behavior and are functional 24 h/d (Roelofs et al., 2010), being these radiotelemetric devices more efficient in detecting animals in estrus (100 *vs.* 73%, using the device or observational detection of estrus, respectively) (Stevenson et al., 1996). However, due to the high variability in duration and intensity of the expressed estrus signs among individuals and the great influence of several different factors, detecting cows in estrus is still a challenge. During the 21st century, average prices of the last estrus detection devices have considerably decrease and fully automated sensor-based technologies that continuously monitor and record detailed information about the cow have been developed and greatly defined to attenuate further reproductive declines (Reith and Hoy, 2018). With these devices (such as HeatWatch® or DEC®), two different trials found efficiencies of 86.6 and 71.1% for estrus detection based on HeatWatch® in comparison with 54.4 and 54.7% provided by visual observation (At-Taras and Spahr, 2001).

Overall, these systems enhance the estrus detection rates in a lower or greater percentage depending on the farm and the device itself, being also one important aspect for the change in trend of the reproductive efficiency in the dairy cow.

5.2.4 *VWP VOLUNTARY WAITING PERIOD*

The VWP is the time between parturition and the time at which the cow is first eligible for insemination based on the farm management decision protocol in order to maximize efficiency (Inchaisri et al., 2011). The insemination and the conception risk at the end of the VWP are the two major determinants of time to pregnancy during lactation, but the duration of VWP can also influence timing pregnancy, since it determines when cows become eligible for insemination (Stangaferro et al., 2018).

Understanding the decision of a VWP as an essential one also contributes to the general improvement of the reproductive efficiency of our dairy systems. A minimal VWP of 45–60 days postpartum is recommended, because it allows for a complete uterine involution and resumption of normal ovarian cyclicity and, therefore, an improvement of successful conception after AI (Fetrow et al., 2007). These are "physiological" reasons for the VWP. However, we now know that the general objective in farms is not to get cows pregnant as soon as possible after calving, but at the moment when they are efficient as possible. In high-yielding dairy cows, an increase of the VWP to prolong the lactation period is nowadays being studied, since it is beneficial for the global economy of the productive system under some circumstances. First, the negative energy balance (NEB) during early lactation (which has detrimental effects on fertility (Wathes et al., 2007) can be avoided. Second, a longer VWP may prevent drying off during high milk production, which can affect in a negative way the health status of udder during the dry period and the subsequent lactation (Bates and Dohoo, 2016). Third, the transition period is a time when there are more diseases and culling risk is greater for the cows, thus, the replacement of many short lactations with fewer longer ones may improve longevity of cows, as well as decrease the number of Holstein calves, since the use of sexed semen has facilitated the production of replacement heifers (Niozas et al., 2019).

As seen before in this chapter, extending the VWP could be especially important in primiparous cows, which have longer and less peaking lactations, more problems of inactive ovaries (Niozas et al., 2019), and could be relevant after some synchronization protocols such as DO (Tenhagen et al., 2003; Gobikrushanth et al., 2014; Stangaferro et al., 2018). Furthermore, in a study by Stangaferro et al. in which VWP of 60 and 88 days (VWP60 and VWP88, respectively) were compared, an interaction was observed between VWP duration and milk yield at dry-off in primiparous cows, producing significantly more milk the animals in the VWP88 group (2018).

Nevertheless, a longer VWP for multiparous cows could also be optimal for the farms, especially in high-yielding ones. It has been observed an increased in conception rates when the VWP is 120 (48.9%) or 180 (49.6%) days long, compared with VWP of 40 days (36.6%) (Niozas et al., 2019). This could be explained because extending VWP period would provide more time for the animal to recover the uterine health (Gilbert et al., 2005; Gautam et al., 2009; Sheldon et al., 2009) through improved immune status, more time to resolve the inflammatory process establish after calving, or both (LeBlanc, 2014). It would also provide more time to return to an optimal metabolic status and hormone secretion patterns which benefits the resumption of ovarian cyclicity (Cheong et al., 2016). Thus, nowadays research has shown the importance, not only of the VWP itself, but also of adjusting it to each farm and animal in order to be more productive and improve fertility in the herd (Stangaferro et al., 2018; Niozas et al., 2019), and all this new knowledge relative to this issue contributes for sure, as well, to the global improvement in dairy cattle fertility.

5.2.5   PREGNANCY LOSS

Fertility is a multifactorial trait and its deterioration is caused by a network of factors (Souza et al., 2018). Pregnancy loss is one of the main problems that decrease fertility, which generates adverse economic effects for dairy farms (Vanroose et al., 2000) since it decrease milk yield, and the number of calves produced and increase culling rate (Souza et al., 2018). This issue has become relevant with the routinization of an always earlier NPD. The early fetal or pregnancy loss (which occurs during the second and third month of gestation, from day 28–60 in lactating cows once positive diagnoses has occurred at 28–33 days after insemination) (Astiz et al., 2018a). Observing this issue and trying to understand and to compensate it, contributes hugely to the general fertility increase of the dairy system, since the high-yielding cows are even more affected than moderate yielding dairy cows (Vasconcelos et al., 1997).

The first articles regarding pregnancy loss were published in the late 1970s, studying the correlation between pregnancy diagnosis by membrane slip and embryonic mortality (Vaillancourt et al., 1979). Later, in the 1980s and 1990s, more research about pregnancy loss was done (Franco et al., 1987; White et al., 1989), especially related to pregnancy diagnosis, since in the early days it was done by transrectal palpation or 2D transrectal ultrasonography, which, in one of these first articles about early pregnancy loss, it was calculated of about 5% (Vaillancourt et al., 1979). But it was not until this century, that the pregnancy loss has become a usual reproductive index to be taken into account in any dairy cattle herd. Currently almost no reproductive publication can demonstrate reproduction results without having studied the rates for pregnancy loss, and the comprehensive of this issue is still a research question. Nowadays, it is estimated to be about 12%, but there is a substantial variation between farms (García-Ispierto et al., 2006; Wijma et al., 2017). In the 1980s, studies were focused on the effect of the pregnancy diagnosis on the pregnancy loss incidence, but currently it has been studied that pregnancy loss is affected by several causes. In this second group, are specially important the parity of the dam, the semen providing bulls, season, and twin pregnancies in different countries (Labèrnia et al., 1996; Santos et al., 2004; Grimard et al., 2006; López-Gatius, 2012). Heat stress is one of the most important factors, being the early pregnancy loss greater during warm and hot season (Souza et al., 2018) since the oocyte on the day of estrus and the developing embryo during the first three cleavage divisions are extremely sensitive (Moore and Thatcher, 2006), but being also important under this circumstance the pregnancy loss after the day 30 of pregnancy. All things considered, pregnancy loss seems to depend more deeply on the individual genetics, which makes the selection program of the farm a key part of the reproductive efficiency of the herd (Chebel and Ribeiro, 2016). Both, animal welfare and genetics are vital aspects that are being improved in the farms, which also imply an improvement in fertility of the herd.

Having understood that our work in fertility does not end with the conception rate results 30 days after AI and the importance of controlling the level of pregnancy losses in our herds, does strongly contribute to the general improvement of the reproduction outputs.

5.3 NUTRITION

Authors would like to emphasize the fact that, even when not at all our specialty, we did not want to write on the global improvement of fertility in the dairy cattle without acknowledging the enormous contributions of other key fields besides reproductive issues such as nutrition, genetics and welfare. Hence, this and the next parts of the chapter are briefly covered.

Every physiological function in the dairy cattle needs a precise supply of specific nutrients in specific proportion. The relationship between reproduction and nutrition is a topic of increasing importance, and their interaction has long been known to have important implications in fertility, since nutrition affects ovarian follicle development through changes in metabolic and reproductive hormones, as well as via direct effects on the ovary and uterus (Bach, 2019) and also because nutrition determines live weight and body condition score, which are correlated with fertility (D'Occhio et al., 2019). Therefore, this factor also plays a relevant role in the improvement of the reproductive efficiency of the dairy cattle farms nowadays, besides of the general fact of requiring adequately fed animals.

Some more concrete aspects of nutrition more directly related to fertility are the following.

5.3.1   ENERGY

Energy is vital in order to have high pregnancies rates, since it has recently been seen that a NEB during the early postpartum period negatively affects follicular and oocyte quality and, therefore, having a negative impact in fertility, both directly and indirectly because of an altered supply to the oocyte (Bach, 2019). In fact, energy status is generally considered to be the major nutritional factor that influences fertility of animals in general and of dairy cattle in particular (Fahar et al., 2018). Thus, prolonged periods of NEB were associated with suppression of pulsatile LH secretion, a reduction in ovarian responsiveness to LH stimulation and reduced estradiol secretion by the dominant follicle, which affects its ovulation (Butler, 2003). Moreover, mobilization of body fat during NEB increased plasma concentration of non-esterified fatty acid (NEFA) and β-hydroxybutyrate (BHB), both of which were associated in high plasmatic concentrations with reduced fertility (Garnsworthy et al., 2008).

Body condition scoring and its variation is probably the most used management tool in order to provide information related to energy reserves and thereby, the nutritional status of dairy cows (Garnsworthy, 2007). The animals are normally scored on a 5-point scale (1 indicating thin and 5 fat)

(Edmonson et al., 1989). In many investigations, body condition score at different moments like calving or at different points in lactation has been determined in order to see its relationship with fertility (Hoedemaker et al., 2009). However, discrepancies regarding the effects of Body Condition Score (BCS) and body condition change on reproductive fertility are common in the literature, since sometimes this relationship is difficult to evaluate because other factor besides nutrition can be involved (López-Gatius et al., 2003).

Nevertheless, it has been proven the connection of some fertility traits and BCS. For example, in a meta-analysis done by López-Gatius et al. (2003) it has been seen that BCS at parturition was associated with the relative risk of conception in cows showing a low BCS at this moment, with a reduction of 9% in pregnancy rate at first AI in comparison to animals with intermediate BCS, possibly due to a prolonged anovulatory period, which is frequent in thin cows (Beam and Butler, 1999). When relating BCS at parturition and at first AI, a relation was found, with homogeneous results in the literature. Thus, in animals showing a body condition ≥ 3.5 at parturition the number of days open were significantly reduced in comparison to cows with low BCS (5.8 or 11.7 days when compared to intermediate or low body condition score animals, respectively). This relationship can also be found between BCS and first AI, since animals in good condition at this moment had a decrease in days open when compared with animals in the intermediate or low body category (11.9 or 24.1, respectively).

All in all, energy is related to some important fertility traits like days open and pregnancy risk. Given that nutritional status is related the management of the herd, we should paid special attention to the cow's nutritional needs during the peripartum period, to avoid metabolic disorders and fertility decrease (Drackley, 1999). Nevertheless, the better knowledge of these needs has already helped to improve reproductive performance in our farms.

5.3.2 PROTEIN

Proteins and their metabolites are also being studied for their relationship with reproductive performance. Proteins are important for the optimal reproduction of the cow, since proteins, or more specifically amino acids are needed for the proper oocyte development (Bach, 2019). It has be seen that reproductive performance can be impaired if the protein intake exceeds the cow's requirements (62 *vs.* 48% of conception rate with diets with 13–14% or 15–19% of crude protein, respectively) (Yasothai, 2014). However, the effect on fertility of low protein intake has been less studied. It is known that short-term protein deficiencies can be met by body reserves, but long-term deficiencies can lead to a NEB that is detrimental to reproductive performance. Also, adequate protein intake is vital to the proper functioning of the reproductive organs and the development of the fetus (Fahar et al., 2018). Thus, the better understanding of the relation between protein levels in diet and fertility has led to a better formulation, and an improvement of fertility during the last decades.

5.3.3 MINERALS AND VITAMINS

Minerals and vitamins have been found important too, but more research is needed in their behalf, since results are still controversial. For example, some studies have found that Zn, Cu, Mn and Co may improve conception rates (29.6 *vs.* 36.6% conception rate at first service for inorganic inorganic trace minerals (ITM) and partial replacement of ITM for chelated trace minerals (Bach et al., 2015), whereas other reports no changes (Siciliano-Jones et al., 2008).

However, not only the ration itself is important in current dairy cattle nutrition. For instance, nowadays there is an increased understanding of its relationship with the balance of metabolic hormones which act at the brain, making it control of the reproductive endocrine system (Clément, 2016). Another important aspect that is being currently studied and starting to understand is the interaction between nutrition and genetics, which can interact in two ways: the genome (and, therefore, the proteome and metabolome) of the host affects the response to a given diet (nutrigenetics); and the nutrients supply may affect the expression of specific genes (nutrigenomics) (Bach, 2019). More research in this topic may give results that could mean an improvement of dairy cattle fertility in the future.

5.4 GENETICS

Over the past 100 years, the range of traits considered for genetic selection in dairy cattle has progressed to meet the demands of both society and industry. Genetic selection for important traits has aided in the transformation and advancement of dairy farming, being the specific traits considered different over time (Miglior et al., 2017). A potential trait must meet different criteria in order to be considered for selection in dairy cattle population (Shook, 1989). First, it should mean an economic improvement of the farms (reducing production costs or having an economic value as a marketable commodity). Second, the trait must have enough genetic variation and heritability. Third, it should be clearly defined, measurable at low cost and recorded consistently. Finally, an indicator trait may be favored if it has a high genetic correlation with the economically relevant trait, reduces recording costs, has a higher heritability, or it can be measured earlier in the animal's life.

It has been the economic value which has been historically driven the genetic selection. From the 1930s to the 1970s, the focus of selection was exclusively on milk production (Miglior et al., 2017). However, this selection for productive traits was detrimental for fertility in dairy cattle, since there is an antagonistic correlation between female fertility and milk production (VanRaden et al., 2004). At first, this idea was controversial, since some studies reported little or no relationship between traits of yield and reproduction (Weller, 1989), or even if the reported it, it was not significant (Shanks et al., 1978). Later, it became accepted that due to unfavorable genetic correlations selection for higher yields in dairy cattle has possibly led a decline in fertility, since the reproduction physiology of dairy cattle changed in response to genetic selection for milk production (Lucy, 2001).

In general, the inclusion of reproductive measures in the general indices was adopted relatively late, mostly due to data availability, except in the Nordic countries, which started to include reproduction traits in national indices in the late 1970s (Miglior et al., 2017). It was not until the 21st century when more countries (several European countries, Australia, New Zealand, and the United States) included fertility in their national selection indices (Miglior et al., 2005).

Selection for fertility traits is not easy, being a challenge to find relevant, easily measurable, or recordable phenotypes to represent the multiple aspects of fertility and better describe the underlying physiology. In the current practices for fertility selection, direct selection on phenotypes describing fertility and indirect selection for improved fertility can be done. Furthermore, novel fertility phenotypes such as progesterone-based measures, estrus expression and activity traits and improved reporting of current traits can also be used for improving the fertility genetics (Fleming et al., 2019) and, therefore, contribute to the global improvement of fertility in cows.

5.4.1   CURRENT PRACTICES FOR FERTILITY SELECTION

5.4.1.1   DIRECT SELECTION ON PHENOTYPES DESCRIBING FERTILITY

Fertility traits measured in dairy cattle are strongly influenced by a great number of factors, such as environmental and management factors and the animal's physiology. This, in addition to the fact that some traits are measured late in life or over long periods and the low hereditability of these traits, explain why the genetic improvement of fertility traits using the traditional genetic evaluation has been slow over the years. It also has mean low reliability of estimated breeding values, and the influence of the reproductive management applied (Fleming et al., 2019).

Traditional fertility traits used in selection programs are usually measured using time intervals and success or nonsuccess traits. The International Bull Evaluation Service Centre (Interbull, Uppsala, Sweden) used five female traits in order to introduce international genetic evaluation service for fertility across countries in 2007 (Fleming et al., 2019). These traits are (National Genetic Evaluations Info-Interbull Centre, 2017): maiden heifer's ability to conceive, lactating cow's ability to recycle after calving, lactating cow's ability to conceive expressed as a rate trait and lactating cow's measurements of interval traits calving-conception. Nevertheless, the different countries also have their own national defined and emphasized fertility traits, based on the selection criteria applied in the population (Fleming et al., 2019).

Nowadays, the availability of genomic data like single nucleotide polymorphisms (SNP) markers and whole genome sequence have provided new opportunities for the improvement of dairy fertility using this traditional traits, since several studies identified SNP and deleterious haplotypes related to fertility and reproduction traits (Müller et al., 2017). The inclusion of the information provided by these technologies has also provided better reliability estimates for fertility traits (VanRaden et al., 2017). However, even with the development done during these years in fertility genetics, the selection for improved genetics in dairy cows is still a challenge for breeders, farmers and the industry (Fleming et al., 2019).

5.4.1.2 INDIRECT SELECTION FOR IMPROVED FERTILITY

In order to achieve a pregnancy and give birth to a healthy calf, various additional traits describing a robust animal in good condition to reproduce are necessary. Some traits that are currently under selection in the dairy industry are genetically correlated with the overall reproductive success of the, which means a contribution to the indirect genetic improvement of fertility in selection programs. Given the low hereditability of fertility traits and the difficulty in their evaluation, fertility-correlated traits have been vital for the improvement of cow fertility. Future traits currently under investigation could help to further this cause (Fleming et al., 2019).

Calving traits such as calving ease, calf size, and stillbirth are usually evaluated in reproduction trait indices (Miglior et al., 2017). Longevity and other similarly defined traits related to ability of or length of time a cow can remain in the herd is usually evaluated worldwide, since it means a decline in involuntary and premature culling. Because infertility is one of the most important reasons for early disposal of the dams, using longevity as a trait favorably selects fertility (Wall et al., 2003). Body condition score is also included in many national genetic evaluations (Fleming et al., 2019). The relationship between energy balance and fertility is a strong subject of interest, as explained before in the previous part of this chapter, and additional indicators traits of energy balance that may relate to reproductive performance are being investigated (McParland et al., 2015) as a new way to enhance fertility. Health traits are now frequently evaluated in dairy cows selection programs using clinical health information (Fleming et al., 2019), since it has been studied that clinical ketosis, dystocia, retained placenta, locomotion disorders, and metritis events influenced days to first service and conception rates (Fourichon et al., 2000). Later, Köck et al. (2014) reported significant genetics correlations between retained placenta, metritis, and cystic ovaries and female fertility traits. Nevertheless, like fertility traits, health traits typically have low heritability estimates but, even so, they are still selected, since cow health is economically important and has welfare implications (Fleming et al., 2019).

Thus, indirect selection for improved fertility could be advantageous to the improvement of fertility, being one of the tools used nowadays. However, more research should be done in order to fully understand the genetic traits utilized, which could be important in order to improve fertility in our farms.

5.4.2   NOVEL FERTILITY TRAITS

To ensure continuous progress and to develop breeding aims that coup with the producer and consumer expectations, the introduction of novel traits should be considered (Miglior et al., 2017), since the current traits used have many disadvantages. In fact, many new phenotypes have been proposed to better express the underlying biology or cattle reproduction (Fleming et al., 2019). Rapid advancement in technology, data sources, and methodology related to dairy industry have permitted the apparition of better opportunities to both, better characterize and improve the accuracy of current traits and potentially collect novel phenotypes at a national level (Crowe et al., 2018; Fleming et al., 2018). In particular, the implementation of genomic selection accelerated progress in novel trait selection, as well as the use of MIR spectroscopy in routine milk testing. This has led to the selection of novel traits that, even though are not directly related to fertility, could help to boost it, like feed efficiency, heat stress, hoof health, or immune response (Miglior et al., 2017). Focusing on fertility traits and phenotypes, nowadays there are a great number of them that describe many different aspects of dairy cows. Some of the most important novel fertility phenotypes are progesterone-based measures, estrous expression, and activity traits. It is also relevant in the development of dairy cattle genetics the improvement of reports of current traits.

Endocrine-level phenotypes largely focused on progesterone (P4) levels have been pointed out as indicators of fertility in dairy cattle because they describe more directly cow's physiology, being less shifting. However, the applications of P4-based measures in genetic evaluation is nowadays limited by the cost and labor associated with obtaining enough P4 samples to generate the phenotypes on large numbers of cows. Advancing on farm technologies may produce data useful in the evaluation of P4 reproduction traits, and that could be an advantage in genetic selection for improved fertility in the future (Fleming et al., 2019).

On the other hand, as seen before in this chapter, many reproductive management strategies rely on estrus behavioral signs. Thus, assessing the ability and strength of estrous expression in dairy cows could improve reproductive efficiency. Thanks to the trend among toward the uptake of new technologies by farmers for detecting estrus that accurately identify individual cows by continuously monitoring with minimal labor involve (e.g., pedometers and activity tags), more phenotypes that are secondary signs of estrus are being recorded. Thus, the interval to first high activity may in the future be applicable to genetic evaluation for improved fertility and reproduction in dairy cattle (Fleming et al., 2019).

In addition to the boosting in understanding the usefulness of new fertility phenotypes, the development of technology has facilitated the use of current fertility traits. For example, pregnancy loss is one of the most important factors affecting fertility in dairy cattle. So, using it as a fertility trait could be vital in enhancing fertility in cows (Fleming et al., 2019). Other aspect in which genetics is focusing is the reproductive management strategies. New reproductive management tools, such as estrus synchronization and TAI are used worldwide at present. Nevertheless, data related to reproductive strategies related to reproductive phenotypes is scarce, and if this new technologies are not taken into account during the selection process, it might benefit cows that are merely good responders to synchronization protocols (Berry et al., 2016). Relatedly, it has been reported low to moderate maternal heritability for number of flushed ova, transferable embryos, degenerated embryos, unfertilized oocytes, and percentage of transferable embryos when superovulation protocols have been studied as a fertility trait (Miglior et al., 2017). Recent studies have investigated the genetics components of various traits related to reproductive technologies and found many regions of the genome associated with them (Gaddis et al., 2017). However, more investigation in this behalf is needed in order to fully understand the relationship between these technologies and genetics.

As reported in this chapter, the interaction nutrition-genetics can also improve fertility in dairy cattle. This interaction can be especially important during development (both pre- and postnatal), since it may result in permanent changes in body composition and metabolic function of the offspring (fetal programming), which primarily involve modifications in the chromatin structure through acetylation of histones or methylation of DNA (Wu et al., 2006). The understanding of the effects and mechanism of this process in reproduction could be beneficial in the improvement of dairy cattle fertility (Bach, 2019).

Therefore, a deeper knowledge of genetics and genomics, together with the evolution and improvement in the selection schemes of our dairy sires and cows worldwide are key factors for the general reproductive improvement in the dairy sector.

5.5 DAIRY CATTLE WELFARE

Animal welfare is a very recent discipline, being the first paper using these terms published in 1983. However, care for the well-being of production animals was an issue much before that year, and was first entered in the social media by the 1960s (von Keyserlingk and Weary, 2017).

Animal welfare bas been defined by the World Organization for Animal Health (OIE) as "the physical and mental state of an animal in conditions in which it lives and dies" (World Organisation for Animal Health, 2015). To describe the right for welfare of animals under human control, five conditions known as the Five Freedoms were published in 1965 (freedom from hunger, malnutrition and thirst, freedom from fear and distress, freedom from physical and thermal discomfort, freedom from pain, injury, and disease, and freedom to express normal patterns of behavior) (Farm Animal Welfare Council—5 Freedoms, 2009), and are nowadays used worldwide to describe animal welfare.

This discipline has been growing in importance during the last years, both in a scientific and social way. During this period, hundreds of papers have been published on this regard, and different legislations has been developed worldwide (von Keyserlingk and Weary, 2017). Some initiatives have also been created in order to control and evaluate the well-being of the farm animals, like the Welfare Quality® project in Europe (Welfare Quality Network, 2018). Moreover, it has been seen that animal welfare is vital in animal farming, not only because of ethical issues regarding the animal, but also because of its impact in productivity. For example, as have been reviewed before in this chapter, dairy cattle has been selected only for milk production for a long time, which has driven to an intensification of production and a change in the farming system which sometimes has had a detrimental impact in animal welfare, also implying less production and fertility (McInerney, 2004).

Thus, animal welfare is a broad subject, and its understanding is complicated (von Keyserlingk and Weary, 2017). But nowadays, there is more and more knowledge about the effect of stress in production and fertility (and also the effect of lowering those stress levels in farm animals) (Von Borell et al., 2007; Whitfield, 2017).

Stress has been defined in different ways over the years. For instance, it was defined by Ewing et al. (1999) as the unfitness to adapt to the environment and reproduce effectively, which gives us the idea that fertility is linked to stress (and, therefore, to animal welfare). The detailed ways in which stress influences reproduction are still not well understood, but may involve a number of endocrine, paracrine, and neural systems (Tilbrook et al., 2000). It is known that stress blocks or delays the preovulatory LH surge in cattle, resulting in a prolonged follicular wave, as well as an atretic follicle if the dominant follicle is not able to reach the ovulatory capacity and reduce estradiol production (Dobson and Smith, 2000). It has also been demonstrated that stress interfere with the onset cycling in the postpartum cow, delaying the process and causing a worsening of the fertility parameters of the animal (Huszenicza et al., 2005; Sheldon, 2004). Stress can induce a premature luteolysis of the CL, resulting in short inter-estrus intervals (Huszenicza et al., 2005).

Thus, the studying of stress, stressors, and their management have been crucial in order to guarantee better welfare of cattle, improving its milk yield and fertility, being another reason for the change in trend in fertility traits during the last two decades. Stressor could be categorized into stress caused by environmental conditions (heat, cold, wind, humidity…), and management-related stressors (social interactions, interspecies interaction, manipulation, transportation…) (Moberg, 1985). This classification of stressor can be useful, since it separates those stressor in which farmers and veterinarians have less control (environment) and those where the sector professionals can work in harder in order to achieve the animal welfare (Whitfield, 2017).

Since the topic of animal welfare is so broad, only two selected themes will be treated in the present chapter: environmental enrichment and heat stress.

5.5.1 ENVIRONMENTAL ENRICHMENT

Almost all dairy cattle is nowadays kept indoors during, at least, some part of their lives, being the number of cows being housed indoors throughout the year increasing in the last years (Van Vuuren and Van Den Pol-Van Dasselaar, 2006; Winsten et al., 2010; March et al., 2014). Thus, the facilities where the cow will spend most of her life are critical in order to achieve optimal levels of cow welfare or cow comfort. Housing management is an important decision for dairy producers, since it will have considerable influence on productivity, health, milk quality, reproduction, animal well-being, and profitability (Bewley et al., 2017).

In continuous indoor housing, also known as zero-grazing systems, cows are kept in tie-stalls, freestalls, or loose-housing cowsheds, being the access to pasture limited or absent (Mandel et al., 2016). Keeping animals indoors has some important welfare benefits, like protection from predators and toxic plants and reduced exposure to extreme weather conditions (Schütz et al., 2010). It also enables the farmer to give the cattle a nutritional balanced diet during the year (Aarhus University, 2009). However, animals also confront a great number of challenges, including abiotic environmental sources of stress, confinement-specific stressor (more related to indoor systems) (Morgan and Tromborg, 2007), higher incidence of lameness (Haskell et al., 2006), and increasing risk for claw or foot problems, teat trampling, mastitis, metritis, dystocia, ketosis, retained placenta, and bacterial infections (Aarhus University, 2009), diseases that have important effects not only in animal welfare itself, but also in its productivity and fertility (e.g., recent studies show that lame cows have 3.5 times greater odds of not resuming cyclicity within 60 days of calving compare to nonlame cows and that preventing lameness would decrease the number of cows with delayed cyclicity by 71% (Garbarino et al., 2004). Once housed, animals are also forced to drastically change their behavior which, when the environment is too impoverished or too small may result in frustration and, therefore, stress (Newberry, 1993).

In order to help animals cope with stressors in their surroundings, prevent frustration and increase the fulfillment of behavioral needs, the enrichment of the environment can be done (Mandel et al., 2016). Environmental enrichment is defined as an improvement in the biological functioning of confined animals, resulting from modifications to their environment. Biological functions are referred as increase fitness in a direct or indirect way, as well as correlation of both (that would be health). Thus, by environmental enrichment, lifetime reproductive success can be improved (Newberry, 1995).

There are five categories of environmental enrichment: social, occupational, physical, sensory, and nutritional. The understanding of each during the last 20 years has caused not only an improvement of cattle welfare, but also of its fertility.

In relation to social enrichment, more concretely with the cow-human interaction, it has been recently seen that by practicing positive handling from an early age, farmers can help animals to reduce stress levels in some intrusive procedures such as AI, which is positively correlated with conception rates (Hemsworth et al., 2000). Also the better understanding of the relationship of cows with their herd mates can be translated in better welfare levels, since now it is now that cows that change their group experience high levels of stress due to destabilization of social dynamics (von Keyserlingk et al., 2008), so other management methods such as using familiar pens for regrouping the cows (Schirmann et al., 2011) or grouping during the evening hours (Boyle et al., 2012) are being used.

Occupational enrichment is also vital, and it is highly related to the type of facilities the animals are maintained in. The decision of one system or other is important, having consequences in the cow lifestyle and, therefore, in its welfare and production (Bewley et al., 2017; Cook, 2019; House, 2019). For example, some studies suggested that freestall and loose housing systems had better reproductive results than tie-stalls (a mean of 2.33 inseminations were required to get pregnant the cows in tie-stalls, compared with 2.32 in freestalls and 1.96 loose housing facilities) (Konggaard, 1977), that could be explained by the fact that tie-stall kept animals are more prone lameness and sole disorders than other systems, as well as more stressed due to the lack of exercise (Bewley et al., 2017; Mandel et al., 2016; Bielfeldt et al., 2005).

Physical enrichment refers to the one applicated in the farm facilities. Thus, when designing housing and husbandry systems, the complex cognitive abilities of cows should also be considered (Nawroth et al., 2019). In zero-grazing systems, facilities are usually designed to provide constant visual and physical contact between conspecifics (Mandel et al., 2016). However, recent research shows that cows prefer to isolate themselves in some moments, like calving or during times of illness (Proudfoot et al., 2014). Lowering stress levels during calving could be beneficial to fertility traits in the farm (Borchers and Bewley, n. d.), being vital the adequate design of the maternity pen (Proudfoot, 2019). Also, the bedding material plays an important part in animal welfare and it is being studied in order to give animals maximum levels of comfort. One of the bedding materials investigated in relationship with fertility traits is the compost bedding. It has been reported no differences in pregnancy after first insemination, mortality rate, or incidence of clinical metritis and endometriosis when comparing compost-bedding and straw-bedding systems. However, they observed positive effects on udder health (Astiz et al., 2014), which can correlate with better fertility and longevity, being one good method to further improve fertility in dairy cattle. In other study, it has been observed that cows in compost-bedded barns had a better claw health status than cows in freestall cubicle barns (Burgstaller et al., 2016).

Sensory enrichment is defined as stimulation designed to trigger one or more of animal's senses (Wells, 2009) through visual, auditory, olfactory, tactile, or taste (Mandel et al., 2016; Bloomsmith et al., 1991). Very few studies have been conducted in each subfield of sensory enrichment (Mandel et al., 2016), and there is none or very little information regarding its relationship with fertility, which could be a good research are for the future.

Lastly, nutritional enrichment can be done through presenting varied or novel food types or by changing the method of food delivery (Bloomsmith et al., 1991). This second idea is more important for high yielding cow fertility. Thus, fenceline feeding of TMR, which is the most common food location in zero-grazing systems (Newberry, 1993) has been seen related with increased agonistic interactions, which is not the case on pasture, where the animals are more spaced out from each other (Miller and Wood-Gush, 1991; DeVries, 2019). Providing animals with a larger feeding space allows for a 57% reduction of aggressive interactions (DeVries et al., 2004), being this change also associated with an increase in feeding activity, especially in subordinate cows (Mandel et al., 2016). This could be related with an improvement of overall body condition score, which is correlated with fertility (Pryce et al., 2001).

All things considered, environmental enrichment methods that are aimed to help cattle to cope better with stressors in their environment, prevent frustration, and increase the fulfillment of behavioral needs will help in the improvement of animal welfare and, indirectly, of animal production and fertility (Mandel et al., 2016).

5.5.2   HEAT STRESS

Escalating global temperatures (Schär et al., 2004), combined with global increases in the number of production animals and the intensification of agriculture (Renaudeau et al., 2012) has resulting in heat stress becoming an important challenge facing the global dairy industry and a major concern for dairy produces because of its association with decrease in milk production and fertility (Polsky and von Keyserlingk, 2017). Given that high milk yielding cows already have elevated internal heat loads, the effects of cumulative incremental heat are exacerbated when humidity and temperature values are increased in their surroundings (West, 2003).

Heat stress is defined as the sum of forces acting on an animal that provokes an increases in its body temperature and is responsible of a physiological (increased respiratory rate, panting, sweating, and reduced milk yield and reproductive performance) or behavioral response (increased water intake, shifting feeding times, increase shade seeking) (Rensis and Scaramuzzi, 2003; West, 2003; Dikmen et al., 2008; Schütz et al., 2008).

In the last years, the effect of exposure to high environmental temperatures in reproduction has been studied, being outlined its effect in compromising steredoigenesis and viability of oocytes (Zeron et al., 2001), reduction of oocyte quality (Hansen, 2002) and reduction of fertilization rate (Sartori et al., 2002), and therefore, being one of the main problems that could explained the low fertility rates in dairy cattle. For example, it has been reported that cows exposed to heat stress prior to AI were 31–33% less likely to conceive than control ones (Chebel et al., 2004). This is in consonance with the results obtained by Pereira et al. which shows a conception rate decline from 21 to 15% when rectal temperature is greater than 39°C during AI (Pereira et al., 2013). Other studies shows a decrease in conception rates during summer season that could be up to 30%, with evident seasonal patterns of estrus detection (Rensis and Scaramuzzi, 2003). Thus, heat stress affects reproduction in multiple ways, which are nowadays still being studied, since they are not fully understood (Fig. 5.6) (Rensis and Scaramuzzi, 2003).

At the present moment, various cooling options for dairy cows are being studied, based on the principles of convection, conduction, radiation, and evaporation (Polsky and von Keyserlingk, 2017). Fan installation have been used in order to decrease environment temperature with good results in animal welfare (decrease of respiratory rate and rectal temperature and increase in dry matter intake; Armstrong, 1994; Mondaca, 2019). A modification of fans is to add high pressure mist injector into them (which function to cool the microclimate air that the cow inspires), or large water droplets that completely soak the hair coat of the cow (Van Os, 2019). Both systems have shown to improve conception rates. For example, in an experiment conducted in summer in Israel, fans with mist injectors were used, being the conception rates of 57 *vs.* 17% for cooled and not cooled cows (Flamenbaum and Galon, 2010). Some recent works has looked at providing cows with self-controlled showers (operated by the animals using pressure-sensitive floors), but more research is needed in order to fully understand this method and its implication in reproductive physiology (Legrand et al., 2011). Physical structures that provide shade (trees, roofs, or cloth) are also vital to avoid heat stress, since they create more hospitable microclimates for cows (Polsky and von Keyserlingk, 2017) that can be beneficial for fertility (44.4 *vs.* 25.3% conception rates for shade and no shade available, respectively) (Roman-Ponce et al., 1977). Nowadays, various intervention techniques are being investigated to improve the coping abilities of heat stress cows, like selection of genes like the slick hair gene (SLICK), that controls hair length and could, therefore, control evaporative heat loss and efficient transfer of heat to the environment (Dikmen et al., 2008), which can, in a future, help with the decrease of fertility during the hot season.

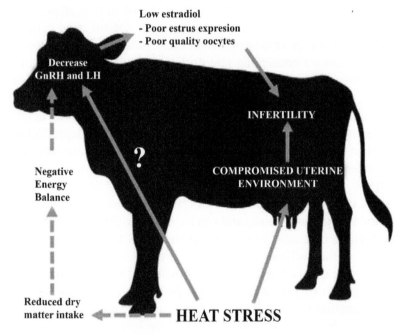

FIGURE 5.6   A schematic representation of possible mechanism for effect of heat stress on reproduction in the lactating dairy cow. Heat stress reduces dry matter intake, which inhibits GnRH and LH secretion (dashed lines). It may also influence the hypothalamus-hypophysis system (solid line), reducing the GnRH and LH secretion. Heat stress can also compromise the uterine environment (solid thick line) to cause embryo loss and infertility. (Modified from Rensis and Scaramuzzi, 2003).

So, welfare is a critical area of research. The better understanding of dairy cattle behavior and the increased consideration toward its well-being has helped to the increase of cow fertility in the last years. However, more effort must be done in order to fully understand animal welfare and its implication in productive and reproductive traits.

5.6 CONCLUSIONS

Nowadays, there is much more knowledge about dairy cattle, which has driven to a major change in veterinary practices in farms, from individual treatment of the animals to the consideration of the farms as a complex system in which the cow is just another element interacting with the facilities, the farm staff, the feeding system. The deeper understanding of cow's physiology has driven to the improvement of reproductive, nutrition, and breeding management practices, as well as to a major consideration of animal welfare. The development of technology during this last decade also plays a key role in the improvement of dairy fertility, since it has allowed a better data recording, allowing for better consideration of some aspects of production and reproduction. All in all, thanks to the effort of all the professionals implicated, plus the advancement in research have permitted us to deal with high-yielding cows much better than before. Being able even to change the trend of dairy cow fertility!

KEYWORDS

- hormonal synchronization programs
- early non-pregnancy diagnosis
- pregnancy loss
- oestrus detection accuracy
- cattle parity.

REFERENCES

Animal Welfare at a Glance: OIE—World Organisation for Animal Health http://www.oie. int/en/animal-welfare/animal-welfare-at-a-glance/ (accessed Feb 23, 2019).

Armstrong, D. V. Heat Stress Interaction with Shade and Cooling. *J. Dairy Sci.* **1994**, *77* (7), 2044–2050.

Astiz, S.; Fargas, O. Pregnancy Per AI Differences Between Primiparous and Multiparous High-Yield Dairy Cows After Using Double Ovsynch or G6G Synchronization Protocols. *Theriogenology* **2013**, *79* (7), 1065–1070.

Astiz, S.; Sebastian, F.; Fargas, O.; Fernández, M.; Calvet, E. Enhanced Udder Health and Milk Yield of Dairy Cattle on Compost Bedding Systems During the Dry Period: A Comparative Study. *Livest. Sci.* **2014**, *159*, 161–164.

Astiz, S.; Gonzalez-Martin, J. V.; Fargas, O.; Sebastian, F.; Gonzalez-Bulnes, A.; Patrón, R.; Pesántez-Pacheco, J. L. *Management Strategies to Enhance Production Efficiency in High Yielding Dairy Farms*; ACVIM: Seattle, **2018a**.

Astiz, S.; Fargas, O.; Sebastian, F.; Heras, J.; Patrón, R.; Pesantez-Pacheco, J. L. *Reproduction in High Yielding Dairy Farm: Learning from Their Own Data*; ACVIM: Seattle, **2018b**.

At-Taras, E. E.; Spahr, S. L. Detection and Characterization of Estrus in Dairy Cattle with an Electronic Heatmount Detector and an Electronic Activity Tag. *J. Dairy Sci.* **2001**, *84* (4), 792–798. Bach, À.; Pinto, A.; Blanch, M. Association Between Chelated Trace Mineral Supplementation and Milk Yield, Reproductive Performance, and Lameness in Dairy Cattle. *Livest. Sci.* **2015**, *182*, 69–75.

Bach, À. Effects of Nutrition and Genetics on Fertility in Dairy Cows. *Reprod. Fertil. Dev.* **2019**, *31* (1), 40.

Barberg, A. E.; Endres, M. I.; Salfer, J. A.; Reneau, J. K. Performance and Welfare of Dairy Cows in an Alternative Housing System in Minnesota. *J. Dairy Sci.* **2007**, *90* (3), 1575–1583.

Bates, A. J.; Dohoo, I. Risk Factors for Peri-Parturient Farmer Diagnosed Mastitis in New Zealand Dairy Herds: Findings from a Retrospective Cohort Study. *Prev. Vet. Med.* **2016**, *127*, 70–76.

Beam, S. W.; Butler, W. R. Effects of Energy Balance on Follicular Development and First Ovulation in Postpartum Dairy Cows. *J. Reprod. Fertil. Suppl.* **1999**, *54*, 411–424.

Bello, N. M.; Steibel, J. P.; Pursley, J. R. Optimizing Ovulation to First GnRH Improved Outcomes to Each Hormonal Injection of Ovsynch in Lactating Dairy Cows. *J. Dairy Sci.* **2006**, *89* (9), 3413–3424.

Berry, D. P.; Friggens, N. C.; Lucy, M.; Roche, J. R. Milk Production and Fertility in Cattle. *Annu. Rev. Anim. Biosci.* **2016**, *4*, 269–290.

Bewley, J. M.; Robertson, L. M.; Eckelkamp, E. A. A 100-Year Review: Lactating Dairy Cattle Housing Management. *J. Dairy Sci.* **2017**, *100* (12), 10418–10431.

Bielfeldt, J. C.; Badertscher, R.; Tölle, K. H.; Krieter, J. Risk Factors Influencing Lameness and Claw Disorders in Dairy Cows. *Livest. Prod. Sci.* **2005**, *95* (3), 265–271.

Bisinotto, R. S.; Ribeiro, E. S.; Martins, L. T.; Marsola, R. S.; Greco, L. F.; Favoreto, M. G.; Risco, C. A.; Thatcher, W. W.; Santos, J. E. P. Effect of Interval Between Induction of Ovulation and Artificial Insemination (AI) and Supplemental Progesterone for Resynchronization on Fertility of Dairy Cows Subjected to a 5-d Timed AI Program. *J. Dairy Sci.* **2010**, *93* (12), 5798–5808.

Bisinotto, R. S.; Ribeiro, E. S.; Santos, J. E. P. Synchronisation of Ovulation for Management of Reproduction in Dairy Cows. *Animal* **2014**, *8* (s1), 151–159.

Bloomsmith, M. A.; Brent, L. Y.; Schapiro, S. J. Guidelines for Developing and Managing an Environmental Enrichment Program for Nonhuman Primates. *Lab. Anim. Sci.* **1991**, *41* (4), 372–377.

Bisinotto, R. S.; Lean, I. J.; Thatcher, W. W.; Santos, J. E. P. Meta-Analysis of Progesterone Supplementation during Timed Artificial Insemination Programs in Dairy Cows. *J. Dairy Sci.* **2015**, *98* (4), 2472–2487.

Borchardt, S.; Schüller, L.; Wolf, L.; Wesenauer, C.; Heuwieser, W. Comparison of Pregnancy Outcomes Using Either an Ovsynch or a Cosynch Protocol for the First Timed AI with Liquid or Frozen Semen in Lactating Dairy Cows. *Theriogenology* **2018**, *107*, 21–26.

Boyle, A. R.; Ferris, C. P.; O'Connell, N. E. Are There Benefits in Introducing Dairy Heifers to the Main Dairy Herd in the Evening Rather than the Morning? *J. Dairy Sci.* **2012**, *95* (7), 3650–3661.

Bridges, G. A.; Helser, L. A.; Grum, D. E.; Mussard, M. L.; Gasser, C. L.; Day, M. L. Decreasing the Interval Between GnRH and PGF$_2\alpha$ from 7 to 5 Days and Lengthening Proestrus Increases Timed-AI Pregnancy Rates in Beef Cows. *Theriogenology* **2008**, *69* (7), 843–851.

Britt, J. H.; Huertasvega, E.; Ulberg, L. C. Managing Reproduction in Dairy Cattle: I. Progestogens for Control of Estrus in Dairy Cows. *J. Dairy Sci.* **1972**, *55* (5), 598–605.

Britt, J. H.; Cox, N. M.; Stevenson, J. S. Advances in Reproduction in Dairy Cattle. *J. Dairy Sci.* **1981**, *64* (6), 1378–1402.

Britt, J. H.; Scott, R. G.; Armstrong, J. D.; Whitacre, M. D. Determinants of Estrous Behavior in Lactating Holstein Cows. *J. Dairy Sci.* **1986**, *69* (8), 2195–2202

Burgstaller, J.; Raith, J.; Kuchling, S.; Mandl, V.; Hund, A.; Kofler, J. Claw Health and Prevalence of Lameness in Cows from Compost Bedded and Cubicle Freestall Dairy Barns in Austria. *Vet. J. Lond. Engl.* **2016**, *216*, 81–86.

Butler, W. R. Review: Effect of Protein Nutrition on Ovarian and Uterine Physiology in Dairy Cattle. *J. Dairy Sci.* **1998**, *81* (9), 2533–2539.

Butler, W. R. Energy Balance Relationships with Follicular Development, Ovulation and Fertility in Postpartum Dairy Cows. *Livest. Prod. Sci.* **2003**, *83* (2), 211–218.

Carvalho, P. D.; Fuenzalida, M. J.; Ricci, A.; Souza, A. H.; Barletta, R. V.; Wiltbank, M. C.; Fricke, P. M. Modifications to Ovsynch Improve Fertility during Resynchronization: Evaluation of Presynchronization with Gonadotropin-Releasing Hormone 6 d before Initiation of Ovsynch and Addition of a Second Prostaglandin F$_2\alpha$ Treatment. *J. Dairy Sci.* **2015**, *98* (12), 8741–8752.

Carvalho, P. D.; Santos, V. G.; Giordano, J. O.; Wiltbank, M. C.; Fricke, P. M. Development of Fertility Programs to Achieve High 21-Day Pregnancy Rates in High-Producing Dairy Cows. *Theriogenology* **2018**, *114*, 165–172.

Chebel, R. C.; Santos, J. E. P.; Reynolds, J. P.; Cerri, R. L. A.; Juchem, S. O.; Overton, M. Factors Affecting Conception Rate after Artificial Insemination and Pregnancy Loss in Lactating Dairy Cows. *Anim. Reprod. Sci.* **2004**, *84* (3–4), 239–255.

Chebel, R. C.; Santos, J. E. P.; Cerri, R. L. A.; Rutigliano, H. M.; Bruno, R. G. S. Reproduction in Dairy Cows Following Progesterone Insert Presynchronization and Resynchronization Protocols. *J. Dairy Sci.* **2006**, *89* (11), 4205–4219.

Chebel, R. C.; Ribeiro, E. S. Reproductive Systems for North American Dairy Cattle Herds. *Vet. Clin. North Am. Food Anim. Pract.* **2016**, *32* (2), 267–284.

Cheong, S. H.; Filho, O. G. S.; Absalón-Medina, V. A.; Pelton, S. H.; Butler, W. R.; Gilbert, R. O. Metabolic and Endocrine Differences Between Dairy Cows That Do or Do Not Ovulate First Postpartum Dominant Follicles. *Biol. Reprod.* **2016**, *94* (1).

Clément, F. Multiscale Mathematical Modeling of the Hypothalamo-Pituitary-Gonadal Axis. *Theriogenology* **2016**, *86* (1), 11–21.

Colazo, M. G.; Ambrose, D. J. Neither Duration of Progesterone Insert nor Initial GnRH Treatment Affected Pregnancy per Timed-Insemination in Dairy Heifers Subjected to a Co-Synch Protocol. *Theriogenology* **2011**, *76* (3), 578–588.

Colazo, M. G.; Ambrose, D. J. Effect of Initial GnRH and Duration of Progesterone Insert Treatment on the Fertility of Lactating Dairy Cows. *Reprod. Domest. Anim. Zuchthyg.* **2015**, *50* (3), 497–504.

Cook, N. B. Optimizing Resting Behavior in Lactating Dairy Cows Through Freestall Design. *Vet. Clin. North Am. Food Anim. Pract.* **2019**, *35* (1), 93–109.

Cooper, M. J., Hammond, D., Harker, D.R., Jackson, P. S. 1976. Control of Bovine Oestrous Cycle with ICI 80996 (Cloprostenol). Field Results in 3810 Beef Cattle. In Proc. VIII th Int. Cong. Anim. Reprod. and IA. Krakow. pp. 449–451.

Crowe, M. A.; Hostens, M.; Opsomer, G. Reproductive Management in Dairy Cows—the Future. *Ir. Vet. J.* **2018**, *71*, 1.

D'Occhio, M. J.; Baruselli, P. S.; Campanile, G. Influence of Nutrition, Body Condition, and Metabolic Status on Reproduction in Female Beef Cattle: A Review. *Theriogenology* **2019**, *125*, 277–284.

De Kruif, A. Factors Influencing the Fertility of a Cattle Population. *J. Reprod. Fertil.* **1978**, *54* (2), 507–518.

De Rensis, F.; López-Gatius, F.; García-Ispierto, I.; Techakumpu, M. Clinical Use of Human Chorionic Gonadotropin in Dairy Cows: An Update. *Theriogenology* **2010**, *73* (8), 1001–1008.

Denis-Robichaud, J.; Cerri, R. L. A.; Jones-Bitton, A.; LeBlanc, S. J. Performance of Automated Activity Monitoring Systems Used in Combination with Timed Artificial Insemination Compared to Timed Artificial Insemination Only in Early Lactation in Dairy Cows. *J. Dairy Sci.* **2018**, *101* (1), 624–636.

DeVries, T. J.; von Keyserlingk, M. A. G.; Weary, D. M. Effect of Feeding Space on the Inter-Cow Distance, Aggression, and Feeding Behavior of Free-Stall Housed Lactating Dairy Cows. *J. Dairy Sci.* **2004**, *87* (5), 1432–1438.

DeVries, T. J. Feeding Behavior, Feed Space, and Bunk Design and Management for Adult Dairy Cattle. *Vet. Clin. North Am. Food Anim. Pract.* **2019**, *35* (1), 61–76.

Dikmen, S.; Alava, E.; Pontes, E.; Fear, J. M.; Dikmen, B. Y.; Olson, T. A.; Hansen, P. J. Differences in Thermoregulatory Ability Between Slick-Haired and Wild-Type Lactating Holstein Cows in Response to Acute Heat Stress. *J. Dairy Sci.* **2008**, *91* (9), 3395–3402.

Diskin, M. G.; Sreenan, J. M. Expression and Detection of Oestrus in Cattle. *Reprod. Nutr. Dev.* **2000**, *40* (5), 481–491.

Dobson, H.; Smith, R. F. What Is Stress, and How Does It Affect Reproduction? *Anim. Reprod. Sci.* **2000**, *60*–61, 743–752.

Drackley, J. K. Biology of Dairy Cows During the Transition Period: The Final Frontier? *J. Dairy Sci.* **1999**, *82* (11), 2259–2273.

Edmonson, A. J.; Lean, I. J.; Weaver, L. D.; Farver, T.; Webster, G. A Body Condition Scoring Chart for Holstein Dairy Cows. *J. Dairy Sci. 72* (1), 68–78.

Erb, H. N.; Grohn, Y. T. Epidemiology of Metabolic Disorders in the Periparturient Dairy Cow. *J. Dairy Sci.* **1988**, *71* (9), 2557–2571.

European Commission EUFADN 2010 Report, 2013; pp 1–216.

Ewing, S. A.; Lay, D. C.; Von Borell, E. *Farm Animal Well-Being: Stress Physiology, Animal Behavior, and Environmental Design*; Prentice Hall: Upper Saddle River, NJ, **1999**.

Fahar, I.; Nawab, A.; Li, G.; Mei, X.; An, L.; Naseer, G. Effect of Nutrition on Reproductive Efficiency of Dairy Animals. *Med. Weter.* **2018**, *74* (6), 356–361.

Farm Animal Welfare Council—5 Freedoms https://webarchive.nationalarchives.gov. uk/20121010012427/http://www.fawc.org.uk/freedoms.htm (accessed Feb 23, 2019).

Feijoo, P., Pesántez, J., Mesías, J., Heras-Molina, A., Sanz, V., Patrón, R., Pérez, N., Vázquez-Gómez, M., Garcia-Contreras, C., Fargas, O., Astiz, S. Ten Years Evolution of Dairy Cattle Herds: Fertility, Production and Management. Book of abstracts, 69th Annual Meeting of the European Federation of Animal Science, Dubrovnik, Croatia, **2018**.

Fetrow, J.; Stewart, S.; Eicker, S.; Rapnicki, P. *Reproductive Health Programs for Dairy Herds: Analysis of Records for Assessment of Reproductive Performance*. In *Current Therapy in Large Animal Theriogenology*; Elsevier, **2007**; pp 473–489.

Flamenbaum, I.; Galon, N. Management of Heat Stress to Improve Fertility in Dairy Cows in Israel. *J. Reprod. Dev.* **2010**, *56 Suppl*, S36–S41.

Fleming, A.; Abdalla, E. A.; Maltecca, C.; Baes, C. F. Invited Review: Reproductive and Genomic Technologies to Optimize Breeding Strategies for Genetic Progress in Dairy Cattle. *Arch. Anim. Breed.* **2018**, *61* (1), 43–57.

Fleming, A.; Baes, C. F.; Martin, A. A. A.; Chud, T. C. S.; Malchiodi, F.; Brito, L. F.; Miglior, F. Symposium Review: The Choice and Collection of New Relevant Phenotypes for Fertility Selection. *J. Dairy Sci.* **2019**.

Foote, R. H. Estrus Detection and Estrus Detection Aids. *J. Dairy Sci.* **1975**, *58* (2), 248–256.

Fourichon, C.; Seegers, H.; Malher, X. Effect of Disease on Reproduction in the Dairy Cow: A Meta-Analysis. *Theriogenology* **2000**, *53* (9), 1729–1759.

Franco, O. J.; Drost, M.; Thatcher, M.-J.; Shille, V. M.; Thatcher, W. W. Fetal Survival in the Cow after Pregnancy Diagnosis by Palpation per Rectum. *Theriogenology* **1987**, *27* (4), 631–644.

Fricke, P. M. Scanning the Future Ultrasonography as a Reproductive Management Tool for Dairy Cattle. *J. Dairy Sci.* **2002**, *85* (8), 1918–1926.

Galvão, K. N.; Sá Filho, M. F.; Santos, J. E. P. Reducing the Interval from Presynchronization to Initiation of Timed Artificial Insemination Improves Fertility in Dairy Cows. *J. Dairy Sci.* **2007**, *90* (9), 4212–4218.

Galvão, K. N.; Santos, J. E. P. Factors Affecting Synchronization and Conception Rate after the Ovsynch Protocol in Lactating Holstein Cows. *Reprod. Domest. Anim.* **2010**, *45* (3), 439–446.

Galvão, K. N.; Federico, P.; De Vries, A.; Schuenemann, G. M. Economic Comparison of Reproductive Programs for Dairy Herds Using Estrus Detection, Timed Artificial Insemination, or a Combination. *J. Dairy Sci.* **2013**, *96* (4), 2681–2693.

Garbarino, E. J.; Hernandez, J. A.; Shearer, J. K.; Risco, C. A.; Thatcher, W. W. Effect of Lameness on Ovarian Activity in Postpartum Holstein Cows. *J. Dairy Sci.* **2004**, *87* (12), 4123–4131.

García-Ispierto, I.; López-Gatius, F.; Santolaria, P.; Yániz, J. L.; Nogareda, C.; López-Béjar, M.; De Rensis, F. Relationship Between Heat Stress During the Peri-Implantation Period and Early Fetal Loss in Dairy Cattle. *Theriogenology* **2006**, *65* (4), 799–807.

Garnsworthy, P. C. Body Condition Score in Dairy Cows: Targets for Production and Fertility. Recent Adv. *Anim. Nutr.* **2007**, *2006* (1), 61–86.

Garnsworthy, P. C.; Sinclair, K. D.; Webb, R. Integration of Physiological Mechanisms that Influence Fertility in Dairy Cows. *Animal* **2008**, *2* (08), 1144–1152.

Gautam, G.; Nakao, T.; Yusuf, M.; Koike, K. Prevalence of Endometritis during the Postpartum Period and Its Impact on Subsequent Reproductive Performance in Two Japanese Dairy Herds. *Anim. Reprod. Sci.* **2009**, *116* (3–4), 175–187.

Gilbert, R. O.; Shin, S. T.; Guard, C. L.; Erb, H. N.; Frajblat, M. Prevalence of Endometritis and its Effects on Reproductive Performance of Dairy Cows. *Theriogenology* **2005**, *64* (9), 1879–1888.

Gobikrushanth, M.; De Vries, A.; Santos, J. E. P.; Risco, C. A.; Galvão, K. N. Effect of Delayed Breeding during the Summer on Profitability of Dairy Cows. *J. Dairy Sci.* **2014**, *97* (7), 4236–4246.

Grimard, B.; Freret, S.; Chevallier, A.; Pinto, A.; Ponsart, C.; Humblot, P. Genetic and Environmental Factors Influencing First Service Conception Rate and Late Embryonic/ Foetal Mortality in Low Fertility Dairy Herds. *Anim. Reprod. Sci.* **2006**, *91* (1), 31–44.

Gröhn, Y. T.; Rajala-Schultz, P. J. Epidemiology of Reproductive Performance in Dairy Cows. *Anim. Reprod. Sci.* **2000**, *60–61*, 605–614.

Gulliksen, S. M.; Lie, K. I.; Løken, T.; Østerås, O. Calf Mortality in Norwegian Dairy Herds. *J. Dairy Sci.* **2009**, *92* (6), 2782–2795.

Hansel, W. Estrous Cycle and Ovulation Control in Cattle1. *J. Dairy Sci.* **1961**, *44* (12), 2307–2314.

Hansen, P. J. Embryonic Mortality in Cattle from the Embryo's Perspective. *J. Anim. Sci.* **2002**, *80* (2), 33–44.

Haskell, M. J.; Rennie, L. J.; Bowell, V. A.; Bell, M. J.; Lawrence, A. B. Housing System, Milk Production, and Zero-Grazing Effects on Lameness and Leg Injury in Dairy Cows. *J. Dairy Sci.* **2006**, *89* (11), 4259–4266.

Helmer, S. D.; Britt, J. H. Mounting Behavior as Affected by Stage of Estrous Cycle in Holstein Heifers1. *J. Dairy Sci.* **1985**, *68* (5), 1290–1296.

Hemsworth, P. H.; Coleman, G. J.; Barnett, J. L.; Borg, S. Relationships Between Human-Animal Interactions and Productivity of Commercial Dairy Cows. *J. Anim. Sci.* **2000**, *78* (11), 2821–2831.

Herlihy, M. M.; Giordano, J. O.; Souza, A. H.; Ayres, H.; Ferreira, R. M.; Keskin, A.; Nascimento, A. B.; Guenther, J. N.; Gaska, J. M.; Kacuba, S. J.; et al. Presynchronization with Double-Ovsynch Improves Fertility at First Postpartum Artificial Insemination in Lactating Dairy Cows. *J. Dairy Sci.* **2012**, *95* (12), 7003–7014.

Hoedemaker, M.; Prange, D.; Gundelach, Y. Body Condition Change Ante- and Postpartum, Health and Reproductive Performance in German Holstein Cows. *Reprod. Domest. Anim.* **2009**, *44* (2), 167–173.

House, H. K.; Anderson, N. G. Maximizing Comfort in Tiestall Housing. *Vet. Clin. North Am. Food Anim. Pract.* **2019**, *35* (1), 77–91.

Huang, C.; Tsuruta, S.; Bertrand, J. K.; Misztal, I.; Lawlor, T. J.; Clay, J. S. Trends for Conception Rate of Holsteins Over Time in the Southeastern United States. *J. Dairy Sci.* **2009**, *92* (9), 4641–4647.

Hurnik, J. F.; King, G. J.; Robertson, H. A. Estrous and Related Behaviour in Postpartum Holstein Cows. *Appl. Anim. Ethol.* **1975**, *2* (1), 55–68.

Huszenicza, G.; Jánosi, S.; Kulcsár, M.; Kóródi, P.; Reiczigel, J.; Kátai, L.; Peters, A. R.; Rensis, F. D. Effects of Clinical Mastitis on Ovarian Function in Post-Partum Dairy Cows. *Reprod. Domest. Anim.* **2005**, *40* (3), 199–204.

Inchaisri, C.; Jorritsma, R.; Vos, P. L. A. M.; van der Weijden, G. C.; Hogeveen, H. Analysis of the Economically Optimal Voluntary Waiting Period for First Insemination. *J. Dairy Sci.* **2011**, *94* (8), 3811–3823.

Kerbrat, S.; Disenhaus, C. A Proposition for an Updated Behavioural Characterisation of the Köck, A.; Miglior, F.; Jamrozik, J.; Kelton, D. F.; Schenkel, F. S. *Genetic Relationships of Fertility Disorders with Reproductive Traits in Canadian Holsteins*; Vancouver, BC, Canada, **2014**; pp 17–22.

Konggaard, S. P. Comparison Between Conventional Tie-Barn and Loose Housing Systems with Respect to Milk Production, Feed Conversion and Reproductive Performance of Dairy Cows. *Livest. Prod. Sci.* **1977**, *4* (1), 69–77.

Labèrnia, J.; López-Gatius, F.; Santolaria, P.; López-Béjar, M.; Rutllant, J. Influence of Management Factors on Pregnancy Attrition in Dairy Cattle. *Theriogenology* **1996**, *45* (6), 1247–1253.

LeBlanc, S. J. Reproductive Tract Inflammatory Disease in Postpartum Dairy Cows. Anim. Int. *J. Anim. Biosci.* **2014**, *8* Suppl 1, 54–63.

Legrand, A.; Schütz, K. E.; Tucker, C. B. Using Water to Cool Cattle: Behavioral and Physiological Changes Associated with Voluntary Use of Cow Showers. *J. Dairy Sci.* **2011**, *94* (7), 3376–3386.

Lopes, G.; Giordano, J. O.; Valenza, A.; Herlihy, M. M.; Guenther, J. N.; Wiltbank, M. C.; Fricke, P. M. Effect of Timing of Initiation of Resynchronization and Presynchronization with Gonadotropin-Releasing Hormone on Fertility of Resynchronized Inseminations in Lactating Dairy Cows. *J. Dairy Sci.* **2013**, *96* (6), 3788–3798.

López-Gatius, F.; Santolaria, P.; Yániz, J.; Rutllant, J.; López-Béjar, M. Factors Affecting Pregnancy Loss from Gestation Day 38 to 90 in Lactating Dairy Cows from a Single Herd. *Theriogenology* **2002**, *57* (4), 1251–1261.

López-Gatius, F.; Yániz, J.; Madriles-Helm, D. Effects of Body Condition Score and Score Change on the Reproductive Performance of Dairy Cows: A Meta-Analysis. *Theriogenology* **2003**, *59* (3), 801–812.

López-Gatius, F. Factors of a Noninfectious Nature Affecting Fertility after Artificial Insemination in Lactating Dairy Cows. A Review. *Theriogenology* **2012**, *77* (6), 1029–1041.

López-Helguera, I.; López-Gatius, F.; Garcia-Ispierto, I. The Influence of Genital Tract Status in Postpartum Period on the Subsequent Reproductive Performance in High Producing Dairy Cows. *Theriogenology* **2012**, *77* (7), 1334–1342.

Lucy, M. C. Reproductive Loss in High-Producing Dairy Cattle: Where Will It End? *J. Dairy Sci.* **2001**, *84* (6), 1277–1293.

Macmillan, K. L.; Thatcher, W. W. Effects of an Agonist of Gonadotropin-Releasing Hormone on Ovarian Follicles in Cattle. *Biol. Reprod.* **1991**, *45* (6), 883–889.

Macmillan, K. L.; Burke, C. R. Effects of Oestrous Cycle Control on Reproductive Efficiency. *Anim. Reprod. Sci.* **1996**, *42* (1), 307–320.

Macmillan, K.; Loree, K.; Mapletoft, R. J.; Colazo, M. G. Short Communication: Optimization of a Timed Artificial Insemination Program for Reproductive Management of Heifers in Canadian Dairy Herds. *J. Dairy Sci.* **2017**, *100* (5), 4134–4138.

Mandel, R.; Whay, H. R.; Klement, E.; Nicol, C. J. Invited Review: Environmental Enrichment of Dairy Cows and Calves in Indoor Housing. *J. Dairy Sci.* **2016**, *99* (3), 1695–1715.

March, M. D.; Haskell, M. J.; Chagunda, M. G. G.; Langford, F. M.; Roberts, D. J. Current Trends in British Dairy Management Regimens. *J. Dairy Sci.* **2014**, *97* (12), 7985–7994.

McInerney, P. J. Animal Welfare, Economics and Policy. *Anim. Welf.* **2004**, 80.

McParland, S.; Kennedy, E.; Lewis, E.; Moore, S. G.; McCarthy, B.; O'Donovan, M.; Berry, D. P. Genetic Parameters of Dairy Cow Energy Intake and Body Energy Status Predicted Using Mid-Infrared Spectrometry of Milk. *J. Dairy Sci.* **2015**, *98* (2), 1310–1320.

Meikle, A.; Kulcsar, M.; Chilliard, Y.; Febel, H.; Delavaud, C.; Cavestany, D.; Chilibroste, P. Effects of Parity and Body Condition at Parturition on Endocrine and Reproductive Parameters of the Cow. *Reproduction* **2004**, *127* (6), 727–737.

Mellado, M.; Lopez, E.; Veliz, F. G.; De Santiago, M. A.; Macias-Cruz, U.; Avendaño-Reyes, L.; Garcia, J. E. Factors Associated with Neonatal Dairy Calf Mortality in a Hot-Arid Environment. *Livest. Sci.* **2014**, *159*, 149–155.

Miglior, F.; Muir, B. L.; Van Doormaal, B. J. Selection Indices in Holstein Cattle of Various Countries. *J. Dairy Sci.* **2005**, *88* (3), 1255–1263.

Miglior, F.; Fleming, A.; Malchiodi, F.; Brito, L. F.; Martin, P.; Baes, C. F. A 100-Year Review: Identification and Genetic Selection of Economically Important Traits in Dairy Cattle. *J. Dairy Sci.* **2017**, *100* (12), 10251–10271.

Miller, K.; Wood-Gush, D. G. M. Some Effects of Housing on the Social Behaviour of Dairy Cows. *Anim. Sci.* **1991**, *53* (3), 271–278.

Moberg, G. P. *Influence of Stress on Reproduction: Measure of Well-Being*. In *Animal Stress*; Moberg, G. P., Ed.; Springer New York: New York, NY, 1985; pp 245–267.

Mondaca, M. R. Ventilation Systems for Adult Dairy Cattle. *Vet. Clin. North Am. Food Anim. Pract.* **2019**, *35* (1), 139–156.

Moore, K.; Thatcher, W. W. Major Advances Associated with Reproduction in Dairy Cattle. *J. Dairy Sci.* **2006**, *89* (4), 1254–1266.

Moreira, F.; de la Sota, R. L.; Diaz, T.; Thatcher, W. W. Effect of Day of the Estrous Cycle at the Initiation of a Timed Artificial Insemination Protocol on Reproductive Responses in Dairy Heifers. *J. Anim. Sci.* **2000**, *78* (6), 1568–1576.

Morgan, K. N.; Tromborg, C. T. Sources of Stress in Captivity. *Appl. Anim. Behav. Sci.* **2007**, *102* (3–4), 262–302.

Müller, M.-P.; Rothammer, S.; Seichter, D.; Russ, I.; Hinrichs, D.; Tetens, J.; Thaller, G.; Medugorac, I. Genome-Wide Mapping of 10 Calving and Fertility Traits in Holstein Dairy Cattle with Special Regard to Chromosome 18. *J. Dairy Sci.* **2017**, *100* (3), 1987–2006.

National Animal Health Monitoring Service (NAHMS). Reproduction Practices on U.S. Dairy Operations, 2007 https://www.aphis.usda.gov/animal_health/nahms/dairy/downloads/dairy07/Dairy07_is_ReprodPrac.pdf (accessed Dec 15, 2018).

National Genetic Evaluations Info-Interbull Centre http://www.interbull.org/ib/geforms (accessed Feb 22, 2019).

National Milk Producers Federation (NMPF) Centennial Booklet https://issuu.com/nmpf01/docs/nmpf_2015_centennial_booklet_68 (accessed Dec 15, 2018).

Newberry, R. C. Environmental Enrichment: Increasing the Biological Relevance of Captive Environments. Appl. *Anim. Behav. Sci.* **1995,** *44* (2), 229–243.

Niozas, G.; Tsousis, G.; Steinhöfel, I.; Brozos, C.; Römer, A.; Wiedemann, S.; Bollwein, H.; Kaske, M. Extended Lactation in High-Yielding Dairy Cows. I. Effects on Reproductive Measurements. *J. Dairy Sci.* **2019,** *102* (1), 799–810.

Norman, H. D.; Wright, J. R.; Hubbard, S. M.; Miller, R. H.; Hutchison, J. L. Reproductive Status of Holstein and Jersey Cows in the United States. *J. Dairy Sci.* **2009,** *92* (7), 3517–3528.

Palmer, M. A.; Olmos, G.; Boyle, L. A.; Mee, J. F. Estrus Detection and Estrus Characteristics in Housed and Pastured Holstein–Friesian Cows. *Theriogenology* **2010,** *74* (2), 255–264.

Pancarci, S. M.; Jordan, E. R.; Risco, C. A.; Schouten, M. J.; Lopes, F. L.; Moreira, F.; Thatcher, W. W. Use of Estradiol Cypionate in a Presynchronized Timed Artificial Insemination Program for Lactating Dairy Cattle. *J. Dairy Sci.* **2002,** *85* (1), 122–131.

Parker Gaddis, K. L.; Dikmen, S.; Null, D. J.; Cole, J. B.; Hansen, P. J. Evaluation of Genetic Components in Traits Related to Superovulation, *in Vitro* Fertilization, and Embryo Transfer in Holstein Cattle. *J. Dairy Sci.* **2017,** *100* (4), 2877–2891.

Patron, R.; López-Helguera, I.; Sebastián, F.; Pesantez-Pacheco, J. L.; Pérez-Villalobos, N.; Vicente González Martín, J.; Fargas, O.; Astiz, S. Influence of Practitioner Expertise during Early Pregnancy Diagnosis on Pregnancy Loss Rate: A Controlled, Blinded Trial. *Reprod. Domest. Anim. Zuchthyg.* **2017,** *52* (6), 1145–1148.

Patron-Collantes, R.; Lopez-Helguera, I.; Pesantez-Pacheco, J. L.; Sebastian, F.; Fernández, M.; Fargas, O.; Astiz, S. Early Postpartum Administration of Equine Chorionic Gonadotropin to Dairy Cows Calved during the Hot Season: Effects on Fertility after First Artificial Insemination. *Theriogenology* **2017,** *92*, 83–89.

Patron, R.; Lopez-Helguera, I.; Pesantez-Pacheco, J. L.; Perez-Villalobos, N.; Heras, J.; Vicente Gonzalez, J.; Fargas, O.; Astiz, S. Resynchronization with the G6G Protocol: A Retrospective, Observational Study of Second and Later Timed Artificial Inseminations on Commercial Dairy Farms. *Reprod. Domest. Anim. Zuchthyg.* **2018.**

Pereira, M. H. C.; Rodrigues, A. D. P.; Martins, T.; Oliveira, W. V. C.; Silveira, P. S. A.; Wiltbank, M. C.; Vasconcelos, J. L. M. Timed Artificial Insemination Programs during the Summer in Lactating Dairy Cows: Comparison of the 5-d Cosynch Protocol with an Estrogen/Progesterone-Based Protocol. *J. Dairy Sci.* **2013,** *96* (11), 6904–6914.

Peters, M. W.; Pursley, J. R. Fertility of Lactating Dairy Cows Treated with Ovsynch after Presynchronization Injections of PGF$_2\alpha$ and GnRH. *J. Dairy Sci.* **2002,** *85* (9), 2403–2406.

Plunkett, S. S.; Stevenson, J. S.; Call, E. P. Prostaglandin F$_2$ Alpha for Lactating Dairy Cows with a Palpable Corpus Luteum but Unobserved Estrus. *J. Dairy Sci.* **1984,** *67* (2), 380–387.

Polsky, L.; von Keyserlingk, M. A. G. Invited Review: Effects of Heat Stress on Dairy Cattle Welfare. *J. Dairy Sci.* **2017,** *100* (11), 8645–8657.

Progressive Dairy Operators (POD). Dairy Labour and Milking System Survey, Ontario, Canada, **2016.**

Proudfoot, K. L.; Jensen, M. B.; Weary, D. M.; von Keyserlingk, M. A. G. Dairy Cows Seek Isolation at Calving and When Ill. *J. Dairy Sci.* **2014,** *97* (5), 2731–2739.

Pryce, J. E.; Coffey, M. P.; Simm, G. The Relationship Between Body Condition Score and Reproductive Performance. *J. Dairy Sci.* **2001,** *84* (6), 1508–1515.

Pursley, J. R.; Mee, M. O.; Wiltbank, M. C. Synchronization of Ovulation in Dairy Cows Using PGF$_2\alpha$ and Gnrh. *Theriogenology* **1995**, *44* (7), 915–923.

Pursley, J. R.; Kosorok, M. R.; Wiltbank, M. C. Reproductive Management of Lactating Dairy Cows Using Synchronization of Ovulation. *J. Dairy Sci.* **1997a**, *80* (2), 301–306.

Pursley, J. R.; Wiltbank, M. C.; Stevenson, J. S.; Ottobre, J. S.; Garverick, H. A.; Anderson, L. L. Pregnancy Rates per Artificial Insemination for Cows and Heifers Inseminated at a Synchronized Ovulation or Synchronized Estrus. *J. Dairy Sci.* **1997b**, *80* (2), 295–300.

R.C. Newberry. The Space-Time Continuum, and its Relevance to Farm Animals. *Etología* **1993**, *3*, 219–234.

Reith, S.; Hoy, S. Review: Behavioral Signs of Estrus and the Potential of Fully Automated Systems for Detection of Estrus in Dairy Cattle. *Animal* **2018**, *12* (02), 398–407.

Renaudeau, D.; Collin, A.; Yahav, S.; Basilio, V. de; Gourdine, J. L.; Collier, R. J. Adaptation to Hot Climate and Strategies to Alleviate Heat Stress in Livestock Production. *Animal* **2012**, *6* (5), 707–728.

Rensis, F. D.; Scaramuzzi, R. J. Heat Stress and Seasonal Effects on Reproduction in the Dairy Cow—a Review. *Theriogenology* **2003**, *60* (6), 1139–1151.

Roelofs, J. B.; van Eerdenburg, F. J. C. M.; Soede, N. M.; Kemp, B. Various Behavioral Signs of Estrous and Their Relationship with Time of Ovulation in Dairy Cattle. *Theriogenology* **2005**, *63* (5), 1366–1377.

Roelofs, J.; López-Gatius, F.; Hunter, R. H. F.; van Eerdenburg, F. J. C. M.; Hanzen, C. When is a Cow in Estrus? Clinical and Practical Aspects. *Theriogenology* **2010**, *74* (3), 327–344.

Roman-Ponce, H.; Thatcher, W. W.; Buffington, D. E.; Wilcox, C. J.; Van Horn, H. H. Physiological and Production Responses of Dairy Cattle to a Shade Structure in a Subtropical Environment. *J. Dairy Sci.* **1977**, *60* (3), 424–430.

Rutigliano, H. M.; Lima, F. S.; Cerri, R. L. A.; Greco, L. F.; Vilela, J. M.; Magalhães, V.; Silvestre, F. T.; Thatcher, W. W.; Santos, J. E. P. Effects of Method of Presynchronization and Source of Selenium on Uterine Health and Reproduction in Dairy Cows. *J. Dairy Sci.* **2008**, *91* (9), 3323–3336.

Santos, J. E. P.; Thatcher, W. W.; Chebel, R. C.; Cerri, R. L. A.; Galvão, K. N. The Effect of Embryonic Death Rates in Cattle on the Efficacy of Estrus Synchronization Programs. *Anim. Reprod. Sci.* **2004**, *82–83*, 513–535.

Santos, J. E. P.; Narciso, C. D.; Rivera, F.; Thatcher, W. W.; Chebel, R. C. Effect of Reducing the Period of Follicle Dominance in a Timed Artificial Insemination Protocol on Reproduction of Dairy Cows. *J. Dairy Sci.* **2010**, *93* (7), 2976–2988.

Sanz, A.; Macmillan, K.; Colazo, M. G. Revisión de Los Programas de Sincronización Ovárica Basados En El Uso de GnRH y Prostaglandina F$_2\alpha$ Para Novillas de Leche y de Carne. ITEA-Inf. Tec. Econ. Agrar. 2019. *115*(4), 326-341.

Sartori, R.; Sartor-Bergfelt, R.; Mertens, S. A.; Guenther, J. N.; Parrish, J. J.; Wiltbank, M. C. Fertilization and Early Embryonic Development in Heifers and Lactating Cows in Summer and Lactating and Dry Cows in Winter. *J. Dairy Sci.* **2002**, *85* (11), 2803–2812.

Schär, C.; Vidale, P. L.; Lüthi, D.; Frei, C.; Häberli, C.; Liniger, M. A.; Appenzeller, C. The Role of Increasing Temperature Variability in European Summer Heatwaves. *Nature* **2004**, *427* (6972), 332–336.

Schirmann, K.; Chapinal, N.; Weary, D. M.; Heuwieser, W.; von Keyserlingk, M. A. G. Short-Term Effects of Regrouping on Behavior of Prepartum Dairy Cows. *J. Dairy Sci.* **2011**, *94* (5), 2312–2319.

Schmitt, E. J.; Diaz, T.; Drost, M.; Thatcher, W. W. Use of a Gonadotropin-Releasing Hormone Agonist or Human Chorionic Gonadotropin for Timed Insemination in Cattle. *J. Anim. Sci.* **1996,** *74* (5), 1084.

Schütz, K. E.; Cox, N. R.; Matthews, L. R. How Important is Shade to Dairy Cattle? Choice Between Shade or Lying Following Different Levels of Lying Deprivation. *Appl. Anim. Behav. Sci.* **2008,** *114* (3), 307–318.

Schütz, K.; Clark, K.; Cox, N.; Matthews, L.; Tucker, C. Responses to Short-Term Exposure to Simulated Rain and Wind by Dairy Cattle: Time Budgets, Shelter Use, Body Temperature and Feed Intake. *Anim. Welf.* **2010,** 9.

Scientific Report on the Effects of Farming Systems on Dairy Cow Welfare and Disease1—Research—AarhusUniversityhttp://pure.au.dk/portal/en/persons/lene-munksgaard(520c323f-66f6-4db8-a49e-df802e406bb3)/publications/scientific-report-on-the-effects-of-farming-systems-on-dairy-cow-welfare-and-disease1(6b2dcef0-ff59-11de-8775-000ea68e967b)/export.html (accessed Mar 16, 2019).

Seppä-Lassila, L.; Sarjokari, K.; Hovinen, M.; Soveri, T.; Norring, M. Management Factors Associated with Mortality of Dairy Calves in Finland: A Cross Sectional Study. *Vet. J.* **2016,** *216,* 164–167.

Shanks, R. D.; Freeman, A. E.; Berger, P. J.; Kelley, D. H. Effect of Selection for Milk Production and General Health of the Dairy Cow. *J. Dairy Sci.* **1978,** *61* (12), 1765–1772.

Sheldon, I. M. The Postpartum Uterus. *Vet. Clin. North Am. Food Anim. Pract.* **2004,** *20* (3), 569–591.

Sheldon, I. M.; Cronin, J.; Goetze, L.; Donofrio, G.; Schuberth, H. J. Defining Postpartum Uterine Disease and the Mechanisms of Infection and Immunity in the Female Reproductive Tract in Cattle. *Biol. Reprod.* **2009,** *81* (6), 1025–1032.

Shook, G. E. Selection for Disease Resistance. *J. Dairy Sci.* **1989,** *72* (5), 1349–1362.

Siciliano-Jones, J. L.; Socha, M. T.; Tomlinson, D. J.; DeFrain, J. M. Effect of Trace Mineral Source on Lactation Performance, Claw Integrity, and Fertility of Dairy Cattle. *J. Dairy Sci.* **2008,** *91* (5), 1985–1995.

Somers, J. G. C. J. Claw Disorders and Disturbed Locomotion in Dairy Cows: The Effect of Floor Systems and Implications for Animal Welfare. Dissertation, 2004.

Sood, P.; Nanda, A. S. Effect of Lameness on Estrous Behavior in Crossbred Cows. *Theriogenology* **2006,** *66* (5), 1375–1380.

Souza, A. H.; Ayres, H.; Ferreira, R. M.; Wiltbank, M. C. A New Presynchronization System (Double-Ovsynch) Increases Fertility at First Postpartum Timed AI in Lactating Dairy Cows. *Theriogenology* **2008,** *70* (2), 208–215.

Souza, F.; Carneiro, L. C.; Cesar, J.; dos Santos, R. M. Non-Infectious Causes That Increase Early and Mid-to-Late Pregnancy Loss Rates in a Crossbreed Dairy Herd. *Trop. Anim. Health Prod.* **2018.**

Squires, E. J. *Applied Animal Endocrinology*, 2nd ed.; CABI, 2010.

Stangaferro, M. L.; Wijma, R.; Masello, M.; Thomas, M. J.; Giordano, J. O. Extending the Duration of the Voluntary Waiting Period from 60 to 88 Days in Cows That Received Timed Artificial Insemination after the Double-Ovsynch Protocol Affected the Reproductive Performance, Herd Exit Dynamics, and Lactation Performance of Dairy Cows. *J. Dairy Sci.* **2018,** *101* (1), 717–735.

Stevenson, J. S.; Call, E. P. Fertility of Postpartum Dairy Cows after Administration of Gonadotropin-Releasing Hormone and Prostaglandin F_2: A Field Trial. *J. Dairy Sci.* **1988,** *71* (7), 8.

Stevenson, J. S.; Smith, M. W.; Jaeger, J. R.; Corah, L. R.; LeFever, D. G. Detection of Estrus by Visual Observation and Radiotelemetry in Peripubertal, Estrus-Synchronized Beef Heifers. *J. Anim. Sci.* **1996,** *74* (4), 729–735.

Stevenson, J. S.; Pulley, S. L. Pregnancy per Artificial Insemination after Presynchronizing Estrous Cycles with the Presynch-10 Protocol or Prostaglandin $F_2\alpha$ Injection Followed by Gonadotropin-Releasing Hormone before Ovsynch-56 in 4 Dairy Herds of Lactating Dairy Cows. *J. Dairy Sci.* **2012,** *95* (11), 6513–6522.

Stevenson, J. S.; Pulley, S. L.; Mellieon, H. I. Prostaglandin $F_2\alpha$ and Gonadotropin-Releasing Hormone Administration Improve Progesterone Status, Luteal Number, and Proportion of Ovular and Anovular Dairy Cows with Corpora Lutea before a Timed Artificial Insemination Program. *J. Dairy Sci.* **2012,** *95* (4), 1831–1844.

Stevenson, J. S. Synchronization and Artificial Insemination Strategies in Dairy Herds. *Vet. Clin. North Am. Food Anim. Pract.* **2016,** *32* (2), 349–364.

Stevenson, J. S.; Britt, J. H. A 100-Year Review: Practical Female Reproductive Management. *J. Dairy Sci.* **2017,** *100* (12), 10292–10313.

Taylor, V. J.; Beever, D. E.; Bryant, M. J.; Wathes, D. C. Metabolic Profiles and Progesterone Cycles in First Lactation Dairy Cows. *Theriogenology* **2003,** *59* (7), 1661–1677.

Tenhagen, B. A.; Vogel, C.; Drillich, M.; Thiele, G.; Heuwieser, W. Influence of Stage of Lactation and Milk Production on Conception Rates after Timed Artificial Insemination Following Ovsynch. *Theriogenology* **2003,** *60* (8), 1527–1537.

Thatcher, W.; de la Sota, R. L.; Schmitt, E.; Diaz, T.; Badinga, L.; Simmen, F.; Staples, C.; Drost, M. Control and Management of Ovarian Follicles in Cattle to Optimize Fertility. *Reprod. Fertil. Dev.* **1996,** *8* (2), 203.

Thatcher, W. W. A 100-Year Review: Historical Development of Female Reproductive Physiology in Dairy Cattle. *J. Dairy Sci.* **2017,** *100* (12), 10272–10291.

Tilbrook, A. J.; Turner, A. I.; Clarke, I. J. Effects of Stress on Reproduction in Non-Rodent Mammals: The Role of Glucocorticoids and Sex Differences. *Rev. Reprod.* **2000,** *5* (2), 105–113.

Tsai, S. J.; Wiltbank, M. C. Prostaglandin $F_2\alpha$ Regulates Distinct Physiological Changes in Early and Mid-Cycle Bovine Corpora Lutea. *Biol. Reprod.* **1998,** *58* (2), 346–352.

Ulberg, L. C.; Christian, R. E.; Casida, L. E. Ovarian Response in Heifers to Progesterone Injections. *J Anim Sci.* **1951,** *10*, 752–759.

USDA ERS—Dairy Data https://www.ers.usda.gov/data-products/dairy-data/ (accessed Mar 30, 2019).

Vaillancourt, D.; Bierschwal, C. J.; Ogwu, D.; Elmore, R. G.; Martin, C. E.; Sharp, A. J.; Youngquist, R. S. Correlation Between Pregnancy Diagnosis by Membrane Slip and Embryonic Mortality. *J. Am. Vet. Med. Assoc.* **1979,** *175* (5), 466–468.

Van Arendonk, J. A.; Liinamo, A. E. Dairy Cattle Production in Europe. *Theriogenology* **2003,** *59* (2), 563–569.

Van der Leek, M. L. Beyond Traditional Dairy Veterinary Services: 'It's Not Just about the Cows!' *J. S. Afr. Vet. Assoc.* **2015,** *86* (1).

Van Os, J. M. C. Considerations for Cooling Dairy Cows with Water. *Vet. Clin. North Am. Food Anim. Pract.* **2019,** *35* (1), 157–173.

Van Vliet, J. H.; Van Eerdenburg, F. J. C. M. Sexual Activities and Oestrus Detection in Lactating Holstein Cows. *Appl. Anim. Behav. Sci.* **1996,** *50* (1), 57–69.

Van Vuuren, A. M.; Van Den Pol-Van Dasselaar, A. Grazing Systems and Feed Supplementation. In *Fresh Herbage for Dairy Cattle*; Elgersma, A., Dijkstra, J., Tamminga, S., Eds.; Springer Netherlands: Dordrecht, 2006; Vol. 18, pp 85–101.

VanRaden, P. M.; Sanders, A. H.; Tooker, M. E.; Miller, R. H.; Norman, H. D.; Kuhn, M. T.; Wiggans, G. R. Development of a National Genetic Evaluation for Cow Fertility. *J. Dairy Sci.* **2004,** *87* (7), 2285–2292.

VanRaden, P. M.; Tooker, M. E.; O'Connell, J. R.; Cole, J. B.; Bickhart, D. M. Selecting Sequence Variants to Improve Genomic Predictions for Dairy Cattle. *Genet. Sel. Evol. GSE* **2017,** *49* (1), 32–32.

Vanroose, G.; de Kruif, A.; Van Soom, A. Embryonic Mortality and Embryo–Pathogen Interactions. *Anim. Reprod. Sci.* **2000,** *60–61,* 131–143.

Vasconcelos, J. L. M.; Silcox, R. W.; Lacerda, J. A.; Pursley, J. R.; Wiltbank, M. C. Pregnancy Rate, Pregnancy Loss, and Response to Head Stress after AI at 2 Different Times from Ovulation in Dairy Cows. *Biol. Reprod.* **1997,** 230–230.

Vasconcelos, J. L. M.; Silcox, R. W.; Rosa, G. J. M.; Pursley, J. R.; Wiltbank, M. C. Synchronization Rate, Size of the Ovulatory Follicle, and Pregnancy Rate after Synchronization of Ovulation Beginning on Different Days of the Estrous Cycle in Lactating Dairy Cows. *Theriogenology* **1999,** *52* (6), 1067–1078.

Von Borell, E.; Dobson, H.; Prunier, A. Stress, Behaviour and Reproductive Performance in Female Cattle and Pigs. *Horm. Behav.* **2007,** *52* (1), 130–138.

Von Keyserlingk, M. a. G.; Olenick, D.; Weary, D. M. Acute Behavioral Effects of Regrouping Dairy Cows. *J. Dairy Sci.* **2008,** *91* (3), 1011–1016.

Von Keyserlingk, M. A. G.; Weary, D. M. A 100-Year Review: Animal Welfare in the Journal of Dairy Science-The First 100 Years. *J. Dairy Sci.* **2017,** *100* (12), 10432–10444.

Wall, E.; Brotherstone, S.; Woolliams, J. A.; Banos, G.; Coffey, M. P. Genetic Evaluation of Fertility Using Direct and Correlated Traits. *J. Dairy Sci.* **2003,** *86* (12), 4093–4102.

Wathes, D. C.; Fenwick, M.; Cheng, Z.; Bourne, N.; Llewellyn, S.; Morris, D. G.; Kenny, D.; Murphy, J.; Fitzpatrick, R. Influence of Negative Energy Balance on Cyclicity and Fertility in the High Producing Dairy Cow. *Theriogenology* **2007,** *68,* S232–S241.

Weigel, K. A. Prospects for Improving Reproductive Performance through Genetic Selection. *Anim. Reprod. Sci.* **2006,** *96* (3–4), 323–330.

Welfare Quality Network. Assessment Protocols http://www.welfarequalitynetwork.net/en-us/reports/assessment-protocols/ (accessed Feb 23, 2019).

Weller, J. I. Genetic Analysis of Fertility Traits in Israeli Dairy Cattle. *J. Dairy Sci.* **1989,** *72* (10), 2644–2650.

Wells, D. L. Sensory Stimulation as Environmental Enrichment for Captive Animals: A Review. *Appl. Anim. Behav. Sci.* **2009,** *118* (1–2), 1–11.

West, J. W. Effects of Heat-Stress on Production in Dairy Cattle. *J. Dairy Sci.* **2003,** *86* (6), 2131–2144.

White, M. E.; Lafaunce, N.; Mohammed, H. O. Calving Outcomes for Cows Diagnosed Pregnant or Nonpregnant by Per Rectum Examination at Various Intervals after Insemination. *Can. Vet. J. Rev. Veterinaire Can.* **1989,** *30* (11), 867–870.

Whitfield, L. Fertility in the Face of Stress in Dairy Cattle. *Livestock* **2017,** *22* (3), 118–122.

Wijma, R.; Stangaferro, M. L.; Masello, M.; Granados, G. E.; Giordano, J. O. Resynchronization of Ovulation Protocols for Dairy Cows Including or Not Including Gonadotropin-Releasing Hormone to Induce a New Follicular Wave: Effects on Re-Insemination Pattern, Ovarian Responses, and Pregnancy Outcomes. *J. Dairy Sci.* **2017,** *100* (9), 7613–7625.

Wilson, D. J.; Mallory, D. A.; Busch, D. C.; Leitman, N. R.; Haden, J. K.; Schafer, D. J.; Ellersieck, M. R.; Smith, M. F.; Patterson, D. J. Comparison of Short-Term Progestin-Based Protocols to Synchronize Estrus and Ovulation in Postpartum Beef Cows. *J. Anim. Sci.* **2010,** *88* (6), 2045–2054.

Winsten, J. R.; Kerchner, C. D.; Richardson, A.; Lichau, A.; Hyman, J. M. Trends in the Northeast Dairy Industry: Large-Scale Modern Confinement Feeding and Management-Intensive Grazing. *J. Dairy Sci.* **2010,** *93* (4), 1759–1769.

Wu, G.; Bazer, F. W.; Wallace, J. M.; Spencer, T. E. Intrauterine Growth Retardation: Implications for the Animal Sciences. *J. Anim. Sci.* **2006,** *84* (9), 2316–2337.

Yousuf, M. R.; Martins, J. P. N.; Ahmad, N.; Nobis, K.; Pursley, J. R. Presynchronization of Lactating Dairy Cows with PGF$_2\alpha$ and GnRH Simultaneously, 7 Days before Ovsynch have Similar Outcomes Compared to G6G. *Theriogenology* **2016,** *86* (6), 1607–1614.

Zeron, Y.; Ocheretny, A.; Kedar, O.; Borochov, A.; Sklan, D.; Arav, A. Seasonal Changes in Bovine Fertility: Relation to Developmental Competence of Oocytes, Membrane Properties and Fatty Acid Composition of Follicles. *Reprod. Camb. Engl.* **2001,** *121* (3), 447–454.

CHAPTER 6

Ovum Pick-Up (OPU) in Cattle: An Update

SALVADOR RUIZ LÓPEZ

Department of Physiology, Faculty of Veterinary Science, International Excellence Campus for Higher Education and Research "Campus Mare Nostrum", University of Murcia, Murcia, Spain

Institute for Biomedical Research of Murcia (IMIB-Arrixaca), Murcia, Spain

E-mail: sruiz@um.es

ABSTRACT

The technique of ultrasound-guided transvaginal follicular aspiration for ovum pick-up (OPU) is a non-invasive procedure for recovering oocytes from antral follicles in live animals, especially in cows and mares. It was originally developed for assisted reproduction in the human species to assist infertility and was used for the first time in cattle in the Netherlands at the end of the decade of the 1980s. OPU does not interfere with the normal reproduction and production cycles of the donor and can be used in adult cows in various physiological states, in old animals with reproductive disorders of non-genetic origin and calves and heifers from 6 months of age. The repeated recovery of oocytes through OPU allows us to obtain the highest possible offspring of animals with high genetic value and speed up processes of animal selection and genetic improvement, while it is an extraordinary source of oocytes for cloning and transgenesis. It has been shown to be a feasible and practical alternative to the MOET (Multiple Ovulation and Embryo Transfer) program and it is being more and more used for commercial applications in the world. However, we must bear in mind that the implementation of an OPU program always requires the support of a specialized laboratory for embryo production.

The aim of this chapter is to describe the most important aspects of the OPU procedure used in cattle considering its historical development, the actual situation of OPU worldwide, the OPU equipment and procedure, technical and biological factors influencing OPU results, other uses of OPU, potential risks and most common sequelae, a brief review about OPU in buffaloes, and finally some considerations about the future of OPU/IVEP (*in vitro* embryo production).

6.1 INTRODUCTION

The association of reproductive efficiency and genetic selection is strategic for the success of dairy and beef industries. Reproductive technologies, such as ovum pick-up (OPU) and *in vitro* embryo production (IVEP), can rapidly enhance genetics of cattle through both female and male linaje (Watabane et al., 2017).

Puncture and aspiration of bovine ovarian follicles have been used for several decades to retrieve oocytes for IVEP. *Cumulus* oocyte complexes (COCs) can be recovered from the ovaries of both slaughtered cows or living donors. The method of oocyte retrieval has an impact on COC morphology, and the importance of "good" quality oocytes as the primary pre-requisite for success in oocyte maturation and *in vitro* development has been considered (Merton et al., 2003). From a practical reproductive perspective, aspiration of immature follicles is particularly interesting when performed on living donors, because the procedure can be repeated, and is highly repeatable (Bols and Stout, 2018). Effectively, one of the fundamental conditions for successful commercial IVEP is the development of an efficient system that allows the recovery of oocytes of living donors of known genetic value that can be used several times with minimal consequences for the animals (Da Silva et al., 2016). The repeated recovery of oocytes through OPU allows to obtain the highest possible offspring of animals with high genetic value and speed up processes of animal selection and genetic improvement (paternal and maternal way), while it is an extraordinary source of oocytes for cloning and transgenesis (Ding et al., 2008).

The technique of ultrasound-guided transvaginal follicular aspiration for OPU is a non-invasive procedure for recovering oocytes from antral follicles in live animals, especially in cows and mares. It was originally developed for assisted reproduction in the human species to assist infertility (Lenz and Lauritsen, 1982), and was used for the first time in cattle in the

Netherlands at the end of the decade of the 80s (Pieterse et al., 1988). The use of OPU routinely in veterinary assisted reproduction began in 1994 (Kruip et al., 1994).

Unlike conventional Multiple Ovulation and Embryo Transfer (MOET), OPU does not interfere with the normal reproduction and production cycles of the donor. It is a technique that can be used in adult cows in various physiological states (cyclical, non-cyclic, in the first third of gestation and in which they do not respond to hormonal stimuli), in old animals with reproductive disorders of non-genetic origin (Galli et al., 2001), in calves and heifers from 6 months (mo) of age (Taneja et al., 2000), and even soon, animals after calving (2–3 weeks) could be a suitable donor. It has been shown to be a feasible and practical alternative to the MOET program (Bousquet et al., 1999), and it is being more and more used for commercial applications in the world (Pontes et al., 2011). However, we must bear in mind that the implementation of an OPU program always requires the support of a specialized laboratory for an embryo production. Moreover, because of the economic value of the calves born, adequate veterinary assistance is recommended to minimize losses owing to the possible incidence of the large offspring syndrome (LOS) or other common perinatal pathologies (Galli et al., 2014).

Altogether, the cost of producing an embryo by OPU in dairy cows in Europe could be 50–100% greater than by MOET. This greater cost and the current breeding context in Europe allow for the use of OPU for a very specialized niche market. Different conditions in other countries offer different opportunities also dictated by economics: for example, the large use in Brazil is certainly determined by the fact that OPU in general works better and it is more cost effective than superovulation in *Bos indicus* beef donors (Galli et al., 2014).

The aim of this chapter is to describe the most important aspects of the OPU procedure used in cattle considering its historical development, actual situation of OPU worldwide, the OPU equipment and procedure, technical and biological factors influencing OPU results, other uses of OPU, potential risks and most common sequelae, a brief review about OPU in buffaloes, and finally some considerations about the future of OPU/IVEP.

6.2 HISTORICAL DEVELOPMENT

The first developed *in vivo* oocyte retrieval procedure was laparotomy that provides full access to the abdominal cavity for the direct manipulation of the internal organs. Despite easy access to the ovaries, all surgery risks were present, like anesthesia, contamination, and problems performing the same procedure several times. Other possibilities were also considered in the past, including colpotomy, small incision in the vagina fornix, with usual risks of surgical procedure and clear limitations, and laparoscopy, via either the transvaginal or paralumbar approach, comparatively less invasive method; however, despite its promising prospects, many articles described technical difficulties in addition to the occurrence of fibroids and ovarian adhesions (reviewed by Da Silva et al., 2016).

All of the oocyte recovery-related challenges in cattle were considered in a new prospective analysis of its successful in women. Effectively, most of the new methodologies proposed in live animals represent adaptations to novelties, which have been developed in human. Of course, these techniques have been adapted in relation to their use and application in animals.

Initially, mature human oocytes were recovered ultrasonically guided percutaneous aspiration through the abdomen under local anesthesia in early 1908s (Lenz and Kauritsen, 1982); subsequently, ultrasound guided transvaginal oocyte aspiration was developed in humans (Dellenbach et al., 1984).

Repeated *in vivo* oocyte collection in cattle was first performed by Canadian researchers who used endoscopy via the right paralumbar fossa (Lambert et al., 1983). Callesen et al. (1987) were the first to use ultrasonography to collect oocytes from living cattle, using an ultrasonographic transducer equipped with a needle guide via a transcutaneous approach. This study was carried out in seven superovulated heifers. By rectal palpation, ovaries and follicles were visualized by ultrasound examination. A total number of 38 follicles were transcutaneously punctured and 16 oocytes were collected that resulted in a recovery rate of 42% (RR = number of oocytes collected/100 follicles punctured) and 2.3 oocytes/heifer.

In vivo oocyte collection by OPU was first established in cattle by a Dutch team, modifying a transvaginal ovum pick-up technique originally developed for use in human reproduction and in cattle. Pieterse et al. (1988) added an extension device to a convex ultrasound transducer that allowed it to be manipulated outside the bovine vagina and enabled nonsurgical oocyte recovery in cattle for the first time. A big advantage of the transvaginal approach in cattle is that it is possible to both secure and manipulate the ovary *per rectum* so that it can be moved around the ultrasound transducer and needle, to present the most optimal position for puncture. In this study, OPU was performed once a week in 10 cows for a total number of 36 transvaginal aspiration procedures, during which 54 oocytes were recovered from 197 punctured follicles. The mean RR was 27.4% and the number of oocytes/cow/sampling was 1.5. The stimulation of the ovaries with pregnant mare serum gonadotropin (PMSG) increased both RR (40 *vs.* 18%) and the number of oocytes/cow/sampling (2.7 *vs.* 1.0). The estrous cycle of these animals was not interrupted due to OPU procedure on the basis of plasma progesterone measurements (reviewed by Boni, 2012). As a result, a minimally invasive method with high repeatability (Pieterse et al., 1991) for repeated oocyte retrieval from living donor cows became available.

Another possibility to collect oocytes from living cows was proposed by Reichenbach et al. (1994), who developed a laparoscopic procedure of oocyte collection (L-OPU). This technique allows the repeated laparoscopic examination of the internal reproductive organs of cows and heifers through the vaginal fornix and visually assisted follicle aspiration. L-OPU showed several advantages with respect to OPU; in particular, the aspiration of primarily superficial follicles; the direct view of the ovary; and the aspiration procedure and a reduced risk of injury to the ovary. L-OPU and OPU techniques were compared by different researchers. Becker et al. (1996) compared transvaginal OPU under ultrasonographic guidance with oocyte retrieval by endoscopic instruments. They concluded that the use of ultrasound resulted in better quality COCs, although it is not entirely clear why endoscopic aspiration should cause more damage to the COCs. Santl et al. (1998) made a comparison of ultrasound-guided (U-OPU) *vs.* L-OPU in Simmental heifers. These researchers found higher proportion of class I oocytes (Grade 1 or A; Oropeza et al., 2004) after U-OPU more than that after L-OPU; these differences also were reflected by the cleavage rate, and morulae and blastocysts rates, attributing to the greater changes in vacuum pressure during L-OPU *vs.* U-OPU as responsible for the difference in oocyte quality.

Finally, as a consequence OPU procedure was easy, repeatable, featured minimal risks, and was developed as a successful technique for retrieving oocytes from selected heifers and cows of high genetic merit (Kruip et al., 1994), to breed large numbers of calves with known production traits, and to shorten the generation interval in cattle breeding programs. Moreover, OPU allowed to obtain embryos in situations of extraovarian infertility that result in the birth of healthy animals, confirming that most cows classified as infertile are able to produce viable gametes (Seneda et al., 2001).

Indeed, the ultimate aim was to produce more embryos and pregnancies per donor cow than was possible through MOET programs (Pieterse et al., 1991). Some advantages of OPU/IVEP over MOET are that multiple offspring for nearly every donor cow can be produced within a limited period, the number of offspring per unit time is significantly larger, and the technology is less dependent on the reproductive status of the donor cow. In addition, several bulls can be used for *in vitro* fertilization (IVF) on oocytes from one collection, rather than one bull as in MOET, thus maximizing genetic gain and minimizing inbreeding (van Wagtendonk-de Leeuw, 2005).

OPU/IVEP, however, requires a more sophisticated and expensive laboratory setting compared to MOET, and the costs per OPU/IVEP embryo are approximately twice those of MOET embryos. Although OPU/IVEP has clear advantages over MOET and artificial insemination (AI) in terms of number of offspring that can be produced per cow per time span (on average for AI 1 calf/year, for MOET 20–25 calves/year, and for OPU/IVEP 80–100 calves/year). The efficiency of reproductive technologies in terms of number of offspring per 100 immature oocytes declines significantly with increased levels of artifice of the technologies, from AI (with 55 live calves on the ground 1 week after birth), MOET (28 calves), until OPU/IVEP (with 11 calves). At the same time, problems associated with calves in terms of birth weight, congenital abnormalities, and perinatal mortality increase. This relative low efficiency in the production of healthy calves together with the relative high cost of compared to MOET in cattle makes its use justifiable mainly for breeding companies and breeders, where the benefits in terms of semen sales from resulting high genetic bulls may outweigh the costs (reviewed by van Wagtendonk-de Leeuw, 2005).

Pontes et al. (2009) investigated why the preferred means to produce bovine embryos in Brazil has changed from *in vivo* to *in vitro*, and compared embryo yield and pregnancy rate between these methods in the same Nelore (*B. indicus*) donor cows. The average number of embryos produced by OPU/IVEP (9.4 ± 5.3) was higher than the MOET method (6.7 ± 3.7). However, pregnancy rates were lower following transfer of *in vitro* produced (IVP) (33.5%) *vs. in vivo* derived (IVD) embryos (41.5%). They concluded that in Nelore cows, with an interval of 15 days between OPU procedures, it was possible to produce more embryos and pregnancies compared to conventional MOET.

6.3 OPU WORLWIDE: ACTUAL SITUATION

According to the International Embryo Transfer Society (IETS) statistics, the number of embryos produced *in vitro* and transferred into recipients has increased in the last years. This outstanding growth of OPU/IVEP seen in the last years is a consequence of a number of factors, such as the significant improvement of *in vitro* culture procedures and the successful use of sex-sorted semen in the IVEP programs enabling the manipulation of the proportion of male and female embryos produced (Blondin, 2015).

In 2016, we could already appreciate an approach between the number of IVD embryos by MOET (516,585) compared with IVP embryos transferred (448,113) (Perry, 2017). In 2017, for the first time in the IETS records, both total production and the number of transfers were greater for IVP than for IVD embryos in cattle. Compared to 2016, there was a 48.9% increase in the number of IVP embryos recorded, whereas the number of IVD embryos collected decrease by 21.7%, resulting in a 2-fold difference between IVP and IVD totals (992,289 *vs.* 495,054, respectively). The main factor driving this change was a remarkable growth of IVEP both in North America and Europe. The development of IVEP in these regions affected the world ET scenario and, for the first time since 1999, the number of IVP embryos in North America was greater than South America (reviewed by Viana, 2018). In 2018, a total of 1,499,367 transferrable embryos were collected or produced, which represents a relative stabilization compared with 2017. In regard to type of embryo, IVD and IVP embryos represented 31.3% (469,967) and 68.7% (1,029,400) of the total, respectively (Viana, 2019) (Fig. 6.1).

In Table 6.1, we refer the data from the IETS Data Retrieval Committee compiled by Joao Viana globally during 2019, for embryo transfer activities in 2018 and presented in the 28th Annual Report, regarding embryos produced *in vitro* by OPU in the different regions worldwide (Viana, 2019). IETS does not have the data for Asia in the period 2016–2018, so the latest data recorded for 2015 has been included (Perry, 2017). In addition, we have included in this table the latest data for embryo transfer activity in Europe in 2018, presented at the last Congress of the Association of Embryo Technology in Europe (AETE) held in Murcia (Spain) (Mikkola, 2019). Finally, in the table we considered OPU sessions or donors, collected oocytes and embryos, as well as the embryo/OPU session index.

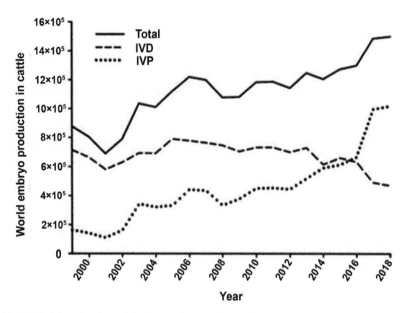

FIGURE 6.1   Number of bovine embryos IVD, IVP, and total recorded in the period 1999–2018. Summary of the International Embryo Transfer Society (IETS) statistical data collected by the Data Retrieval Committee (Viana, 2019).

TABLE 6.1   OPU and Bovine Embryos Produced *In Vitro* Worldwide in 2018.

Regions	Donors	Oocytes	Embryos	Embryos/session
Africa	621	18,486	3741	6.02
Asia (2015)	3177	59,224	9438	2.97
Europe	14,200	148,859	36,832	2.59
North America	118,410	2,004,491	497,511	4.20
Oceania	2,056	35,767	11,997	5.83
South America	78,522	1,256,556	444,537	5.66
Total	216,986	3,523,383	1,004,056	4.63

Source: Adapted from Perry, 2017; Mikkola, 2019; Viana, 2019.

In the last 2 years, USA has become in the world leader in the production of OPU/IVEP bovine embryos relegating Brazil to a second place. According to the data of the IETS for 2018, USA performed 108,827 OPU sessions with a total of 1,843,458 oocytes and an average of 16.94 oocytes/OPU session; 446,028 transferable embryos and an average of 4.1 embryos per OPU session (Viana, 2019).

In contrast, numbers have stabilized in Brazil, increasing the difference between the two countries. According to the data of the IETS for 2018, Brazil made a total of 59,638 OPU sessions with a total of 843,418 recovered oocytes, and an average of 14.14 oocytes/OPU session. As for the obtained embryos, the figure of 341,583, with an average of embryos per session of OPU, is 5.73 (Viana, 2019). However, we must consider that 46.42% OPU sessions in USA were with the stimulation of donors and that in Brazil, the total OPU sessions were in non-stimulation donors. Both in USA and in Brazil, most IVP embryos come from dairy than from beef breeds (53.3% and 62.3%, respectively) (Viana, 2019).

With respect to Europe, AETE updated the data of OPU and embryos produced *in vitro* in Europe for 2018 (Mikkola, 2019). In this statistic, the number of OPU sessions in Europe was 14,200 with a total number of oocytes of 148,859, an average of 10.48 oocytes per session of OPU, 36,832 total *in vitro* produced embryos and 2.59 embryo index per OPU session (Mikkola, 2019).

OPU remains the main source of oocytes for IVF (98.9% of IVP embryos), whereas the number of embryos produced using abattoir-derived oocytes decreased in 2018 (-4.5%) (Viana, 2019).

6.4   OPU EQUIPMENT AND PROCEDURE

The OPU system consists of three major components (Fig. 6.2): an ultrasonographic scanner with an appropriate transducer (probe), a vacuum pump, and a needle guidance system connected to an oocyte collecting tube (Bols and Stout, 2018).

For visualization of the ovarian follicles, native endovaginal probes (5–7.5 MHz) are available essentially for human use. Several manufacturers of ultrasound equipment have provided custom-made plastic holders or handgrips that can house generic convex array transducers together with the needle guide. The use of native endovaginal probes allows the complete replacement, for each donor animal, not only of the probe latex cover, but also of the needle guide together with the needle (Galli et al., 2014). Bols et al. (1995) proposed an OPU device that mounted 19G disposable needles that were connected to silicone tubing by means of a stainless-steel connector. This system was inserted into a stainless-steel tube, creating a rigid structure that allowed the needle to move back and forth. At present, there are already several commercial companies

(Minitube, IMV Technologies, etc.) that manufacture specific holders for OPU in cattle.

Inside the handgrip close to the transducer, the puncture needle can be visualized on the ultrasound screen when it is advanced into the sonographic field to enter a follicle and to facilitate visualization; it is helpful to have a biopsy guide on the ultrasound screen. This biopsy line programmed into the scanner's software is displayed on the screen and indicates where the follicle needs to be positioned for successful puncture.

The needle is in turn connected to a vacuum pump by silicone or Teflon tubing such that follicular contents are aspirated as soon as aspiration pressure is applied via the vacuum pump. The vacuum pump usually provides a vacuum set at flow rate between 15 and 25 ml/min to ensure maximum recovery with the least damage to the COCs. Flow rates are more indicative than vacuum pressure because the gauge of the needle and the length of the tubing can make a big difference (Galli et al., 2001).

The washing and oocyte collection medium consist in phosphate-buffered saline (PBS) supplemented with heparin (2.2 IU/ml), to prevent clotting, and fetal bovine serum (1%) (Ruiz et al., 2013b).

The follicular fluid and oocytes are collected into a collection device positioned between the needle and the pump. This oocyte collection device can be a regular embryo filter or a simple Falcon tube sealed with a stopper, into which an afferent tube delivers the follicle aspirate and from which an efferent line is connected to the vacuum pump that applies the aspiration pressure.

Prior to OPU cows can be sedated with xylazine (i.m.), treated with carprofen (s.c.) to prevent pain, to ensure comfort, and thus to improve reproductive efficiency; finally, epidural anesthesia is induced using lidocaine 2% (Ruiz et al., 2013b). Subsequently, the feces are removed from the rectum; the tail has been fixed to one side; the vulva and perineum are thoroughly cleaned and disinfected before the OPU device, containing the transducer and the needle guidance system, is inserted into the vagina.

While the OPU handgrip can be manipulated with one hand outside the cow, the head of the ultrasound transducer is positioned cranio-dorsally to the left or right of the cervix, depending on which ovary is to be collected from. Using the other hand, normally left hand in a right-handed person, per rectum, the operator fixes the ovary and positions it against the head of the transducer such that the ovary and follicles can be visualized on the ultrasound screen. The operator then advances the needle slowly forward until the vaginal wall is pierced and the needle is visualized entering the ultrasound field. By monitoring the needle's position and simultaneously manipulating the ovary transrectally, the needle can be directed into a follicle. Once the needle enters the follicle, the aspiration pump is activated using the foot pedal and the follicular fluid, and COCs are collected into the embryo filter that contains oocyte collection medium. An assistant should wash the system every time and 3–4 follicles are punctured to avoid excessive oocyte loss and improve the RR.

Subsequently, the filter contents are washed and transferred to a Petri dish and the oocytes are identified using a stereomicroscope, captured using a glass pipette, and placed into maturation medium. After 24 h of *in vitro* maturation (IVM), they will be fertilized *in vitro* and cultured for 7 days *in vitro* to reach the blastocyst stage (reviewed by Bols and Stout, 2018).

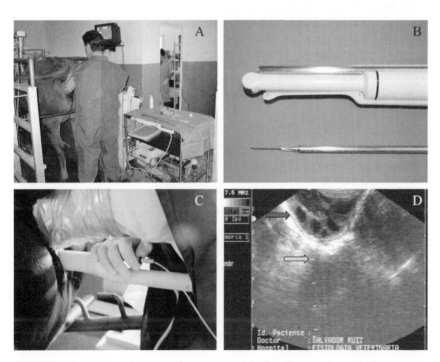

FIGURE 6.2 OPU equipment and procedure. (**A**) Cow in restraint with the operator cleaning rectum and all the equipment prepared for OPU session. (**B**) Detail of endovaginal scanner (5–7.5 MHz), handgrip, needle guidance system, and 18G (1.2 × 40 mm) needle. (**C**) Introducing handgrip and needle guidance system in cow. (**D**) Ovary ecographic image surrounding by operator's fingers. Red arrow: Ovarian follicles between 6 and 10 mm diameter. Yellow arrow: Biopsy line.

6.5   FACTORS AFFECTING OPU RESULTS

OPU success requires consideration of the technical aspects such as transducer type and frequency, needle puncture, vacuum pressure, and operator experience. The biological aspects are also important and include individual variations, breed and age of the donor, physiological status and body conditions of the donors, frequency and timing of follicle puncture, and hormonal stimulation to prepare donor for OPU.

The issue is obviously complex considering differences in breeds, reproductive statuses, operator ability, and other factors. In addition, technical improvements increase the number of aspirated oocytes even with the use of an OPU system with or without hormonal stimulation. The knowledge of the technical variables is essential for maximizing follicle aspiration efficiency (Da Silva et al., 2016).

The implementation of an OPU program requires always the support of a specialized laboratory for embryo production. Moreover, because of the economic value of the calves born, adequate veterinary assistance is recommended to minimize losses owing to the possible incidence of the large offspring syndrome or other common perinatal pathologies (Galli et al., 2014).

6.5.1   TECHNICAL FACTORS

OPU success rate is quantified first in terms of the oocyte RR, which is influenced by factors including needle diameter, aspiration pressure ultrasound equipment, operator experience, and another technical factors. As a result, RRs have been reported to vary between 7% and 70% for different OPU teams. For example, Galli et al. (2001) obtained an oocyte RR of 55–60% of the follicles punctured with their particular conditions of work: needles 17G-55 cm and 19G-7 cm; vacuum pump set at 115 mm Hg (flow rate: 20–25 ml/min); and as ultrasound scanners a Toshiba Capasee and a Medison Sonovet 600 equipped with a 6 MHz endovaginal probes with a custom-made holder.

Over the years, many different needle diameters and aspiration pressures have been used in either experimental or commercial bovine OPU programs, which makes it difficult to directly compare recovery rates. A final very important factor determining OPU outcome is the experience of the operator or the team that is retrieving the oocytes (reviewed by Bols and Stout, 2018).

6.5.1.1 FOLLICULAR ASPIRATION NEEDLES

Transvaginal oocyte recovery in cattle was first performed using long needles (55–60 cm) with an outer diameter of 1–1.5 mm designed specific for follicular aspiration in cows (Pieterse et al., 1988). Despite the good efficiency of the long needles, their high cost represented an obstacle to the regular use of OPU worldwide; moreover, another major disadvantage of these needles is that they become blunt quite quickly and, even with regular re-sharpening, never regain their original sharpness, and contained a large dead space. Due to their price, the same needle was commonly used in several animals and the bevel had reduced ability to penetrate the ovary, forcing to the operator to use greater force during the puncture. This situation presented two problems: one was the possibility of damage to the ovarian stroma, especially in animals with repeated punctures; and the second one referred to low oocyte recovery resulting from re-used needles causing abrupt follicular rupture, which increases the risk of oocytes falling into the abdominal cavity (Da Silva et al., 2016). Alternative OPU systems were achieved, when the long needles were successfully replaced with disposable hypodermic needles (Bols et al., 1995).

The needle inner diameter is another important aspect to consider. Needles with diameters larger than 18G are associated with higher recovery rates as well as higher percentages of denuded oocytes. The reason for this is that a large diameter needle enables quick flow of the oocytes and granulosa cells from the *cumulus oophorus*, which may easily detach from the zona pellucida. Another problem is the large ovarian area that is damaged during the puncture, which also increases the degree of blood aspiration. On the other hand, a needle with too small a diameter (<21G) provides a low speed flow, which increases the possibility of the oocyte lost during the procedure and falling into the abdominal cavity. Bols et al. (1996) studied the effects of aspiration vacuum and three different needle diameters (18, 19, and 21G) on the morphology of COCs and developmental capacity of the oocyte after IVF using a disposable OPU needle guidance system whose construction permits its use *in vitro*. The highest oocyte RR were obtained when using the thickest needle (18G) and the thinner needles result in a higher proportion of recovered COCs with a compact *cumulus*, regardless of the aspiration vacuum. Considering all these aspects, it is well accepted that the best diameters are 18–20G (reviewed by Da Silva et al., 2016).

Another important point related to the needle is the bevel length. Bols et al. (1997) studied the effects of needle tip bevel on the morphology and developmental capacity of bovine COCs, testing three different diameters (18, 19, and 20G) and two different needle bevels (long and short). The results showed that the length of the needle bevel has a significant effect on oocyte recovery, in favor of the long-beveled needle. The probable explanation for this is the sharp edge of long bevel allows rapid follicular penetration, whereas short bevels are usually less sharp.

Regarding the needle length, 40–75 mm is considered ideal. Needles <40 mm do not cover the ovary during the puncture, and excessive manipulation is required to reach all follicles; on the other hand, needles >75 mm are too flexible and bend easily.

Finally, a further increase in oocyte recovery can be obtained by twisting the needle within the follicle. This technique showed a significant improvement of approximately 30% of the RR (Sasamoto et al., 2003) due to a better detachment of the COC by curettage of the follicular wall during the follicle aspiration.

6.5.1.2   VACUUM PUMP

A combination of needle diameter and vacuum pressure contributes to oocyte efficiency and quality. Considering the vacuum itself, some studies have linked low pressure such as 50 mmHg with low aspiration efficiency because there is not enough suction to collect the oocytes when the puncture is performed. However, higher pressure such as 120 mmHg may cause damage to oocytes or full loss of *cumulus oophorus* cells. As soon as higher aspiration vacuum is used, a decrease of the number of compact CCOs can be observed resulting in a higher proportion of naked oocytes. There is large variation among studies with values of 40–400 mmHg (Bols et al., 1996).

The exact aspiration pressure exerted through the tip of the needle depends on the aspiration device, the length and diameter of the tubing, the size and type of collection vessel, as well as on the needle diameter. To make comparisons possible, the aspiration pressure needs to be expressed in terms of the amount of fluid (in ml) that can be aspirated per minute, rather than in mmHg exerted from the vacuum pump. Effectively, we must considerer that a modest change in needle diameter can triple the rate of fluid aspiration without any change in aspiration pressure (Bols and Stout, 2018). Considerable variation 4.4–40 ml/min has been reported, although the range of 15–25 ml/min has been most widely used since it demonstrated high efficiency of oocyte recovery and minimal damage to the *cumulus oophorus* during OPU (Bungartz et al., 1995; Galli et al., 2001).

Many vacuum pumps have been considered viable options for OPU in cows. Theoretically, any vacuum machine featuring pressure control could be used. OPU can be performed using aspiration machines that are commonly used for several health applications such as dentistry, abdominal surgery, or controlled infusion. Currently, many devices designed specifically for OPU in cows are commercially available (reviewed by Da Silva et al., 2016).

6.5.1.3 ULTRASONOGRAPHY

Transducer frequency and sensitivity of the ultrasound equipment constitute a significant variable in the oocyte recovery process and represent another parameter of extreme relevance for the OPU efficiency. Reports involve frequencies of 3.5–7.5 MHz. The first study on OPU in The Netherlands used a 5.0 MHz sector scanner probe allowing the visualization of follicles larger than 3 mm. The passage to a 6.5 MHz curved array probe significantly improved either the number of visible follicles or the number of the collected oocytes (Kruip et al., 1994). A comparison between a linear array and a mechanical multiple angle sector (MAP) transducer for OPU was made by Bols et al. (2004). A significant difference was found for the ability to visualize smaller follicles in favor of the MAP transducer.

Considering that the operator will manipulate the ovary very close to the transducer, the adoption of high frequencies of 6–8 MHz is recommended since they provide the best image definition of follicles and other ovarian structures (Da Silva et al., 2016).

The vast majority of OPU procedures are performed with convex or micro convex transducers, which are commonly used in humans as well. Linear probes, the most versatile transducer type in veterinary medicine, present a lower OPU efficiency; approximately, 10–20% of follicles cannot be reached due to limited space between the ovary and needle (Seneda et al., 2003); moreover, the ovary size may represent a critical aspect in the use of a linear transducer.

Galli et al. (2001) made an interesting review about different equipment, scanners and probes, referred in the literature until that moment; we can quote the following: Aloka 500 with a 5 MHz convex array transducer; Hitachi EUB 415 with a 8.5 MHz vaginal curved array; Capasee Toshiba with a 6 MHz human endovaginal probe; Medison Sonovet 600 with an ad hoc endovaginal probe; Hitachi EUB 405 with a 6.5 MHz finger-tip probe and Pie Medical Falco-Vet scanner with a 5–7.5 MHz human endovaginal probe.

At present, several commercial companies have designed their own scanners, transducers, and holders for performing OPU in cows (e.g. *Easi-Scan* from BCF-Technologies, *"All in one"* and *Exago* or *Exapad* from Echo Control Medical-ECM-; both companies form a new imaging division "IMV Imaging" within the IMV Technology Group).

6.5.1.4   OPU TEAM AND OPERATOR EXPERIENCE

A technique with people involved will always be affected by the performance of those individuals. The OPU technique is performed by either one or two persons and, in certain companies, the same people carry out the development of the technique in a similar way during years, using the same conditions techniques. The experience of the operator in a one-person system or the operator and the assistant (in a system of two people) has a significant effect in the number and quality of collected oocytes (Merton et al., 2003) and in a proper way an adequate selection of operators and/or assistants it can help improve the results. Therefore, in an embryo technology program with only one or two OPU technicians, the overall results of OPU/IVEP will be determined to a substantial extent by the OPU team, as evidenced by an in-depth analysis of 7,800 OPU sessions performed in "Holland Genetics" by Merton et al. (2003).

6.5.2   BIOLOGICAL FACTORS

A substantial body of literature is available on biological factors that might influence the likelihood of blastocyst formation when IVEP is based on COCs recovered via OPU. Now, we are going to review some factors that are directly related to the OPU procedure. Between these biological factors, we can include the frequency and timing of follicle puncture, the physiological status and body condition of the donor, individual variations, the breed and age of the donor, the hormone stimulation to prepare donors for OPU, and finally the influence of climate and season.

6.5.2.1 FREQUENCY AND TIMING OF FOLLICLE PUNCTURE

There are two major OPU systems including non-stimulation and pre-stimulation procedure, the difference is whether the donor will be stimulated with hormone prior to OPU. The original OPU procedure includes no hormone stimulation.

The frequency of sampling represents a crucial point. OPU routinely performs twice-a-week (usually Monday and Thursday), which allows the maximum recovery of oocytes of suitable quality for embryo production in a given time interval compared to once-a-week OPU, because no dominant follicle develops when all visible follicles are aspirated in the OPU process. While in most once-a-week collections, a dominant follicle develops at the successive collection, which causes the regression and degeneration of the subordinate follicles. In a result, oocytes collected by this scheme are relatively less and with low quality in a given time interval. In the once-a-week collection schedule, the donors also can come into estrus while this is never the case in a twice-a-week schedule (Galli et al., 2001).

On a per cow per session basis, there was no difference between "OPU 1/week" and "OPU 2/week" protocols in terms of the average number of follicles aspirated, oocytes retrieved, and blastocysts produced on Day 7. While on a weekly basis, those three indexes were significantly higher in the "OPU 2/week" protocol than those in the "OPU 1/week" (Chaubal et al., 2006).

Viana et al. (2004) evaluated oocyte recovery and embryo yield using these two different ovarian follicular aspiration schedules, once a week (1x) and twice weekly (2x), for nine consecutive weeks in donor non-lactating cows of the Gyr breed. More oocytes were recovered per session in 1x as compared with 2x (8.9 ± 0.8 *vs.* 7.0 ± 0.7), resulting in a greater RR in this group (74.3% *vs.* 58.7%). More COCs of Grade 1 were recovered from 2x (22.6% *vs.* 13.3%). There was no difference in cleavage rate between groups, but the percentage of embryos that reached the blastocyst stage was greater in 2x as compared with 1x (31.8% *vs.* 21.6%). The results from this study demonstrated that the use of shorter intervals (3–4 days, twice week) between successive OPU sessions was the preferred schedule for recovering greater quality COCs and maximizing IVEP in Gyr (*B. indicus*) cows.

Moreover, this system does not interfere with the normal reproduction cycles of the donor; there were no any long-term detrimental effects on the donor cow's fertility even after twice-a-week OPU for over a year (Galli et al., 2001; Chastan-Maillard et al., 2003) performed by experienced operators (reviewed by Qi et al., 2013).

Another aspect of the OPU efficiency is related to its continuity. Petyim et al. (2003) compared the twice-weekly OPU application by using continuous or discontinuous (i.e. restricted to days 0–12 of the estrous cycle) schemes. The mean number of punctured follicles and collected oocytes as well as the oocyte quality and the cleavage rate did not differ per puncture session between the two OPU schemes. The discontinuous OPU scheme permits a normal ovulation and corpus luteum (CL) formation that shows characteristics similar to those of the pre-OPU period. Heifers submitted to continuous OPU scheme barely showed cyclicity with irregular interestrous intervals and weaker signs of estrus (reviewed by Boni, 2012).

In conclusion, twice weekly OPU schedule resulted in an increased follicular wave frequency, and an arrest of the estrous cycle, follicle maturation, and ovulation. Animals submitted to this sampling regimen entered a para-physiological status in which follicular waves were uncoupled from the estrous cycle. However, as soon as OPU sampling ceased, ovulation took place within 6 days (Kruip et al., 1994).

6.5.2.2 PHYSIOLOGICAL STATUS AND BODY CONDITION OF THE DONOR

Each donor's physiological condition, including weight, breed, age, and individual variations has been characterized in several studies. In cattle breeding programs, OPU is generally performed on selected healthy heifers with excellent genetic potential for production traits, which could in themselves be predictive for oocyte yield and the number of blastocysts produced (Merton et al., 2009). The reproductive potential of females can be maximized if OPU/IVEP embryos are applied in the course of non-productive periods such as pregnancy, anestrus, and postpartum. OPU can be performed at various stages of a cow's reproductive life; even pregnancy does not exclude OPU, since oocytes can successfully be retrieved during the first 3 months of gestation (Bungartz et al., 1995). The only exception are pregnant animals after the third or fourth month of pregnancy and animals with severe ovarian hypoplasia or in the immediate post-partum before ovarian activity is restored (Galli et al., 2001).

Takuma et al. (2010) compared the OPU efficiency in pregnant and empty cows between hot and cool seasons. The quality of the collected COCs did not differ in relation to the reproductive phase of the donor cows. Analyzing the two reproductive phases, however, the number of follicles and collected oocytes significant decreased during the hot season, limitedly in empty cows. In addition, when data from the two seasons were combined, pregnant cows showed a significant higher proportion of cleavage and blastocyst rates and freezable embryos than empty cows (reviewed by Boni, 2012).

Few studies of OPU/IVEP embryos were performed in early post-partum period in beef breeds. Perez et al. (2000) observed that the number of follicles aspirated and oocytes recovered were greater from FSH-treated cows at days 25 and 35 postpartum compared to cows not treated with FSH. Kendrick et al. (1999) found that the number of oocytes retrieved by OPU increased linearly from days 30 to 100 postpartum in Holstein cows and the oocyte quality was greatest at 30 days postpartum. However, Lopes et al. (2006) determined that in animals of the same breed there was no effect of days postpartum on the number and quality of oocytes retrieved, although the days postpartum had a positive influence on the blastocyst rate.

Aller et al. (2010) investigated, in early postpartum suckled beef cows with and without FSH pre-stimulation, the influence of the postpartum period on the number and quality of oocytes recovered by OPU, the overall efficiency of the OPU/IVEP embryos from days 30 to 80 postpartum and if repeated OPU negatively affect fertility following a fixed-time artificial insemination (FTAI) protocol. These authors concluded that FSH-treated suckled postpartum cows can be a source of oocytes for IVF, and repeated dominant follicle ablation and OPU applied during postpartum period did not affect the subsequent fertility following FTAI.

Vieira et al. (2014) evaluated the efficacy of superstimulation with p-FSH before OPU on IVEP in lactating and non-lactating Holstein donors. Regardless of treatment, non-lactating cows had a higher blastocyst rate (41.9% *vs.* 13.4%) and produced more transferable embryos per OPU session (3.5 ± 0.5 *vs.* 1.3 ± 0.3) than lactating cows.

In relation to body condition, there is consensus about malnourished donors having reduced capacity for oocytes to develop embryos. Effectively, undernutrition has a negative effect on the developmental competence of recovered oocytes *in vitro*, as illustrated by the decreasing percentage of blastocysts associated with decreasing body condition score of the donor, and an increasing proportion of good quality oocytes with increasing body condition score (reviewed by Bols and Stout, 2018).

Ruiz (2010) performs a brief review on some results of oocytes and embryos obtained by OPU/IVEP in animals in different physiological status with and without pre-stimulation hormonal.

6.5.2.3   INDIVIDUAL VARIATIONS

The donor animal is a major source of variation both the management and genetic point of view. The efficiency of OPU/IVEP techniques has been impaired by the large variability among donors in their response to these procedures (Merton et al., 2003; Pontes et al., 2009). Therefore, the success of IVEP technologies has been associated primarily with physiological characteristics, such as ovarian antral follicle population (AFP) and oocyte competence to reach the blastocyst stage (Taneja et al., 2000; Pontes et al., 2011).

The AFP has been related to several substances, including the concentrations of circulating insulin, insulin-like growth factor I, and anti-Müllerian hormone (AMH) (Batista et al., 2014).

AMH is a dimeric glycoprotein of the inhibitory transforming growth factor-b (TGF-b) superfamily that is expressed only in the gonads. In females, granulosa cells from growing secondary follicles produce AMH during follicle recruitment. It acts as an inhibiting growth factor on the pool of resting follicles. As shown in mice, humans, and cattle, the concentration of AMH in plasma reflects the total number of oocytes in the ovary and the number of follicles, which are involved in preantral and antral follicular activity (reviewed by Vernunft et al., 2015). Therefore, the strong association between the follicle population and the AMH concentration could provide a consistent method for predicting the AFP.

In human medicine, plasma AMH levels have become an important predictive parameter for the success of assistant reproductive technologies, which include OPU/IVEP (Dewailly et al., 2014). However, in veterinary reproductive medicine, this parameter is not used very often. During the last few years, strong linear regressions between plasma AMH levels and the number of antral follicles have also been described in different breeds of cattle (Batista et al., 2014).

From puberty on, the AMH levels of individual heifers stay at a constant level; through the estrous cycle, the plasma AMH levels show only slight dynamics with a decrease one week after ovulation. But that decrease in the AMH level is not big enough, that animals with high AMH levels will reach the plasma AMH levels of animals with low plasma AMH levels (Monnieaux et al., 2012). Therefore, AMH can also be considered as an independent marker of the ovarian follicle reserve in cattle. Recently, it was shown that AMH can be used as a predictive marker for *in vivo* embryo production in cattle (Monnieaux et al., 2010; Rico et al., 2012).

Guerreiro et al. (2014) evaluated the association between plasma AMH concentration and IVEP from *B. taurus* (Holstein) and *B. indicus* (Nelore) donors. They found a positive correlation between the plasma AMH and number of *in vitro* embryos produced from Holstein and Nelore donors. The results revealed that females classified as having high AMH presented a greater number of visible aspirated follicles and a greater number of recovered COCs. Moreover, donors classified as having high AMH yielded a greater number of embryos produced per OPU compared with those classified as having low AMH. Concluding that although the plasma AMH concentration did not alter the ability of the COC to reach the blastocyst stage, the AMH concentration in plasma can be an accurate endocrine marker for the *in vitro* embryo yield from either *B. taurus* (Holstein) or *B. indicus* (Nelore) donors, and it becomes in a promising tool to enhance the overall efficiency of OPU/IVEP programs in the field as a selective criterion for high embryo producing donors.

In opposition, Vernunft et al. (2015) analyzed the plasma AMH levels in Holstein–Friesian heifers and their results suggest that correlations between AMH and outcomes of an OPU/IVEP program are too low to use AMH as a precise predictive parameter for the success of a particular OPU procedure in cattle. However, AMH can help identify groups of very good or very poor oocyte donors.

In conclusion, more studies must be conducted to clarify these different results and to determine the role of AMH levels in OPU/IVEP procedures in cattle.

6.5.2.4   DONOR BREED

The OPU efficiency did not show a significant variation among cow breeds as long as *B. taurus* breeds are concerned (Kruip et al., 1994). If this evaluation is extended to *B. indicus* breeds and *indicus-taurus* donor significant differences were observed.

There are physiological similarities, as well as differences, between *B. indicus* and *B. taurus* breeds. For instance, Nelore cows are similar to other *B. indicus* and *B. taurus* breeds when comparing the average embryo production by MOET (reviewed by Pontes et al., 2009). However, *B. indicus* breeds tend to have, on average, more follicular waves (Figueiredo et al., 1997) as well as a greater number of follicles >5 mm per wave compared to *B. taurus* breeds. Because there is a greater efficiency of oocyte recovery from follicles <4 mm in diameter (Seneda et al., 2001), it is another reason that more oocytes are obtained from *B. indicus* than from *B. taurus* donors. It was also reported that Nelore cows have smaller dominant follicles and CL, and shorter estrus than *B. taurus* breeds. Other reproductive characteristics, such as the LH surge, seem to be specific to Nelore females. However, the physiological basis for the number of follicles in Nelore cattle has not been established and despite the physiological importance of these differences, the high number of oocytes obtained via OPU seems to be a unique characteristic of Nelore cows (Pontes et al., 2009).

Pontes et al. (2010) reported a large-scale commercial program for IVEP from dairy *B. taurus*, *B. indicus*, and *indicus-taurus* donors, using sexed sperm. The number of viable oocytes per OPU session was 12.1 ± 3.9 for Gyr cows, 8.0 ± 2.7 for Holstein, 16.8 ± 5.0 for 1/4 Holstein x 3/4 Gyr, and 24.3 ± 4.7 for 1/2 Holstein–Gyr crossbred females. The mean number of embryos produced by OPU/IVEP and the pregnancy rates were 3.2 and 40% for Gyr cows, 2.1 and 36% for Holstein, 3.9 and 37% for 1/4 Holstein x 3/4 Gyr, and 5.5 and 37% for 1/2 Holstein–Gyr (reviewed by Boni, 2012).

Another study from Pontes et al. (2011) developed an OPU/IVEP program using Nelore cattle donors. They reported data from 656 OPU/IVEP procedures, performed on 317 Nelore cows, without hormone stimulation or control of ovarian follicular waves. The average number of total and viable oocytes produced per OPU session was 30.84 ± 0.88 (ranged between groups from 58.94 ± 2.04 to 10.26 ± 0.57) and 23.35 ± 0.7 (ranged from 47.06 ± 1.6 to 6.31 ± 0.389), with an average of 8.1 ± 0.3 embryos (from 15.06 ± 0.86 to 2.42 ± 0.25) and 3.0 ± 0.1 pregnancies on day 30 (from 5.62 ± 0.86 to 0.92 ± 0.13) per OPU/IVEP procedure. Oocyte production varied widely among donor so that the number of viable oocytes recovered ranged from 0 to 128. Since donors with numerous viable oocytes produced many viable embryos and pregnancies, oocyte production was useful for donor selection. However, there was no significant effect of the number of OPU sessions per donor on mean numbers of oocytes produced. The authors confirmed field reports of high oocyte production by some Nelore donors and demonstrated individual variation in oocyte yield, which was associated with embryo production and pregnancy rates. Highly contrasting results have been reported in Belgian Blue donors with impaired fertility, which yielded an average of only 3.1 oocytes and 0.5 embryos per puncture session (Bols et al., 1996).

Despite the great differences in total of oocytes retrieved per OPU procedure across breeds, outstanding donors can be found in all breeds and the number of oocytes retrieved per individual donor seems consistent across time. In fact, it was previously shown the occurrence of high within-cow repeatability in oocyte production over time (Monteiro et al., 2017). However, contrasting results were shown across genetic groups. For *B. taurus*, the number of recovered oocytes seemed fairly constant, even up to 32 consecutive OPU sessions (Petyim et al., 2003). Conversely, in *B. indicus* cattle, decreased numbers of recovered oocytes following consecutive OPU sessions have been reported (Gimenes et al., 2015); it appears to be an issue particularly within donors with high numbers of COCs retrieved at the beginning of the program (Monteiro et al., 2017). Despite that, donors classified as high COC resulted in increased blastocyst production per OPU. More importantly, the high repeatability efficiency in terms of COC retrieved is a remarkable finding that has major implications to IVEP labs worldwide (reviewed by Watanabe et al., 2017).

In conclusion, breed donor influences the OPU process because different breeds have various numbers of follicles in the ovary during the follicular wave cycle. *Bos indicus* cows tend to have more numerous follicular waves and a larger number of smaller follicles than *B. taurus*. This feature has resulted in very fast OPU/IVEP popularity growth in Brazil, since the Brazilian herd is around 200 million animals about 80–85% of which are Nelore breeds. Although *in vivo* embryo production continues to be widely used in *indicus* donors, the use of OPU/IVEP enables the production of more embryos in the same period (reviewed by Da Silva et al., 2016).

6.5.2.5　DONOR AGE

Age is a commonly discussed factor. The very young and very old donor ages are generally reported as problematic situations. Prepubertal and aging donors commonly have poor-quality oocytes. Elderly cows also have fewer available gametes (Da Silva et al., 2016).

Virtually, all female cattle starting from 2 mo of age can be oocyte donors by follicular aspiration. The only exception are pregnant animals after the third or fourth month of pregnancy and animals with severe ovarian hypoplasia or in the immediate post-partum before ovarian activity is restored. Calves of about 2–3 mo can be oocyte donors. But for an efficient collection without side effects the procedure requires a laparotomy under general anesthesia. The ovaries are exposed through the incision and the oocytes are recovered by follicular aspiration (Galli et al., 2001).

Presicce et al. (1997) designed a study to determine the acquisition of developmental competence of oocytes using prepubertal heifers as a model. Oocytes were collected by OPU from calves at 5, 7, 9, and 11 mo of age that had or had not received gonadotropin stimulation. Numbers of oocytes recovered from unstimulated heifers decreased with age. Embryo development to morula and blastocyst stages were poorer for oocytes collected from unstimulated calves at 5–9 mo of age than for those from the age-matched but gonadotropin-stimulated groups. In calves 11 mo of age, embryo development to morula and blastocyst stages was similar with and without gonadotropin stimulation and was comparable to that of adult cow oocytes. The authors concluded that the acquisition of oocyte competence for normal embryo development in prepubertal calves is influenced by animal age and hormonal treatment.

The possibility of producing embryos from oocytes repeatedly collected by OPU from unstimulated calves before and after puberty was compared in the same animals, determining that oocytes can be collected by repeated OPU in calves 7–10 mo old without affecting their growth or the onset of puberty. The correlation observed for the number of follicles punctured before and after puberty suggests that this parameter is determined before puberty (Majerus et al., 1999).

The major problem with prepubertal donors is the impaired *in vitro* developmental capacity of the recovered oocytes (Taneja et al., 2000), resulting in a low overall efficiency of the procedure.

Rizos et al. (2005) reported that a significantly higher number of total oocytes (4.7 *vs.* 2.8) and grade 1-2 oocytes recovered/animal from heifers than from cows (3.0 *vs.* 1.8); while there was no significant difference in the percentage of oocytes cleaving after fertilization, or in the percentage reaching the blastocyst stage between heifers and cows.

Jin et al. (2016) investigated the effect of age (3-6 and 7-9 years) and number of parities (2-3 and 4-7) on the potential of the Korean native cow (Hanwoo breed) as oocyte donor in OPU and subsequent IVEP. With advancement in age and parity of animals, there was an increase in number of ovarian follicles. The total number of recovered COCs was increased in old cows with increased number of parities. The authors concluded that repeated OPU of cows resulted in significant decrease in the *in vitro* production of embryos in young compared with old cows.

6.5.2.6   HORMONAL STIMULATION

Several investigators have used gonadotropin stimulation in OPU protocols ranging from a full superovulatory dose to shorter treatments for 2–3 days with one or two injections per day in presence of a progesterone releasing device or a CL. The positive effect of the gonadotropins can be attributed to the increase in size of small follicles and to the acquisition of a higher developmental competence of the oocytes as it occurs with *in vivo* matured oocytes (Merton et al., 2003).

In prepubertal calves, gonadotropin stimulation is required to obtain an acceptable level of developmental competence (Taneja et al., 2000; Galli et al., 2001). However, use of gonadotropin stimulation does not seem to be effective in *B. indicus* donors; it is not used in large scale programs (Pontes et al., 2009; 2010).

Many attempts of hormonal stimulation have been evaluated in order to improve follicle population in animals submitted to OPU. Now, we are going to refer the most important studies in the last years.

Pieterse et al. (1988) treated cows with 1000–3000 IU of PMSG in the presence of an active mid-cycle CL 2 days before OPU. The mean number of aspirated follicles significantly increased in stimulated compared to non-stimulated donors and the treatment decreased the RR value.

Bungartz et al. (1995) compared the OPU efficiency, twice weekly (3–4 days intervals), on Holstein–Friesian lactating cows, which were or were not stimulated 4-day prior to OPU aspiration with a single injection of 100 mg of porcine FSH (p-FSH). The number of aspirated follicles was higher in the treated group (10.6 ± 0.7 *vs.* 8.9 ± 0.5); however, the number of collected oocytes, RR, percentage of viable oocytes, cleavage, and morula/blastocyst rates did not differ between treated and non-treated groups. The authors concluded that repeated aspiration of viable COC at short intervals was possible and additional FSH treatment did not increase oocyte yields.

Goodhand et al. (1999) studied in Simmental heifers the effects of frequency of follicular aspiration and treatment of donor cattle with FSH on *in vivo* oocyte recovery and *in vitro* embryo production. The oocyte donors were aspirated once a week, twice a week, or once a week following treatment with FSH (total dose 9.0 mg ovine-FSH, o-FSH) for 3 days prior to aspiration. Significantly more oocytes per heifer per week recovered from animals treated with FSH were graded Class 1. FSH treatment of bovine oocyte donors aspirated once a week enabled a similar number of transferable embryos to be produced per donor week as aspiration twice a week without FSH treatment. These two treatments produced twice as many transferable embryos per donor week as aspiration once a week without FSH treatment.

One year later, the same authors (Goodhand et al., 2000) studied *in vivo* oocyte recovery (once weekly) and IVEP from bovine oocyte donors treated with progestagen plus estradiol 17b or FSH. Treatment with steroid had no significant effect on any follicular, oocyte or embryo production variate other than to reduce the number and the diameter of large follicles >10 mm present at aspiration. FSH increased numbers of medium (6–10 mm) and large follicles and there was a corresponding decrease in the number of small follicles (2–5 mm). The total number of follicles at aspiration increased from 17.7 ± 1.60 for animals not treated with FSH to 23.6 ± 1.97 following multiple dose treatment with FSH. Significantly, more follicles were aspirated following FSH treatment (no FSH 9.7 ± 1.09, single dose FSH 13.6 ± 1.30, multiple dose FSH 17.3 ± 1.52) and numbers of oocytes recovered per cow per week increased, but the differences were not significant. Significantly, more good oocytes (Grade 1) were recovered from animals treated with FSH. There was no overall significant effect of FSH on embryo production rate or the total number of transferable embryos produced but the number of transferable embryos was highest following administration of multiple doses of FSH.

De Roover et al. (2005) applied an ovarian superstimulation protocol prior to OPU, tailored to the individual donor response, to evaluate its advantages and disadvantages in terms of follicle numbers and diameters, the numbers of retrieved oocytes and day 7 cultured blastocysts. 10 adult non-lactating Holstein cows were superstimulated with p-FSH and subjected to OPU-IVF six times at 2-week intervals. The total dose of p-FSH prior to the first OPU session was 300 mg/animal (total p-FSH dose was unchanged, increased or reduced (±50 mg), according to the percentage of follicles >11 mm, present in the previous session of that particular donor. The mean number of punctured follicles per session was 11.9 ± 7.7, with a mean of 5.6 ± 4.1 COCs (RR = 47%). Finally, all COCs were subjected to IVEP, which resulted in a mean of 2.0 ± 2.3 blastocysts on 7 D. The changes in p-FSH dose influenced the sizes but not the numbers of follicles, the latter parameter was influenced by the individual donor and OPU session.

Chaubal et al. (2006) evaluated the effects of once *vs.* twice-weekly OPU, dominant follicle removal (DFR) and FSH stimulation (once weekly 200 mg, divided in 80 mg i.m. and 120 mg s.c.) prior OPU on five groups of 3 cows each (Angus-cross cows); each group was allotted to a treatment protocol, which was repeated every week for 10 consecutive weeks. Treatment with FSH, followed by twice-weekly OPU, failed to show any synergistic effect of FSH and increased aspiration frequency. When FSH was given 36 h after DFR, followed by OPU 48 h later, more follicles, oocytes and embryos were obtained during each session, but not on a weekly basis. Pooled results over 10 weeks showed an overall improved performance for the treatment groups with twice-weekly OPU sessions, due to the doubled number of OPU sessions performed. However, the protocol that consisted of DFR, FSH treatment and a subsequent single OPU per week was considered the most productive and cost-effective (reviewed by Boni, 2012).

Some authors have studied the effect during ovarian stimulation of the presence or absence of a progesterone-releasing intravaginal device (CIDR), and i.v. treatment with LH 6 h prior to OPU (yes *vs.* no), on oocyte competence, judged by blastocyst development rates following IVF. Presence of CIDR during superstimulation had no effect on the follicular response. Administration of LH 6 h prior to OPU increased the oocytes of higher morphological grades, and in the absence of a CIDR, improved blastocyst development rate, resulted in 2.89 ± 0.4 blastocysts per cow per OPU session (1.3–1.5 better than the rest of experimental groups) (Chaubal et al., 2007).

De Roover et al. (2008) published a retrospective study about the effects of OPU frequency and FSH stimulation of beef cattle (Belgium Blue) IVEP. Data from 7 years of work were analyzed comparing number of follicles, COCs and IVP embryos obtained from 1,396 non-stimulated OPU sessions on 81 donor animals (2-weekly OPU scheme) with 640 sessions following FSH-LH superstimulation, on 112 donors (OPU once every 2 weeks). The stimulation protocol started with the insertion of an ear implant (3 mg norgestomet) 8 days before puncture. The dominant follicle was ablated by OPU on day 6. On day 3 and 2, cows were injected with FSH twice daily (total dose: 160 mg FSH and 40 mg LH) per donor per stimulation cycle and animals were punctured 48 h after the last FSH injection (day 0). Progesterone implants were removed day +1. Results demonstrated that, expressed per session, FSH stimulation prior to OPU increases production efficiency with significantly more follicles punctured and oocytes retrieved. However, when overall results during comparable 2-week periods are considered (4 non-stimulated sessions *vs.* 1 stimulated), more follicles are punctured and more oocytes are retrieved using the non-stimulated protocol. The absence of significant differences between these two regimens in the number of *in vitro* produced embryos within the 2-week period suggests a positive effect on *in vitro* oocyte developmental competence in the treated animals.

Sendag et al. (2008) compared the ovarian response, oocyte yields per animal, and the morphological quality of oocytes collected by OPU from Holstein cows treated either with FSH (500 IU) or eCG (3000 IU). Recovered oocytes were graded morphologically based on the *cumulus* investment. Average follicle number in ovaries was higher in FSH group than eCG group. Oocyte yields per animal did not differ between FSH and eCG groups but the proportion of oocytes Grade 1 was higher in the FSH group in the than eCG group. These results suggest that ovarian response, follicle number in ovaries, and oocyte quality are affected by the type of gonadotropin, and FSH is better alternative than eCG for OPU treatment.

Aller et al. (2010) studied, in early postpartum suckled beef cows (Angus) with and without FSH pre-stimulation, the influence of the post-partum period on the number and quality of oocytes recovered by OPU, the overall efficiency of OPU/IVP embryos (days 30 to 80 postpartum) and if repeated OPU negatively affect fertility following a FTAI protocol. Treatments included DFR, FSH treatment (total doses 9 mg s.c. once a day over 2 days at equal doses) and OPU procedure 5 days after DFR. In both groups, OPU was repeated four times (days 35, 49, 63, and 77 postpartum). The numbers of follicles visible and aspirated in FSH-treated cows were greater than in non-treated cows (10.6 ± 0.6 and 8.4 ± 0.4 *vs.* 8.0 ± 0.5 and 4.6 ± 0.3). Following FSH treatment, the number of recovered oocytes per cow per OPU session and percentage of viable oocytes were greater in the treated than in non-treated animals (3.0 ± 0.1 and 39.5% *vs.* 1.5 ± 0.1 and 30.0%). The cleavage, embryo development and pregnancy rates after FTAI were not different among groups. The authors concluded that FSH-treated suckled postpartum cows can be a source of oocytes for IVF and repeated DFR/OPU applied during postpartum period did not affect the subsequent fertility following FTAI.

Vieira et al. (2014) evaluated the efficacy of superstimulation with p-FSH before OPU on IVEP in lactating and non-lactating Holstein donors. On a random day of the estrous cycle (day 0), all cows received an intravaginal progesterone device and estradiol benzoate (EB) (2.0 mg, i.m.). Cows in the p-FSH group received a total dosage of 200 mg of p-FSH on days 4 and 5 (in four decreasing doses 12 h apart). On day 7, the progesterone device was removed, and OPU was conducted in both groups (40 h after the last p-FSH injection in the p-FSH treated group). There was no difference between groups in the numbers of follicles that were aspirated per OPU session; however, p-FSH-treated cows had a higher percentage of medium-sized follicles (6–10 mm) at the time of the OPU (55.1%) than control cows (20.8%). Although RR was lower (60.0% *vs.* 69.8%), p-FSH-treated cows had a higher blastocyst production rate (34.5% *vs.* 19.8%) and more transferable embryos per OPU session were produced in the p-FSH group (3.0 ± 0.5 *vs.* 1.8 ± 0.4).

Two years later, this same group of authors (Vieira et al., 2016) evaluated the efficacy of a single injection of p-FSH (i.m.) in hyaluronan (HA) prior to OPU in Holstein cattle. Plasma FSH profiles, IVEP after OPU, and establishment of pregnancy with IVP embryos were compared in untreated Holstein oocyte donors and those superstimulated with multiple injections or a single injection of p-FSH in HA (200 or 300 mg p-FSH in 5 or 7.5 ml, respectively of a 0.5% HA). A greater proportion of medium-sized (6–10 mm) follicles were observed in cows receiving p-FSH, regardless of the treatment group. Also, numbers of follicles, COCs retrieved and matured cleavage rates and blastocysts produced per OPU session were greater in cows receiving p-FSH, regardless of the treatment group. Cows in 200 mg FSH group had a greater RR, number of COCs cultured, and blastocysts produced per OPU session than cows in the 300 mg FSH group. Similar pregnancy rates were observed 50–60 days after transferring IVP embryos from donors in the different treatment groups. They concluded that a single injection of p-FSH combined in 0.5% HA resulted in similar plasma FSH profiles as twice-daily p-FSH treatments. Treatment of non-lactating donors with p-FSH, with or without HA, resulted in increased IVEP over untreated controls. A single dose of 200 mg of p-FSH in 0.5% HA resulted in greater IVEP than 300 mg p-FSH in HA and finally, pregnancy rates with IVP embryos were similar, regardless donor treatment.

Some researchers have employed hormonal treatments to improve the ovarian follicular wave synchronization prior to OPU. In this way, Barboza da Silva et al. (2017) evaluated the effects of FSH treatment (200 mg p-FSH) on ovarian follicle stimulation and *in vitro* oocyte competence for IVEP in non-lactating Holstein cows with synchronized follicular wave emergence. On random days of the estrous cycle (day 0), received a progesterone (P4)-releasing intravaginal device and 2 mg of EB, and on day 3, 0.530 mg $PGF_2\alpha$. FSH was split in 4 or 6 administrations (day 4 or 3, respectively). On day 7 (36 h of "coasting" period for FSH-treated groups), the P4 devices were removed and cows were subjected to OPU. Although FSH treatment did not increase the total number of follicles, FSH4 and FSH6 hormonal stimulation regimens increased the number of medium follicles and reduced the number of small follicles. Also, FSH treatment did not increase the number of viable oocytes, RR and the number of IVP blastocyst. The authors concluding that FSH stimulation protocol proposed is effective to stimulate the growth of small antral follicle (6–10 mm) population prior to OPU, but it was ineffective to improve *in vitro* oocyte competence for IVEP in non-lactating Holstein cows with synchronized follicular wave emergence.

Cavalieri et al. (2017) also evaluated the effects of the synchronization of ovarian follicular wave emergence on the efficiency of OPU/IVEP in Nelore (*B. indicus*) cows. However, they concluded that synchronization of the follicular wave prior to OPU showed positive effects on IVEP as well as on pregnancy rates. Animals in the synchronization group received a protocol-based progesterone implant, EB and $PGF_2\alpha$ on a random day of the estrous cycle (day 0) and the OPU was performed on day 5. After IVEP, embryos were transferred to recipients synchronized at a fixed time. An evaluation of the parameters for each OPU session revealed that donors that received the synchronization protocol pre-OPU showed a greater number of embryos (5.9 ± 0.5 *vs*. 4.5 ± 0.4), higher rate of embryo production (45.8% *vs*. 38.5%) and higher mean number of conceptions per group (2.2 ± 0.2 *vs*. 1.6 ± 0.2) in relation to the group that did not receive hormonal treatment.

Recently, some authors in Japan have evaluated the effect of EB (1 mg, one single injection) at luteal phase prior to OPU during IVP of transferable embryos in Japanese Black cattle (Hidaka et al., 2018). The number and proportion of medium-sized follicles (4–6 mm) increased gradually and achieved a peak 72–96 h after EB injection. The OPU was performed 88 h after EB treatment. The stimulation with EB significantly increased the number of follicles aspirated, and good quality COCs. Furthermore, the percentage of transferable embryos was significantly greater than in control group. But nevertheless, we must remember that estradiol (EB) is forbidden in EU countries and in future dates it will be in some countries of South America, like Chile or Argentina.

6.5.2.7   CLIMATE AND SEASON

The influence of temperature and climate during the bovine follicle formation and development may also interfere with oocyte quality and embryonic development. Heat stress suppresses follicular dominance, causing follicle growth-related changes (Qi et al., 2013). Zeron et al. (2001) reported that the number of follicles 3–8 mm in diameter per ovary was higher in winter (19.6) compared with summer (12.0) and 7.5 oocytes per ovary were found in winter and 5.0 oocytes per ovary in summer after aspiration of follicles.

Bos indicus cattle have shown better reproductive performance than *B. taurus* in tropical and subtropical regions. This adaptation may involve different mechanisms. A severe decrease in the quality of Holstein cow oocytes was observed in the warmer season compared to the cold season, whereas no differences were detected in the oocytes obtained from Brahman cows (*B. indicus*) in different seasons (Rocha et al., 1998). On the other hand, lymphocytes of Brahman and Senepol cows were less susceptible to apoptosis induced by the heat, suggesting a mechanism of protection of cells in *B. indicus* animals (Paula-Lopes et al., 2003). Some of these mechanisms are shock proteins thermal type chaperones (HSP), which promote cellular protection against damage by heat, avoiding the denaturation of proteins and the blocking of apoptosis. The transcription of these HSPs increases during thermal shock, which may be an indicator of stress in bovine embryos (reviewed by De Ondiz and Ruiz, 2011).

Camargo et al. (2007) analyzed and quantified the relative expression of the protein Hsp 70.1 in immature oocytes, obtained by OPU, of Holstein cows and Gyr by real-time PCR after reverse transcription. The rate of embryonic division was higher for Gyr cows than in Holstein cows and blastocyst production was 19.6% compared to 10.8%, respectively, although the pregnancy rates were not statistically different after the transfer to the receptors. The immature Holstein oocytes had a higher relative expression level of Hsp 70.1 than the oocytes obtained from Gyr cows. In conclusion, oocytes obtained from Gyr cows in a tropical region were less susceptible to heat stress and more favorable to development after IVF, than Holstein oocytes.

6.6   OTHER USES OF OPU IN CATTLE

OPU can be used as a tool for interfering with follicle dynamics in order to advance our knowledge in its regulatory mechanisms and for technology or therapeutic purposes. Also, OPU has been employed as a source of oocytes for research purposes and as an implement in reproductive biotechnology for the recovery and conservation of endangered bovine breeds; moreover, OPU is an extraordinary source of oocytes for cloning and transgenesis.

The continuous application of OPU twice-weekly doubles the frequency of follicular waves, which becomes uncoupled from the estrous cycle because of inhibition of ovulation. In addition, the absence of a CL avoids interference of the progesterone on follicle growth. This particular condition together with the removal of each follicle larger than 2 mm makes easier to study either the growth or the replacement of follicles (Boni, 2012).

Viana et al. (2010) evaluated ovarian follicular dynamics during intervals between successive OPU and determined its effects on the number and quality of recovered COCs in Gyr cows (*B. indicus*), finding that, repeated follicle aspirations altered ovarian follicular dynamics, that follicular dominance could be established in cows undergoing twice-a-week OPU; and that the presence of a dominant follicle not affect COC quality, except when a codominant follicle was present.

OPU can be used to eliminate the deleterious effect of the presence of a dominant follicle during superovulation in cows, by puncturing the dominant follicle 38–46 h prior to superovulatory treatment (Merton et al., 2003). The OPU application efficiently resets the >2 mm diameter follicular population to zero which in effect guarantees that the new population will be uniformly renewed with less atresia (Boni, 2012).

Torres-Júnior et al. (2008) used OPU to find that long-term exposure of Gyr cows (*B. indicus*) to heat-stress had a delayed deleterious effect on ovarian follicular dynamics and oocyte competence. Following a 28 days' experimental period of heat stress, cows had longer periods of noncyclic activity, as well as shorter estrous cycles, the diameter of the dominant and double-dominant follicles as well as the number of follicles >9 mm in diameter, characterized as follicular codominance, significantly increased.

OPU can have its own therapeutic effect on infertile donors, especially those affected by ovarian cysts. Virtually, all empty donors come on cycle within 2 weeks from the last oocyte collection and can be inseminated successfully (Galli et al., 2001).

Lievaart et al. (2006) treated follicular cyst problems in cows by single transvaginal-guided needle aspiration. After aspiration, 82.1% of the cows showed estrous behavior at 13.3 ± 6.0 days, and the animals were inseminated during the first heat after cyst aspiration with a pregnancy rate of 64.2%. They concluded that single transvaginal-guided needle aspiration of ovarian follicular cysts is an easy and good method for the treatment of follicular cysts; moreover, it is a safe and good alternative method for the manual, active rupturing of cysts during rectal palpation.

OPU has been used as a source of oocytes for studies of IVF (Ruiz et al., 2009; 2013a) or IVEP with sex sorted semen (Pontes et al., 2010; Presicce et al., 2011), *in vitro* embryo production after IVF with frozen-thawed, sex-sorted, re-frozen-thawed bull sperm (Underwood et al., 2010) or using sexed sperm from previously frozen doses (reverse-sorted semen) (Morotti et al., 2014).

Some researchers have employed the OPU technique as a tool together another reproductive biotechnology for the recovery and conservation of endangered bovine breeds (Ruiz et al., 2013b).

Finally, special modifications of OPU have been used to collect ovarian tissue for primary follicle isolation (Aerts et al., 2005).

6.7 DONOR HEALTH: OPU SEQUELAE

During ultrasound-guided oocyte collection, cattle undergo repeated restraint, transrectal palpation, introduction of an intravaginal device, epidural anesthesia and repeated ovarian punctures. Among these manipulations, transrectal palpation and introduction of an intravaginal device, commonly practiced by veterinarians and inseminators, have been shown to induce moderate stress. Epidural anesthesia is a less common practice. However, even repeated associated lesions seem minor and occur in only a few animals. The most questionable aspect of OPU is the multiple transvaginal and transovarian punctures, which constitute the more invasive and the most specific part of the OPU.

The animals subjected to follicular puncture must be evaluated periodically to monitor for the likely procedure-related consequences. Perforation of the vaginal fornix with or without transient irritation of the vagina and cervix is repeatedly one such consequence and the vaginal drilling points can be identified up to 48–72 h post-puncture (reviewed by Da Silva et al., 2016). Bruising in the perivaginal region is also seem, but this consequence seems not to cause major damage to the donor (Viana et al., 2003).

Sequelae noted in the ovaries can indicate significant changes in consistency and or mobility. Ovarian perforation can cause the appearance of adhesions and fibrosis, particularly in cows that are subjected to multiple consecutive puncture sessions, through a prolonged period. It is important to consider the impact of technical variables and the operator' ability to prevent the occurrence of such lesions (reviewed by Da Silva et al., 2016).

Kruip et al. (1994) conducted one experience to examine the efficacy of transvaginal ultrasound-guided puncturing of ovarian follicles for collecting immature oocytes in cattle. They checked daily the health of the cows punctured. The results did not differ between the months of the experiments, indicating that the transvaginal puncturing method can be used successfully over a 5 mo period. Moreover, no detrimental effects were observed after clinical and postmortem examinations, nor did breed, age or reproductive status appear to affect the results.

Viana et al. (2003) evaluated lesions of the genital tract in animals used in different experiments involving OPU technique. The cows evaluated underwent 9–42 puncture sessions with a low prevalence of inflammatory changes in the vagina mucosa. Histopathologic evaluation revealed scar tissue, inflammatory cell infiltration, and presence of luteal tissue dispersed within the ovarian stroma.

Chastant-Maillard et al. (2003) evaluated the impact of repeated follicular puncture used in OPU technique on the welfare of cows. The evaluation relies on the physiological measurement of stress, milk production criteria, immune status, and the histological examination of ovaries. Although the blood cortisol concentrations increased after each session, concentrations were the same in both the control and the punctured groups. The transvaginal puncture did not affect milk production, or blood and milk somatic cell counts. Histological examination of the ovaries 4 days after puncture revealed blood-filled follicles and hemorrhagic foci in ovarian stroma, but the 30-day examination after the last puncture session demonstrated very limited, if any, fibrosis. They concluded that repeated transvaginal follicular puncture on its own did not impact adversely on the welfare of cows.

Finally, Peytim et al. (2007) studied the effects of OPU technique on animal well-being during 4 months of twice-weekly OPU. They measured heart rates and cortisol, vasopressin, and prostaglandin metabolite in blood, as well as reactions to each sub-procedure of OPU ('restraint', 'epidural', 'device in' and 'puncture'); changes in routine behavior, estrous behavior, body temperature, or other clinical traits were recorded. Although there was an insignificant increase in heart rate and cortisol throughout the OPU procedure, both parameters declined to pre-OPU levels 10 min after completion of the procedure. No significant changes were seen in vasopressin or PG-metabolite. Behaviorally, the heifers showed the strongest response to epidural anesthesia, with a tendency for more intense response during the late 4-month sessions. There were no changes in the routine or estrous behavior throughout the experiment and no signs of clinical disorders. No major pathological changes were macroscopically seen in the ovaries and tails subsequent to OPU during 4 mo. They concluded that the heifers showed a response to OPU, mostly to administration of epidural anesthesia; however, this experience has been shown that epidural anesthesia can be administered in a way causing less discomfort (Peytim et al., 2007).

Follicular aspiration is a technique with pros and cons. The risk of sequelae must be considered. The procedure must be performed carefully to minimize the possible damage that allows the results to outweigh the expected results (Da Silva et al., 2016).

6.8   OPU IN BUFFALOES

Some countries are very interested in the reproduction biotechnologies in buffaloes as Italy, Argentina, China, India, etc. (Galli et al., 2001; Liang et al., 2008; Manjunatha et al., 2008; Galli et al., 2014; Konrad et al., 2017). In the buffalo, OPU has great potential because MOET programs have given poor results compared with those in cattle (Carvalho et al., 2002), and it has never made an impact on buffalo breeding programs, both because of the limited number of embryos that can be recovered and also because of the low survival after cryopreservation (reviewed by Galli et al., 2014). Because of these limits, the OPU technology has always been of great interest also in buffalo breeding.

The procedure is performed exactly in the same way as in cows. Oocyte recovery, embryo production, and offspring obtained have been described in several publications (Galli et al., 2001; Neglia et al., 2011; Konrad et al., 2017) but only about 10–15% of the oocytes recovered develop to transferable embryos (Galli et al., 2014).

In general, the ovaries of buffalo cows and heifers are small; in addition, the follicles tend to be fewer and of small diameter. Therefore, few follicles are available for OPU and the follicular population is influenced by the seasonality reported in the buffalo (Neglia et al., 2011; Di Francesco et al., 2012).

Gonadotrophin stimulation might be beneficial (Presicce et al., 2002; Gimenes et al., 2015) for increasing the small size and paucity of follicles found especially in anestrous donors.

Because of the great value of the female offspring in buffalo herds, the combination of OPU with sexed semen (Liang et al., 2008) and cryopreservation offer the opportunity to accelerate the genetic gain in the buffalo industry (reviewed by Galli et al., 2014).

6.9 OPU/IVEP IN THE FUTURE

The bovine genome is being sequenced and bovine genes for traits of economic interest becoming totally available in few years. OPU/IVEP will prove invaluable in rapidly multiplying rare genes or Quantitative Trait Loci (QTL) of high value. This will require a cost effective and efficient methods for embryo biopsy and genotyping that allow Marker Assisted Selection or Gene Assisted Selection (MAS/GAS) at the embryo level (Bredbacka, 2001). OPU/IVEP is being used for breeding of bulls with the desired genes/QTL that code for animal productivity traits such as health and fertility and more importantly for cow herd population in the case of genes for milk composition traits. Juvenile OPU/IVEP will further accelerate gene dissemination as will have sexed semen and embryo cloning. The MAS/GAS schemes, in combination with sib testing, may, partially, replace conventional progeny testing schemes and provide opportunities for customizing animals to different markets. MAS/GAS is already applied at several places in the world, and it can be applied to either reduce the size of the progeny testing scheme and maintain the same level of genetic gain or increase genetic gain at the same level of progeny testing (van Wagtendonk-de Leeuw, 2006).

It is recognized that OPU, and particularly IVEP, provide the basis for more advanced technologies such as cloning and transgenesis (Ding et al., 2008), which are believed to have limited scope due to low efficiencies and animal welfare and public perception issues. This limited scope is likely to remain, until the first convincing examples of positive uses are presented, possibly first from areas outside the farming industry such as the medical or pharmaceutical industry (reviewed by van Wagtendonk-de Leeuw, 2006).

Also, Assisted Reproductive Technologies (ARTs) such as MOET, OPU/IVEP, intracytoplasmic sperm injection (ICSI), cloning by somatic cell nuclear transfer (SCNT) and transgenesis involve several steps that may exert environmental stress on gametes and early embryos. Therefore, there is growing interest in the putative link between these techniques and epigenetic modifications that promote changes in gene expression profiles and might result in developmental disorders. Researchers have been targeting a better understanding of the epigenetic mechanisms and the opportunity of manipulating events, in order to improve the efficiency of ARTs. The current knowledge about epigenetic influence on gametes, embryos and fetus allowed us to view the reproductive process from a new angle. Although the exact time and concentration of some gene products and its specific sites in the genome are already clarify, we are far from fully understanding epigenetic control of reproduction (reviewed by Franco et al., 2016).

6.10 CONCLUDING REMARKS

OPU and IVEP can both be considered mature technologies by now. Obtaining oocytes through *in vivo* follicular aspiration is only the first step of *in vitro* embryo production. Once the oocytes are retrieved, their maturation, fertilization, and embryo development occur in specific IVEP laboratories. The main challenges for the further spread of OPU include the high equipment and the need for technical training. OPU is a livestock service tool. If used properly, it provides satisfactory results that correspond the expectations of the investment. However, if misused, it can cause damage in the donors. It is necessary for a careful analysis of each OPU/IVEP proposal for breeders, farmers and veterinarians as well to achieve the best results using this biotechnology. Although there will be a shift in application of OPU/IVEP over the next years from increasing selection intensity to rapid and smart gene dissemination, this technology has and will continue to make a significant contribution to the cattle industry.

KEYWORDS

- Aspiration of bovine ovarian follicles
- OPU equipment and procedure
- Factors influencing OPU
- OPU and *in vitro* embryo production
- OPU worldwide situation

REFERENCES

Aerts, J. M.; Oste, M.; Bols, P. E. J. Development and Practical Applications Of A Method For Repeated Transvaginal, Ultrasound-Guided Biopsy Collection of The Bovine Ovary. *Theriogenology* **2005**, *64*, 947–957.

Aller, J. F.; Mucci, N. C.; Kaiser, G. G.; Ríos, G.; Callejas, S. S.; Alberio, R. H. Transvaginal Follicular Aspiration and Embryo Development In Superstimulated Early Postpartum Beef Cows And Subsequent Fertility After Artificial Insemination. *Anim. Reprod. Sci.* **2010**, *119*, 1–8.

Barboza da Silva, J. C.; Ferreira, R. M.; Filho, M. M.; Naves, J. R.; Santin, T.; Pugliesi, G.; Madureira, E. H. Use Of FSH In Two Different Regimens For Ovarian Superstimulation Prior To *Ovum Pick Up* And *In Vitro* Embryo Production In Holstein Cows. *Theriogenology* **2017**, *90*, 65–73.

Batista, E. O. S.; Macedo, C. G.; Sala, R. V.; Ortolan, M. D. D. V.; Sá Filho, M. F.; Del Valle, T. A.; Jesus, E. F.; Lopes, R. N. V. R.; Renno F. P.; Baruselli, P. S. Plasma Antimullerian Hormone as a Predictor of Ovarian Antral Follicular Population in *B. indicus* (Nelore) and *B. taurus* (Holstein) Heifers. *Reprod. Dom. Anim.* **2014**, *49*, 448–452.

Becker, F.; Kanitz, W.; Nürnberg, G.; Kurth, J.; Spitschak, M. Comparison Of Repeated Transvaginal Ovum Pick-Up In Heifers By Ultrasonographic And Endoscopic Instruments. *Theriogenology* **1996**, *46*, 999–1007.

Blondin, P. Status Of Embryo Production In The World. *Anim. Reprod.* **2015**, *12*, 356–358.

Bols, P. E. J.; Vandenheede, J. M. M.; Van Soom, A.; de Kruif, A. Transvaginal Ovum Pick Up (OPU) In The Cow: A New Disposable Needle Guidance System. *Theriogenology* **1995**, *43*, 677–687.

Bols, P. E. J.; Van Soom, A.; Ysebaert, M. T.; Vandenheede, J. M. M.; de Kruif, A. Effects Of Aspiration Vacuum And Needle Diameter On *Cumulus* Oocyte Complex Morphology And Developmental Capacity Of Bovine Oocytes. *Theriogenology* **1996**, *45*, 1001–1014.

Bols, P. E. J.; Ysebaeti M. T.; Van Soom, A.; de Kruif, A. Effects Of Needle Tip Bevel And Aspiration Procedure On The Morphology And Developmental Capacity Of Bovine Compact *Cumulus* Oocyte Complexes. *Theriogenology* **1997**, *47*, 1221–1236.

Bols, P. E. J.; Leroy, J. L.; Vanholder, T.; Van Soom, A. A Comparison Of A Mechanical Sector And A Linear Array Transducer For Ultrasound-Guided Transvaginal Oocyte Retrieval (OPU) In The Cow. *Theriogenology* **2004**, *62*, 906–914.

Bols, P. E. J.; Stout, T. A. E. Transvaginal Ultrasound-Guided Oocyte Retrieval (OPU: Ovum Pick-Up) in Cows and Mares. In *Animal Biotechnology 1: Reproductive Biotechnologies;* Niemann, H.; Wrenzycki, C., Eds.; Springer: Cham, **2018**; pp 209–234.

Boni, R. Ovum Pick-Up In Cattle: A 25 Yr Retrospective Analysis. *Anim. Reprod.* **2012**, *9*, 362–369.

Bousquet. D.; Twagiramungu, H.; Morin, N.; Brisson, C.; Carboneau, G.; Durocher, J. *In Vitro* Embryo Production In The Cow: An Effective Alternative To The Conventional Embryo Production Approach. *Theriogenology* **1999**, *51*, 59–70.

Bredbacka, P. Progress On Methods Of Gene Detection In Preimplantation Embryos. *Theriogenology* **2001**, *55*, 23–34.

Bungartz, L.; Lucas-Hahn, A.; Rath, D.; Niemann, H. Collection Of Oocytes From Cattle Via Follicular Aspiration Aided By Ultrasound With Or Without Gonadotropin Pretreatment And In Different Reproductive Stages. *Theriogenology* **1995**, *43*, 667–675.

Callesen, H.; Greve, T.; Christensen, F. Ultrasonically Guided Aspiration Of Bovine Follicular Oocytes. *Theriogenology* **1987**, *27*, 217.

Camargo, L. S. A.; Viana, J. H. M.; Ramos, A. A; Serapião, R. V.; de Sa, W. F.; Ferreira A. M.; Guimarães M. F. M.; do Vale Filho, V. R. Developmental Competence And Expression Of The Hsp 70.1 Gene In Oocytes Obtained From *B. Indicus* And *B. Taurus* Dairy Cows In A Tropical Environment. *Theriogenology* **2007**, *68*, 626–632.

Carvalho, N. A.; Baruselli, P. S.; Zicarelli, L.; Madureira, E. H.; Visintin, J. A.; D'Occhio, M. J. Control Of Ovulation With A GnRH Agonist After Superstimulation Of Follicular Growth In Buffalo: Fertilization And Embryo Recovery. *Theriogenology* **2002**, *58*, 1641–1650.

Cavalieri, F. L. B.; Morotti, F.; Seneda, M. M.; Colombo, A. H. B.; Andreazzi, M. A.; Emanuelli, I. P.; Rigolon, L. P. Improvement Of Bovine *In Vitro* Embryo Production By Ovarian Follicular Wave Synchronization Prior To Ovum Pick-Up. *Theriogenology* **2018**, *117*, 57–60.

Chastant-Maillard, S.; Quinton, H.; Lauffenburger, J.; Cordonnier-Lefort, N.; Richard, C.; Marchal, J.; Mormede P.; Renard, J. P. Consequences Of Transvaginal Follicular Puncture On Well-Being In Cows. *Reproduction* **2003**, *125*, 555–563.

Chaubal, S. A.; Molina, J. A.; Ohlrichs, C. L.; Ferre, L. B.; Faber, D. C.; Bols, P. E. J.; Riesen, J. W. X.; Tian, X.; Yang, X. Comparison Of Different Transvaginal Ovum Pick-Up Protocols To Optimise Oocyte Retrieval And Embryo Production Over A 10-Week Period In Cows. *Theriogenology* **2006**, *65*, 1631–1648.

Chaubal, S. A.; Ferre, L. B.; Molina, J. A.; Faber, D. C.; Bols, P. E. J.; Rezamand, P.; Tian, X.; Yang, X. Hormonal Treatments For Increasing The Oocyte And Embryo Production In An OPU-IVP System. *Theriogenology* **2007**, *67*, 719–728.

Da Silva, C. B.; Machado, F. Z.; González S. M.; Seneda, M. M. Ovum Pick-Up. In *Recent Trends in Biotechnology. Biotechnology of Animal Reproduction;* Seneda, M.M.; Silva-Santos, K.C.; Marinho, L.S.R., Eds.; Nova Science Publishers: New York, **2016**; pp 157–169.

Dellenbach, P.; Nisand, I.; Moreau, L.; Feger, B.; Plumere, C.; Gerlinger, P.; Brun, B.; Rumpler, Y. Transvaginal Sonographically Controlled Ovarian Follicle Puncture For Egg Retrieval. *Lancet* **1984**, *1*, 1467.

De Ondiz, A.; Ruiz, S. *Aspiración folicular transvaginal guiada por ultrasonografía (OPU), producción in vitro de embriones (PIV) y semen sexado en la reproducción bovina.* In *Innovación y Tecnologías en la ganadería doble propósito;* González-Stagnaro, C.; Madrid, N.; Soto, E., Eds.; Astrodata: Maracaibo, **2011**; pp 797–805.

De Roover, R.; Genicot, G.; Leonarda, S.; Bols, P. E. J.; Dessy, F. Ovum Pick Up And *In Vitro* Production In Cows Superstimulated With An Individually Adapted Superstimulation Protocol. *Anim. Reprod. Sci.* **2005**, *86*, 13–25.

De Roover, R.; Feugang, J. M. N.; Bols, P. E. J.; Genicot, G.; Hanzen, C. Effects of Ovum Pick-Up Frequency and FSH Stimulation: A Retrospective Study on Seven Years of Beef Cattle *In Vitro* Embryo Production. *Reprod. Dom. Anim.* **2008**, *43*, 239–245.

Dewailly, D.; Andersen, C.Y; Balen, A.; Broekmans, F.; Dilaver, N.; Fanchin, R.; Griesinger, G.; Kelsey, T. W.; La Marca, A.; Lambalk, C.; Mason, H.; Nelson, S. M.; Visser, J. A.; Wallace, W. H.; Anderson, R. A. The Physiology And Clinical Utility Of Anti-Mullerian Hormone In Women. *Hum. Reprod. Update* **2014**, *20*, 370–385.

Di Francesco, S.; Suarez Novo, M. V.; Vecchio, D.; Neglia, G.; Boccia, L.; Campanile, G.; Zicarelli, L.; Gasparrini, B. Ovum Pick-Up And *In Vitro* Embryo Production (OPU-IVEP) In Mediterranean Italian Buffalo Performed In Different Seasons. *Theriogenology* **2012**, *77*, 148–154.

Ding, L. J.; Tian, H. B.; Wang, J. J.; Chen, J.; Sha, H. Y.; Chen, J. Q.; Cheng, G. X. Different Intervals of Ovum Pick-Up Affect the competence of Oocytes to Support the Preimplantation Development of Cloned Bovine Embryos. *Mol. Reprod. Dev.* **2008**, *75*, 1710–1715.

Figueiredo, R. A.; Barros, C. M.; Pinheiro, O. L.; Sole, J. M. P. Ovarian Follicular Dynamics In Nelore Breed (*Bos Indicus*) Cattle. *Theriogenology* **1997**, *47*, 1489–1505.

Franco, M. M.; Marinho, L. S. R.; Lunardelli, P. A. Epigenetic modifications and their roles in Animal Reproduction. In *Recent Trends in Biotechnology. Biotechnology of Animal Reproduction;* Seneda, M. M.; Silva-Santos, K. C.; Marinho, L. S. R., Eds.; Nova Science Publishers: New York, **2016**; pp 315–341.

Galli, C.; Crotti, G.; Notari, C.; Turini, P.; Duchi, R.; Lazzari, G. Embryo Production By Ovum Pick Up From Live Donors. *Theriogenology* **2001**, *55*, 1341–1357.

Galli, C.; Duchi R.; Colleoni S.; Lagutina, I.; Lazzari, G. Ovum Pick Up, Intracytoplasmic Sperm Injection And Somatic Cell Nuclear Transfer In Cattle, Buffalo And Horses: From The Research Laboratory To Clinical Practice. *Theriogenology* **2014**, *81*, 138–151.

Gimenes, L. U.; Ferraz, M. L.; Fantinato-Neto, P.; Chiaratti, M. R.; Mesquita, L. G.; Sá Filho, M. F.; Meirelles, F. V.; Trinca, L. A.; Rennó, F. P.; Watanabe, Y. F.; Baruselli, P. S. The Interval Between The Emergence Of Pharmacologically Synchronized Ovarian Follicular Waves And Ovum Pickup Does Not Significantly Affect *In Vitro* Embryo

Production In *B. Indicus*, *B. Taurus*, And *Bubalus Bubalis*. *Theriogenology* **2015**, *83*, 385–393.

Guerreiro, B. M.; Batista, E. O. S.; Vieira, L. M.; Sá Filho, M. F.; Rodrigues, C. A.; Castro Netto, A.; Silveira, C. R. A.; Bayeux, B. M.; Dias, E. A. R.; Monteiro, F. M.; Accorsi, M.; Lopes, R. N. V. R.; Baruselli, P. S. Plasma Anti-Mullerian Hormone: An Endocrine Marker For *In Vitro* Embryo Production From *B. Taurus* And *B. Indicus* Donors. *Domest. Anim. Endocrinol.* **2014**, *49*, 96–104.

Goodhand, K. L.; Watt, R. G.; Staines, M. E.; Hutchinson, J. S.; Broadbent, P. J. *In Vivo* Oocyte Recovery And *In Vitro* Embryo Production From Bovine Donors Aspirated At Different Frequencies Or Following FSH Treatment. *Theriogenology* **1999**, *51*, 951–961.

Goodhand, K. L.; Staines, M. E.; Hutchinson, J. S. M.; Broadbent, P. J. *In Vivo* Oocyte Recovery And *In Vitro* Embryo Production From Bovine Oocyte Donors Treated With Progestagen, Oestradiol And FSH. *Anim. Reprod. Sci.* **2000**, *63*, 145–158.

Hidaka, T.; Fukumoto, Y.; Yamamoto, Y.; Ogata, Y.; Horiuchi, T. Estradiol Benzoate Treatment Before Ovum Pick-Up Increases The Number Of Good Quality Oocytes Retrieved And Improves The Production Of Transferable Embryos In Japanase Black Cattle. *Vet. Anim. Sci.* **2018**, *5*, 1–6.

Jin, J. I.; Ghanem, N.; Kim, S. S.; Choi, B. H.; Ha, A. N.; Lee K. L.; Sun D. W.; Lim, H. T.; Lee, J. G.; Kong, I. K. Interaction of donor age, parity and repeated recovery of *cumulus*-oocyte complexes by ovum pick-up on *in vitro* embryo production and viability after transfer. *Lives. Sci.* **2016**, *188*, 43–47.

Kendrick, K. W.; Bailey, T. L.; Garst, A. S.; Pryor, A. W.; Ahmadzadeh, A.; Akers, R. M.; Eyestone, W. E.; Pearson, R. E.; Gwazdauskas, F. C. Effects Of Energy Balance On Hormones, Ovarian Activity And Recovered Oocytes In Lactating Holstein Cows Using Transvaginal Follicular Aspiration. *J. Dairy Sci.* **1999**, *82*, 1731–1740.

Konrad, J.; Clérico, G.; Garrido, M. J.; Taminelli, G.; Yuponi, M.; Yuponi, R.; Crudeli, G.; Sansinena, M. Ovum Pick-Up Interval In Buffalo (*Bubalus Bubalis*) Managed Under Wetland Conditions In Argentina: Effect On Follicular Population, Oocyte Recovery, And *In Vitro* Embryo Development. *Anim. Reprod. Sci.* **2017**, *183*, 39–45.

Kruip, T. A. M.; Boni, R.; Wurth, Y. A.; Roelofsen, M. W.; Pieterse, M. C. Potential Use Of Ovum Pick-Up For Embryo Production And Breeding In Cattle. *Theriogenology* **1994**, *42*, 675–684.

Lambert, R. D.; Bernard, C.; Rioux, J. E.; Béland, R.; D'Amours, D.; Montreuil, A. Endoscopy In Cattle By The Paralumbar Route: Technique For Ovarian Examination And Follicular Aspiration. *Theriogenology* **1983**, *20*, 149–161.

Lenz, S.; Lauritsen, J. G. Ultrasonically Guided Percutaneous Aspiration Of Human Follicles Under Local Anesthesia: A New Method Of Collecting Oocytes For *In Vitro* Fertilization. *Fert. Steril.* **1982**, *38*, 673–677.

Liang, X. W.; Lu, Y. Q.; Chen, M. T.; Zhang, X. F.; Lu, S. S.; Zhang, M.; Pang, C. Y.; Huang, F. X.; Lu, K. H. *In Vitro* Embryo Production In Buffalo (*Bubalus Bubalis*) Using Sexed Sperm And Oocytes From Ovum Pick Up. *Theriogenology* **2008**, *69*, 822–826.

Lievaart, J. J.; Parlevliet, J. M.; Dieleman, S. J.; Rientjes, S.; B.man, E.; Vos, P. L. Transvaginal Aspiration As First Treatment Of Ovarian Follicular Cysts In Dairy Cattle Under Field Circumstances. *Tijdschr. Diergeneeskd.* **2006**, *131*, 438–442.

Lopes, A. S.; Matinusen, T.; Greve, T.; Callesen, H. Effect Of Days Postpartum, Breed And Ovum Pick-Up Scheme On Bovine Oocyte Recovery And Embryo Development. *Reprod. Dom. Anim.* **2006**, *41*, 196–203.

Manjunatha, B. M.; Ravindra, J. P.; Gupta, P. S. P.; Devaraj, M.; Nandi, S. Oocyte Recovery by Ovum Pick Up and Embryo Production in River Buffaloes (*Bubalus bubalis*). *Reprod. Dom. Anim.* **2008**, *43*, 477–480.

Majerus, V.; De Roover, R.; Etienne, D.; Kaidi, S.; Massip, A.; Dessy, F.; Donnay, I. Embryo Production By OPU In Unstimulated Calves Before And After Puberty. *Theriogenology* **1999**, *52*, 1169–1179.

Merton, J. S.; de Roos, A. P. W.; Mullaart, E.; de Ruigh, L.; Kaal, L. Vos, P. L. A. M.; Dieleman, S. J. Factors Affecting Oocyte Quality And Quantity In Commercial Application Of Embryo Technologies In The Cattle Breeding Industry. *Theriogenology* **2003**, *59*, 651–674.

Merton, J. S.; Ask, B.; Onkundi, D. C.; Mullaart, E.; Colenbrander, B.; Nielen, M. Genetic Parameters For Oocyte Number And Embryo Production Within A Bovine Ovum Pick-Up-*In Vitro* Production Embryo-Production Program. *Theriogenology* **2009**, *72*, 885–893.

Mikkola, M. In *Commercial Embryo Transfer Activity in Europe 2018*, Proceedings of the 35th Annual Meeting Association of Embryo Technology in Europe (AETE), Murcia, Spain, Sept 13–14, **2019**; pp 23-28.

Monniaux, D.; Barbey, S.; Rico, C.; Fabre, S.; Gallard, Y.; Larroque, H. Anti-Müllerian hormone: a predictive marker of embryo production in cattle? *Reprod. Fertil. Dev.* **2010**, *22*, 1083–1091.

Monniaux, D.; Drouilhet, L.; Rico, C.; Estienne, A.; Jarrier, P.; Touzé, J. L.; Sapa, J.; Phocas, F.; Dupont, J.; Dalbiès-Tran, R.; Fabre, S. Regulation Of Anti-Müllerian Hormone Production In Domestic Animals. *Reprod. Fertil. Dev.* **2012**, *25*, 1–16.

Monteiro, F. M.; Batista, E. O. S.; Vieira, L. M.; Bayeux, B. M.; Accorsi, M.; Campanholi, S. P.; Dias, E. A. R.; Souza, A. H.; Baruselli, P. S. Beef Donor Cows With High Number Of Retrieved COC Produce More *In Vitro* Embryos Compared With Cows With Low Number Of COC After Repeated Ovum Pick-Up Sessions. *Theriogenology* **2017**, *90*, 54–58.

Morotti, F.; Sanches, B. V.; Pontes, J. H. F.; Basso, A. C.; Siqueira, E. R.; Lisboa, L. A.; Seneda, M. M. Pregnancy Rate And Birth Rate Of Calves From A Large-Scale IVF Program Using Reverse-Sorted Semen In *B. Indicus*, *B. Indicus-Taurus*, And *B. Taurus* Cattle. *Theriogenology* **2014**, *81*, 696–701.

Neglia, G.; Gasparrini, B.; Vecchio, D., Boccia, L.; Varricchio E.; Di Palo, R.; Zicarelli, L.; Campanile, G. Long Term Effect Of Ovum Pick-Up In Buffalo Species. *Anim. Reprod. Sci.* **2011**, *123*, 180–186.

Oropeza, A.; Wrenzycki, C.; Herrmann, D.; Hadeler, K. G.; Nieman, H. Improvement Of The Developmental Capacity Of Oocytes From Prepubertal Cattle By Intraovarian Insulin-Like Growth Factor-I Application. *Biol. Reprod.* **2004**, *70*, 1634–1643.

Paula-Lopes, F. F.; Chase, C. C.; Al-Katanani, Y. M.; Krininger, C. E.; Rivera, R. M.; Tekin, S.; Majewski, A. C.; Ocon, O. M.; Olson, T. A.; Hansen, P. J. Genetic Divergence In Cellular Resistance To Heat Shock In Cattle: Differences Between Breeds Developed In Temperate Versus Hot Climates In Responses Of Preimplantation Embryos, Reproductive Tract Tissues And Lymphocytes To Increased Culture Temperatures. *Reproduction* **2003**, *125*, 285.

Perez, O.; Richard, R.; Green, H. L.; Young, C. R.; Godke, R. A. Ultrasound-Guided Transvaginal Oocyte Recovery From FSH-Treated Post-Partum Beef Cows. *Theriogenology* **2000**, *53*, 364.

Perry, G. 2016 Statistics of Embryo Collection and Transfer in Domestic Farm Animals. *26th Annual Report*. 2017. International Embryo Transfer Society (IETS). pp 1–16.

Petyim, S.; Båge R.; Hallap, T.; Bergqvist, A. S.; Rodríguez-Martínez, H.; Larsson, B. Two Different Schemes Of Twice-Weekly Ovum Pick-Up In Dairy Heifers: Effect On Oocyte Recovery And Ovarian Function. *Theriogenology* **2003**, *60*, 175–188.

Petyim, S.; Båge R.; Madej, A.; Larsson, B. Ovum Pick-up in Dairy Heifers: Does it Affect Animal Well-being? *Reprod. Dom. Anim.* **2007**, *42*, 623–632.

Pieterse, M. C.; Kappen, K. A.; Kruip, T. A. M.; Taverne, M. A. M. Aspiration Of Bovine Oocytes During Transvaginal Ultrasound Scanning Of The Ovaries. *Theriogenology* **1988**, *30*, 751–762.

Pieterse, M. C.; Vos, P. L. A. M.; Kruip, T. A. M.; Willemse, A. H.; Taverne, M. A. M. Characteristics Of Bovine Estrous Cycles During Repeated Transvaginal, Ultrasound-Guided Puncturing Of Follicles For Ovum Pick-Up. *Theriogenology* **1991**, *35*, 401–413.

Pontes, J. H. F.; Nonato-Junior, I.; Sanches, B. V.; Ereno-Junior, J. C.; Uvoa, S.; Barreiros, T. R. R.; Oliveira, J. A.; Hasler, J. F.; Seneda, M. M. Comparison Of Embryo Yield And Pregnancy Rate Between *In Vivo* And *In Vitro* Methods In The Same Nelore (*B. Indicus*) Donor Cows. *Theriogenology* **2009**, *71*, 690–697.

Pontes, J. H. F.; Silva, K. C.; Basso, A. C.; Rigo, A. G.; Ferreira, C. R.; Santos, G. M.; Sanches, B. V.; Porcionato, J. P.; Vieira, P. H.; Faifer, F. S.; Sterza, F. A.; Schenk, J. L.; Seneda, M. M. Large-Scale *In Vitro* Embryo Production And Pregnancy Rates From *Bos Taurus, Bos Indicus,* And *Indicus-Taurus* Dairy Cows Using Sexed Sperm. *Theriogenology* **2010**, *74*, 1349–1355.

Pontes, J. H. F.; Melo Sterza, F. A.; Basso, A. C.; Ferreira, C. R.; Sanches, B. V.; Rubin, K. C. P.; Seneda, M. M. Ovum Pick Up, *In Vitro* Embryo Production, And Pregnancy Rates From A Large-Scale Commercial Program Using Nelore Cattle (*B. Indicus*) Donors. *Theriogenology* **2011**, *75*, 1640–1646.

Presicce, G. A.; Jiang, S.; Simkin, M.; Zhang, L.; Looney, C. R.; Godke, R. A.; Yang, X. Age And Hormonal Dependence Of Acquisition Of Oocyte Competence For Embryogenesis In Prepubertal Calves. *Biol. Reprod.* **1997**, *56*, 386–392.

Presicce, G. A.; Senatore, E. M.; De Santis, G.; Stecco, R.; Terzano, G. M.; Borghese, A.; De Mauro, G. J. Hormonal Stimulation And Oocyte Maturational Competence In Prepuberal Mediterranean Italian Buffaloes (*Bubalus Bubalis*). *Theriogenology* **2002**, *57*, 1877–1884.

Presicce, G. A.; Xu, J.; Gong, G.; Moreno, J. F.; Chaubal, S.; Xue, F.; Bella, A.; Senatore, E. M.; Yang, X.; Tian X. C.; Du, F. Oocyte Source and Hormonal Stimulation for *In Vitro* Fertilization Using Sexed Spermatozoa in Cattle. *Vet. Med. Int.* **2011**, *26*, 1–8.

Qi, M.; Yao, Y.; Ma, H.; Wang, J.; Zhao, X.; Liu, L.; Tang, X.; Zhang, L.; Zhang, S.; Sun, F. Transvaginal Ultrasound-guided Ovum Pick-up (OPU) in Cattle. *J. Biomim. Biomater. Tissue Eng.* **2013**, *18*, 118.

Reichenbach, H. D.; Wiebke, N. H.; Modl, J.; Zhu, J.; Brem, G. Laparoscopy Through The Vaginal Fornix Of Cows For The Repeated Aspiration Of Follicular Oocytes. *Vet. Rec.* **1994**, *135*, 353–356.

Rico, C.; Drouilhet. L.; Salvetti, P.; Dalbiès-Tran, R.; Jarrier, P.; Touzé, J. L.; Pillet, E.; Ponsart, C.; Fabre, S.; Monniaux, D. Determination Of Anti-Müllerian Hormone Concentrations In Blood As A Tool To Select Holstein Donor Cows For Embryo Production: From The Laboratory To The Farm. *Reprod. Fertil. Dev.* **2012**, *24*, 932–944.

Rizos, D.; Burke, L.; Duffy, P.; Wade, M.; Mee J. F., O'Farrel, K. J.; Macsiurtain, M.; Boland, M. P.; Lonergan, P. Comparisons Between Nulliparous Heifers And Cows As Oocyte Donors For Embryo Production *In Vitro*. *Theriogenology* **2005**, *63*, 939–949.

Rocha, A.; Randel, R. D.; Broussard, J. R.; Lim, J. M.; Blair, R. M.; Roussel, J. D.; Godke, R. A.; Hansel, W. High Environmental Temperature And Humidity Decrease Oocyte Quality In *Bos Taurus* But Not In *Bos Indicus* Cows. *Theriogenology* **1998**, *49*, 657.

Ruiz, S.; Zaraza, J.; De Ondiz, A.; Rath, D. Early Fertilization Events in Bovine IVF Employing OPU-Oocytes and Sex-Sorted Frozen/Thawed Sperm. *Reprod. Dom. Anim.* **2009**, *44*, 123.

Ruiz, S. *Ovum Pick Up (OPU) en bovinos: Aplicaciones en Biotecnología de la Reproducción.* Cría y Salud. **2010**, *31*, 58–64.

Ruiz, S.; Camisao, J.; Zaraza, J.; De Ondiz, A.; Romero, J.; Rodrigues, R.; Rath, D. Use Of Sex-Sorted And Unsorted Frozen/Thawed Sperm And *In Vitro* Fertilization Events In Bovine Oocytes Derived From Ultrasound Guided Aspiration. *R. Bras. Zootec.* **2013a**, *42*, 721–727.

Ruiz, S.; Romero, J.; Astiz, S.; Peinado, B.; Almela, L.; Poto, A. Application Of Reproductive Biotechnology For The Recovery Of Endangered Breeds: Birth Of The First Calf Of Murciana-Levantina Bovine Breed Derived By OPU, *In Vitro* Production And Embryo Vitrification. *Reprod. Dom. Anim.* **2013b**, *48*, 81–84.

Santl, B.; Wenigerkind, H.; Schernthaner, W.; Modl, J.; Stojkovic, M.; Prelle, K.; Holtz, W.; Brem, G.; Wolf, E. Comparison Of Ultrasound-Guided *Vs.* Laparoscopic Transvaginal Ovum Pick-Up (OPU) In Simmental Heifers. *Theriogenology* **1998**, *50*, 89–100.

Sasamoto, Y.; Sakaguchi, M.; Katagiri, S.; Yamada, Y.; Takahashi, Y. The Effects Of Twisting And Type Of Aspiration Needle On The Efficiency Of Transvaginal Ultrasound-Guided Ovum Pick-Up In Cattle. *J. Vet. Med. Sci.* **2003**, *65*, 1083–1086.

Sendag, S.; Cetin, Y.; Alan, M.; Hadeler, K. G.; Niemann, H. Effects Of Ecg And FSH On Ovarian Response, Recovery Rate And Number And Quality Of Oocytes Obtained By Ovum Pick-Up In Holstein Cows. *Anim. Reprod. Sci.* **2008**, *106*, 208–214.

Seneda, M. M.; Esper, C. R.; Garcia, J. M.; de Oliveira J. A.; Vantini, R. Relationship Between Follicle Size And Ultrasound-Guided Transvaginal Oocyte Recovery. *Anim. Reprod. Sci.* **2001**, *67*, 37–43.

Seneda, M. M.; Esper, C. R.; Garcia, J. M.; Andrade, E. R.; Binelli, M.; de Oliveira J. A.; Nascimento A. B. Efficacy Of Linear And Convex Transducers For Ultrasound-Guided Transvaginal Follicle Aspiration. *Theriogenology* **2003**, *59*, 1435–1440.

Takuma, T.; Sakai, S.; Ezoe, D.; Ichimaru, H.; Jinnouchi, T.; Kaedei, Y.; Nagai T.; Otoi, T. Effects Of Season And Reproductive Phase On The Quality, Quantity And Developmental Competence Of Oocytes Aspirated From Japanese Black Cows. *J. Reprod. Dev.* **2010**, *56*, 55–59.

Taneja, M.; Bols, P. E. J.; Van de Velde, A.; Ju, J. C.; Schreiber, D.; Tripp, M. W. Developmental Competence Of Juvenile Calf Oocytes *In Vitro* And *In Vivo*: Influence Of Donor Animal Variation And Repeated Gonadotropin Stimulation. *Biol. Reprod.* **2000**, *62*, 206–213.

Torres-Júnior, J. R. S.; Pires, M. F. A.; Sá, W. F.; Ferreira, A. M.; Viana, J. H. M.; Camargo, L. S. A.; Ramos, A. A.; Folhadella, I. M.; Polisseni, J.; Freitas, C.; Clemente, C. A.; Sá Filho, M. F.; Paula-Lopes, F. F.; Baruselli, P. S. Effect Of Maternal Heat-Stress On Follicular Growth And Oocyte Competence In *B. Indicus* Cattle. *Theriogenology* **2008**, *69*, 155–166.

Underwood, S. L.; Bathgate, R.; Pereira, D. C.; Castro, A.; Thomson, P. C.; Maxwell, W. M. C.; Evans, G. Embryo Production After *In Vitro* Fertilization With Frozen-Thawed, Sex-Sorted, Re-Frozen-Thawed Bull Sperm. *Theriogenology* **2010**, *73*, 97–102.

van Wagtendonk-de Leeuw, A. M. Ovum Pick Up and *In Vitro* Production In The Bovine After Use In Several Generations: A 2005 Status. *Theriogenology* **2006**, *65*, 914–925.

Vernunft, A.; Schwerhoff, M.; Viergutz, T.; Diederich, M.; Kuwer, A. Anti-Muellerian Hormone Levels In Plasma Of Holstein-Friesian Heifers As A Predictive Parameter For Ovum Pick-Up And Embryo Production Outcomes. *J. Reprod. Dev.* **2015**, *61*, 74–79.

Viana, J. H. M.; Nascimento, A. A.; Pinheiro, N. L.; Ferreira, A. M.; Camargo, L. S. A.; Sá, W. F.; Júnior, A. P. M. Characterization Of Tissue Damages After Ovum Pick-Up In Bovine. *Pesq. Vet. Bras.* **2003**, *23*, 119–124.

Viana, J. H. M.; Camargo, L. S. A.; Ferreira, A. M.; de Sa, W. F.; Fernandes, C. A. C.; Junior, A. P. M. Short Intervals Between Ultrasonographically Guided Follicle Aspiration Improve Oocyte Quality But Do Not Prevent Establishment Of Dominant Follicles In The Gir Breed (*B. Indicus*) Of Cattle. *Anim. Reprod. Sci.* **2004**, *84*, 1–12.

Viana, J. H. M.; Palhao, M. P.; Siqueira, L. G. B.; Fonseca, J. F.; Camargo, L. S. A. Ovarian Follicular Dynamics, Follicle Deviation, And Oocyte Yield In Gyr Breed (*B. Indicus*) Cows Undergoing Repeated Ovum Pick-Up. *Theriogenology* **2010**, *73*, 966–972.

Viana, J. 2017 Statistics Of Embryo Production And Transfer In Domestic Farm Animals. Is It A Turning Point? In 2017 More *In Vitro*-Produced Than *In Vivo*-Derived Embryos Were Transferred Worldwide. *Embryo Tech. Newsl.* **2018**, *36*, 8–25.

Viana, J. 2018 Statistics Of Embryo Production And Transfer In Domestic Farm Animals. Embryo Industry On A New Level: Over One Million Embryos Produced *In Vitro*. *Embryo Tech. Newsl.* **2019**, 1–26.

Vieira, L. M.; Rodrigues, C. A.; Castro Netto, A.; Guerreiro, B. M.; Silveira C. R. A.; Moreira, R. J. C.; Sá Filho, M. F.; Bó, G. A; Mapletoft, R. J.; Baruselli, P. S. Superstimulation Prior To The Ovum Pick-Up To Improve *In Vitro* Embryo Production In Lactating And Non-Lactating Holstein Cows. *Theriogenology* **2014**, *82*, 318–324.

Vieira, L. M.; Rodrigues, C. A.; Castro Netto, A.; Guerreiro, B. M.; Silveira, C. R. A.; Freitas, B. G.; Bragança, L. G. M.; Marques, K. N. G.; Sá Filho, M. F.; Bó, G. A.; Mapletoft, R. J.; Baruselli, P. S. Efficacy Of A Single Intramuscular Injection Of Porcine FSH In Hyaluronan Prior To *Ovum Pick-Up* In Holstein Cattle. *Theriogenology* **2016**, *85*, 877–886.

Watanabe, Y. F.; de Souza, A. H.; Mingoti, R. D.; Ferreira, R. M.; Batista, E. O. S.; Dayan A.; Watanabe, O.; Meirelles, F. M.; Nogueira, M. F. G.; Ferraz, J. B. S.; Baruselli, P. S. Number Of Oocytes Retrieved Per Donor During OPU And Its Relationship With *In Vitro* Embryo Production And Field Fertility Following Embryo Transfer. *Anim. Reprod.* **2017**, *14*, 635–644.

Zeron, Y.; Ocheretny, A.; Kedar, O. Seasonal Changes In Bovine Fertility: Relation To Developmental Competence Of Oocytes, Membrane Properties And Fatty Acid Composition Of Follicles. *Reproduction* **2001**, *121*, 447–454.

SECTION II
Equine

CHAPTER 7

Clinical Endocrinology of Pregnant Mares

KATY SATUÉ* and MARÍA MARCILLA

Department of Animal Medicine and Surgery, Faculty of Veterinary, University CEU-Cardenal Herrera, Valencia, Alfara del Patriarca, Tirant lo Blanc, 46115 Valencia, Spain

Corresponding author. E-mail: ksatue@uchceu.es

ABSTRACT

The ability to produce a viable foal is critical to the broodmare. The interaction and coordination between the ovary, the placenta, and the fetus guarantee the hormonal secretion necessary to achieve a successful pregnancy. Maternal–fetal interaction is mediated by the fetoplacental unit, the necessary interface for the production and secretion of these steroid hormones. Therefore, both the mare and the fetus adapt to pregnancy through modifications in the maternal endocrine metabolism mediated by feedback mechanisms of fetal origin. In equine clinical practice, the evaluation of hormonal profiles during pregnancy is one of the main determinants of fetal and/or placental involvement. Consequently, measurements of progestogens, estrogens, and relaxin, among others, are useful to monitor the health status of the placenta and fetal viability. Since placental and/ or compromised pathologies or death lead to alterations in the profiles of these hormones, hormonal diagnosis allows the timing and detection of early pathological conditions to establish the appropriate treatment for the maintenance of pregnancy and to reduce the loss of foals. This chapter reviews normal and abnormal hormonal patterns and reviews the available scientific evidence on the possible clinical benefits of the most widely used treatments to improve the pregnancy outcome in the mare.

7.1   INTRODUCTION

Equine pregnancy implies considerable endocrine changes, which can be explained in part by the development of embryonic vesicle, primary and secondary corpus luteums (CLs), endometrial cups, and fetoplacental unit (FPU) development. Both the pregnant mare and the fetus adapt to this development with unique mechanisms, including alterations in maternal endocrine metabolism and hormonal feedback. Since that the ability to produce a viable foal is critical to the broodmare, maintenance of pregnancy entails almost a year of physiological effort on the part of the gravid mare. In this chapter, normal and abnormal endocrine patterns in pregnant are reviewed. Hormonal diagnosis related with placentitis, abortions, recurrent pregnancy loss, and preterm births has also been considered.

7.2   ENDOCRINOLOGY OF PREGNANT MARE

7.2.1   AT THE TIME OF OVULATION

The estral cycle in the mare is under the endocrinological control of the hypothalamic–pituitary–gonadal (HPG) axis. Also, noteworthy is the influence of photoperiod and other factors, such as nutrition and temperature to a lesser extent. In fact, the mare is defined as a seasonal polyester female of long day or positive phototropic, in which the reproductive activity is regulated directly by the photoperiod. The pineal gland is the organ in charge of controlling the activity of the HPG axis, through the synthesis and secretion of melatonin. This hormone is produced during the hours of darkness, exerting an inhibitory effect on the HPG axis, so that as the photoperiod increases, the suppression ceases and allows the hypothalamic synthesis of gonadotropin-releasing hormone (GnRH) and, consequently, follicle-stimulating hormone (FSH) and luteinizing hormone (LH) in the pituitary gland (Davies Morel, 2008). FSH acts at the level of the granulose cells of the preovulatory follicle favoring growth, follicular maturation, and estrogen synthesis. On the other hand, LH acts on theca cells, participating in oocyte maturation, ovulation as well as the establishment, development, and maintenance of the CL and in the synthesis of progesterone (P4). In turn, both steroid hormones (estrogen and P4) have a feedback mechanism on hypothalamic activity, regulating GnRH synthesis (Ginther, 1992; Aurich, 2011).

The follicular waves that occur during the estrous cycle are temporarily associated with the maximum concentration of FSH, with levels decreasing when the largest follicle reaches 13 mm in diameter, giving way to the mechanism of follicular selection or deviation. LH reaches its maximum concentration the day after ovulation, being essential for the synthesis of estradiol-17β (E_2) and ovulation. Thus, the rupture of the preovulatory follicle causes the passage of the oocyte together with the corona radiata, or crown of cells to the oviduct and the formation of CL occurs. During the reproductive season, the estral cycle in the mare lasts 22 days, of which 5–7 days constitute the estrus phase. Luteolysis begins on the 15th postovulation day due to endometrial secretion of prostaglandin $(PG)F_2\alpha$. In addition to PG, other factors such as oxytocin and cyclooxygenase 2 (COX2) are related to the induction of luteolysis, since its endometrial expression increases markedly during this period (Aurich, 2011; Aurich and Budik, 2015).

After ovulation, the luteal tissue from the granulose cells is responsible for the synthesis of P4. The concentrations of this hormone increase progressively during right-handedness, reaching maximum values 5–6 days after ovulation (10 ng/mL). If the oocyte has not been fertilized, P4 drops drastically to basal levels after the CL lysis (<1 ng/mL). However, if the mare becomes pregnant, the production is maintained and this hormone will be in charge of the maintenance of the gestation during the first 50–70 days (Holtan et al., 1979; Davies Morel, 2008; Aurich, 2011).

The endocrinological study of gestation in the mare requires differentiating two fundamental periods: early gestation (from fertilization to the 150th day of gestation) and late gestation (from the 150th day to term) (Davies Morel, 2008). In each of these periods, events take place that deserve special mention, both for their relevance in the term of a successful gestation and for the particularities linked to the equine species.

7.2.2 MAINTENANCE OF GESTATION AND EMBRYO IMPLANTATION

The nutritional support of the embryo before placentation derives entirely from the histotrophic secretions of the luminal epithelium and endometrial glands, the production of which depends mainly on the action of P4. In fact, its main function is to prepare the endometrium to house the embryo, finding specific steroid receptors up to 20 days postovulation. The activity of these receptors is related to the production of histotrophic and growth factors, which stimulate differentiation and development of maternal–fetal tissues at the beginning of pregnancy (Wilsher et al., 2011; Aurich and Budik, 2015; Kalpokas et al., 2018). Likewise, the presence of this hormone is essential for the mobility and fixation of the conceptus at the base of one of the uterine horns and its orientation within the uterus. Specific receptors have also been found in the equine trophoblast itself (Rambags et al., 2008).

In experimental animals, the role of P4 in the oviduct has been demonstrated, acting on the transport mechanisms, as well as on the volume and composition of the oviductal fluid (Akison et al., 2014). In the mare, high concentrations of P4 have been identified in the oviductal tissue and fluid from the ipsilateral horn to ovulation. Although it is not known whether its origin is in systemic circulation, follicular fluid or in the synthesis itself in the oviduct, this finding is supported by local expression of steroidogenic enzymes (Nelis et al., 2015). Together with P4, the progestagens 5α-pregnano-3β,20α-diol (βα-diol) and 3β-dydroxy-5α-pregnan-20ona (3β5P) increase rapidly after ovulation reaching maximum values around the fifth day of gestation and then descend to the formation of secondary CLs and accessories. Although the initial origin of the progestogens derives from luteal tissue, it is also considered that their circulating levels are the result of both luteal and placental synthesis, However, from day 160 of gestation the fetoplacental unit is fully functional and the primary CL, secondary CL, and accessories involute ceasing their secretory function (Daels et al., 1991a; Holtan et al., 1991).

In the maintenance of equine gestation, it is essential to establish a complete and uninterrupted interaction between the uterus and the conceptus to prevent the regression of primary CL as a result of the blocking of luteolysis. Although the mechanisms underlying this phenomenon, known as "maternal recognition of gestation (MGR)," have not been fully clarified, it is widely recognized that the mobility of the conceptus within the uterine lumen between days 11 and 15 is a fundamental condition to prevent lysis of primary CL, condition named as "*first luteal response of pregnancy*" (Ginther, 1992). The continuous movements of the embryonic vesicle along the uterine lumen seem to compensate for the reduced contact surface due to the relatively small size of the equine trophoblast, demonstrating that restriction of movement only partially leads to early embryo loss (Ginther, 1983). The PG synthesized and secreted by the concept itself stimulate myometrial contractions that promote their migration through the uterus, avoiding premature regression of CL. Additionally, the longitudinal direction of the uterine folds, as well as the spherical shape of the embryo due to the persistence of the glycoprotein capsule, contribute to facilitate this movement (Gastal et al., 1998; Ginther, 1998; Stout and Allen, 2001).

On the other hand, the implication of some antiluteolytic factor, not yet identified, secreted by the embryo itself has been postulated (Aurich and Budik, 2015). However, unlike other species, no substance capable of directly inhibiting the endometrial release of prostaglandin $F_2\alpha$ ($PGF_2\alpha$) has been identified (Baker et al., 1991; Raeside et al., 2004). In other domestic species, such as rodents, ruminants, or swine, the concept produces interferons (IFN) during the pre-implantation period and its presence is related to the regulation of uterine receptivity, decidualization, and placental development. In the mare, the expression of a type of IFN has been detected between days 16 and 22 of gestation which rules out its intervention in the GMR, although it could be involved later in the embryo implantation (Aurich and Budik, 2015).

The production of high amounts of estrogen by the equine conceptus from day 10 of gestation onward has given rise to different researches that suggest its implication in the development of the embryonic and endometrial vasculature. In fact, during the mobility phase of the conceptus and its subsequent fixation uterine perfusion is notably increased, being observed simultaneously with a greater expression of the vascular endothelium growth factor (VEGF-A) and its receptor (VEGFR2). The expression of this factor has been demonstrated in endothelium, lumen, glandular epithelium, and stromal cells in pregnant mares (Silva et al., 2011). In experimental animals, estrogen activity on increased uterine permeability is recognized. This action can be direct or indirect, through the stimulation of factors, such as VEGF, which promote the diffusion of nutrients and oxygen in the placental interface (Rowe et al., 2003; Raeside et al., 2004). Additionally, estrogens of embryonic origin exert important local effects on myometrial activity, uterine mobility and endometrial gland secretion (Raeside et al., 2012). Estrone sulfate (E_1S) is the predominant form during this period in vitelline fluid and its increase parallel to the development of the concept is a characteristic finding of equine gestation (Raeside et al., 2004). In fact, several investigations have shown the importance of embryo synthesis in the maintenance of maternal plasma concentrations of this steroid during early gestation, and its measurement can be used as an indicator of embryonic viability. In this way, Hyland et al. (1985) showed that the elimination of an embryo in a twin pregnancy leads to a 50% decrease in maternal E_1S concentrations, while other studies have documented a significant reduction after inducing abortion in mares between 44 and 89 days of gestation (Hyland et al., 1985; Kasman et al., 1988).

7.2.3   THE FORMATION OF ENDOMETRIAL CUPS

Between the 15th and 17th days postovulation, the size reached by the conceptus together with the decrease of the uterine lumen and the increase of the muscular tone result in the cessation of mobility and the subsequent fixation of the embryonic vesicle at the base of one of the uterine horns. The dissolution of the blastocyst capsule exposes the trophoblast to the uterine environment and allows the development of trophoblastic cells on the outer surface of the choriovitelline membrane. In this way, adhesion to the endometrium and absorption of uterine milk is promoted (Ginther, 1983, 1998).

Embryo implantation begins around day 36 postovulation and involves the development of the chorionic band from the trophoblast, whose cells invade the maternal endometrium giving rise to endometrial cups. The development of the invasive trophoblast requires the proliferation and differentiation of the uninuclear cells of the trophoblast into the binuclear cells that will later synthesize the equine chorionic gonadotropin (eCG). It also acquires an invasive character that allows them to penetrate the endometrial luminal epithelium (Antczak et al., 2013). In relation to this last fact, it has been postulated the implication of several growth factors such as the epidermal growth factor (EGF) and the transforming growth factor type β (TGFβ), whose expression in the glandular epithelium increases notably around the 30–40 of gestation (Lennard et al., 1995, 1998). Likewise, VEGF and its receptors are found in the luminal epithelium and glandular endometrium during the development of the chorionic band. This may autocrine stimulate the maturation of the chorionic band cells (Allen et al., 2007). Similarly, hepatocyte growth factor or "scatter factor" is expressed in the mesothelial and mesenchymal allantoid cells underlying the chorion and chorionic band, suggesting that it may act as a mitogenic agent during trophoblastic proliferation (Gerstenberg et al., 1999).

The eCG can be detected in maternal circulation between days 40 and 120 of gestation, although they present their greatest size and functionality around 50–85 postovulation days, with mean plasma values of 64.5 ± 3.7 IU/mL (Wilsher and Allen, 2011). However, blood levels, as well as the total amount secreted during the period of cup activity, are directly related to the endometrial tissue developed, that is, the amount of trophoblastic tissue invading the endometrium. In addition, numerous factors, such as body condition, exercise performance, female size, and uterine environment, among others, may also alter its secretion (Allen et al., 1993, 2002; Allen and Wilsher, 2009; Antczak et al., 2013; Wilsher and Allen, 2011).

Through the lymphatic sinuses that develop in the stroma underlying each gland, gonadotropin reaches the maternal circulation and it induces an increase of primary CL size and functionality. This fact is called the "second luteal response of pregnancy" and involves an increase in plasma levels of P4 similar to the increase in the luteal area. In addition, it coincides temporarily with the detection of circulating eCG. Subsequently, about 38–40 days of pregnancy, the LH activity characteristic of eCG causes "third luteal response of pregnancy" which consists of ovulation or luteinization of ovarian follicles developed during the first half of gestation due to waves of pituitary FSH. In this way, secondary and accessory CLs are formed, respectively, causing an increase in P4 secretion around the 75th day of gestation (Ginther, 1992; Ginther and Santos, 2015). Thus, during this period, two secretion peaks of P4 are described with plasma values ranging around 10 ng/mL first and 12 ng/mL, subsequently, that gradually decreased to undetectable levels at 200 days of gestation (Legacki et al., 2016; Satué et al., 2018).

Ovarian P4 is necessary for the early maintenance of gestation in the mare, which has been demonstrated with the experimental induction of abortion as a consequence of bilateral ovariectomy at 75 days of gestation. On the contrary, if the ovariectomy is performed between 75 and 150 days, the probability of abortion is variable, and after day 150, it no longer occurs, since the CLs have already regressed and the placenta is then the organ in charge of maintaining gestation (Holtan et al., 1979; Davies Morel, 2008). Several studies describe maximum levels of P4 during the second and third month of gestation, followed by a significant decrease to minimum values (<1 ng/mL) from mid-gestation to term (Tsumagari et al., 1991; Naber et al., 1999; Satué et al., 2011). Additionally, the presence of eCG causes a change in luteal steroidogenesis. In this case, CL changes from synthesizing only P4 to secreting also estrogens and androgens, increasing plasma levels rapidly and tripling the basal values (Satué et al., 2019). The origin of both steroids is found in the primary CL, since their increase takes place before the formation of the secondary CL and is absent in mares without functional CL. Although the mechanism by which gonadotropin exerts this activity is unknown, an increase in the expression of the enzyme 17α-hydroxylase in charge of the conversion of pregnenolone (P5) into dehydroepiandrosterone (DHEA) and P4 into androstenedione (A_4) has been described. Both events coincide with the secretion of eCG, they seem to be limited to the first period, since they are not detected toward the middle of gestation (Satué et al., 2019). In contrast, the levels of the enzyme 3β-hydroxideshydrogenase (3β-HSD), which converts P5 into P4, are similar to those of the right-handed. Thus, the increase in P4 responds primarily to the growth of primary CL and develop secondary and accessory CLs without changes in enzyme expression (Albrecht et al., 1997; Bergfelt, 2000) (Fig. 7.1).

During the period of endometrial cups activity, secretion peaks are described for testosterone (T) and A_4 (Daels et al., 1996a, 1998), whose activity may be decisive in uterine processes related to cell transformation associated with decidualization (Kajihara et al., 2014). In addition, estrogen production depends on the increased synthesis and availability of androgens that are subsequently metabolized by the enzyme aromatase present in luteal tissue even before eCG secretion. Thus, total estrogen levels are similar to right-handed during the first 35 days of gestation and increase around day 40 due to follicular development prior to the formation of CL (Ferraz et al., 2001; Tsumagari et al., 1991). Additionally, primary gestational CL produces E_1S in response to eCG stimulation (Satué et al., 2011, 2018), describing values between 3 and 5 ng/mL (Daels et al., 1991a).

Simultaneously to the formation of endometrial cups, a microvillous union with interdigitations between noninvasive cells of the trophoblast and endometrium is initiated. The development of these structures culminates around 120 days of gestation and gives rise to placental microcotyledons. These structures maximize the area of maternal–fetal contact and are composed of fetal and maternal capillaries. In this capillary network, the exchange of nutrients, gases, and waste substances between the mother and fetus takes place, representing the hemotrophic exchange unit during equine gestation. Additionally, the endometrial glands in charge of secreting "uterine milk" remain active during the rest of gestation, releasing their secretions in the remaining spaces between the microcotyledons known as areolas (Allen, 2001a).

Although the exact stimulus that initiates placental interdigitation has not been identified, the implication of various growth factors has been postulated, such as the transforming growth factor β1 (TGFβ1) and EGF. The expression of these factors in the endometrial luminal and glandular epithelium increases around the month of gestation as previously reported (Stewart et al., 1994; Lennard et al., 1998). The endometrial cells covering the apical portions of the glands express this factor at days 35–40 postovulation coinciding with the beginning of interdigitations between the allantocorion and the endometrium to form the microcotyledonary placenta (Lefranc and Allen, 2007). Likewise, the presence of EGF is reduced in pregnant females with placental problems and endometriosis (Gerstenberg et al., 1999; Stewart et al., 1999). On the other hand, VEGF and its receptors are located in the invasive trophoblastic cells of the endometrial cups and in the noninvasive trophoblast of allantocorion (Allen et al., 2007), while plasma levels of placental growth factor increase during the first months of gestation, reaching maximum values in the third month (Satué et al., 2018). This growth factor belongs to the VEGF-A family and binds with high affinity to the VEGFR1 receptor, promoting angiogenesis in women, sows and small ruminants. This action is performed through different mechanisms, such as the mobilization of hematopoietic precursors, smooth muscle cells, fibroblasts, monocytes and macrophages, necessary for the growth, migration and survival of endothelial cells and collateral vessels (De Falco, 2012; Ribatti, 2008; Bairagi et al., 2016).

7.2.4 FETOPLACENTAL ESTEROIDOGENESIS

The regression of the endometrial cups to 100–120 days of gestation causes the cessation of eCG secretion and luteal development, observing a progressive decrease in plasma levels of P4 to reach basal values around 200 days of gestation (Satué et al., 2011, 2018). At this time, all the luteal structures present in the ovary have completely involuted (Ginther, 1992). Although the onset of this process has traditionally been associated with the cellular immune response of the pregnant female, recent research suggests that chorionic band and endometrial calyx cells are capable of modulating the immune response, suppressing lymphocyte proliferation and cytokine expression (Flaminio and Antczak, 2005). It has also been demonstrated that they themselves determine their apoptosis (de Mestre et al., 2011), while the maternal leukocyte reaction would be a physiological response secondary to the presence of already degenerated cups (Lunn et al., 1997). In any case, from this moment onward, various metabolites derived from P4 called progestins increase in systemic circulation, obtaining, in some cases, variable plasma levels between 5 and 50 ng/mL that exceed 500 ng/mL during the last weeks of gestation, which subsequently fall in the 24–48 h prior to birth (Holtan et al., 1991) (Fig. 7.1).

Progestins can be classified in pregnenes and 5α-pregnenes. The first group includes P5, P4 and 5-pregnene-3β,20β-diol (P5ββ), while second group includes 5α-pregnane-3,20-dione (5αDHP), 3β-hydroxy-5α-pregnan-3-one (3β5P), 20α-hydroxy-5α-pregnan-3-one (20α5P), 5α-pregnane-3β,20β-diol (ββ-diol), and 5α-pregnane-3β,20α-diol (βα-diol). Of them, the most important ones in maternal plasma during this period are 5α-dihydroprogesterone (5αDHP) and its derivatives, 20α-hydroxy-5α-pregnan-3-one (20α5P) and 5α-pregnano-3β,20α-diol (βα-diol). The origin of all of them is found in P5, synthesized mainly in the fetal adrenal gland, with a production rate exceeding 10 μmol/min. In the placenta, P5 is converted to P4 and this is transformed into 5αDHP in the endometrium (Hamon et al., 1991; Han et al., 1995). Maternal plasma concentrations of 5αDHP progressively increase from 1.5 ng/mL in the first week of gestation to 38 ng/mL at term. Although at the beginning of gestation the pattern of secretion runs parallel to that of P4 around 90 days of gestation. Subsequently, the onset of P4 decline gives way to fetoplacental synthesis of the different progestogens whose concentrations continue to increase during the second half of gestation. Thus, 20α5P, which is initially at 5 ng/mL, reaches 69 ng/mL at 200 days of gestation and 300 ng/mL at term. On the other hand, the concentrations of βα-diol increase to 484 ng/mL (Legacki et al., 2016), while 3β5P, P5ββ, and ββ-diol reach values of 100, 10, and 100 ng/mL, respectively toward the end of gestation (326–350 days) (Ousey et al., 2005).

Although the activity of progestogens is still the subject of research, it is suggested that they may play a very important role in the maintenance of gestation, acting directly on P4 receptors. In addition, although 5αDHP appears to be less effective than P4 in regulating myometrial contractibility, it has a greater affinity for its receptors (Chavatte-Palmer et al., 2000; Fowden et al., 2008). In fact, a recent study indicates that daily administration of DHP in pregnant females is capable to maintain gestation until day 27 in the absence of luteal P4 (Scholtz et al., 2014).

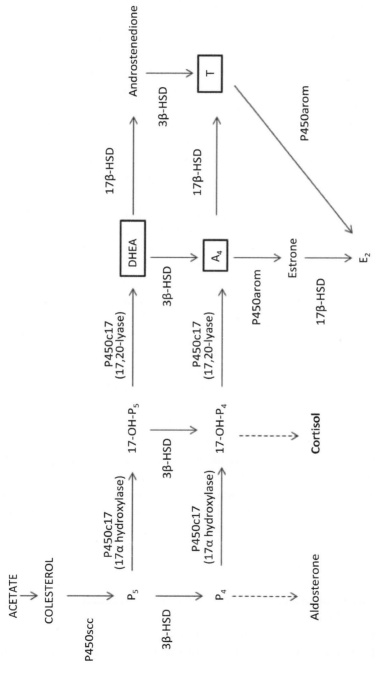

FIGURE 7.1   Steroidogenic pathways. Adapted from Haffner et al. (2010) and Miller and Auchus (2011).

On the other hand, the concentration of these steroids in maternal and umbilical circulation is variable and changes as the time of delivery approaches. This is related to the maintenance of uterine quiescence during this period, during which uterine stress related to increased fetal size may stimulate myometrial contractility. Thus, 5αDHP is found primarily at the uterine level during mid-gestation, but as labor approaches, its distribution changes and is predominantly in fetal circulation. Additionally, this metabolite is an immediate precursor of allopregnanolone, a potent gamma-aminobutyric acid receptor agonist with activity on myometrial relaxation in other species (Holtan et al., 1991; Scholtz et al., 2014; Conley, 2016; Wynn et al., 2018a). Serum levels of allopregnanolone increase similarly to its precursor, reaching maximum values at middle of gestation (16 ng/mL) and a term (20 ng/mL) (Legacki et al., 2016). However, both P4 and DHP prevent weakly myometrial contractions induced by oxytocin *in vitro*, suggesting the intervention of the other hormones in the maintenance of uterine quiescence (Ousey et al., 2000). On the other hand, an umbilical increase of P4 after 300 days of gestation has been described, related to a greater expression in the trophoblast of the enzyme 3β-HSD, necessary for the conversion of P5 into P4 (Ousey et al., 2003).

Simultaneously with the production of progestagens, the FPU synthesizes phenolic estrogens, E_1S and E_2, 17β and 17α, through the aromatization of dihydroandrosterone, DHEA, and its precursors (3β-hydroxyl C-19). The estrogens β-unsaturated, equilin, and echinelin, specific to the equine species, derive from farnesyl pyrophosphate, through a noncholesterol-dependent pathway (Möstl, 1994). In general, the pattern of estrogen secretion during gestation is characterized by a first peak of secretion around day 40 in relation to follicular development prior to the formation of secondary and accessory CLs and a subsequent increase from day 80, reaching maximum levels around 210 days of gestation (Henderson and Stewart, 2000; Henderson and Eayrs, 2004; Fowden et al., 2008). Thus, the initial plasma concentrations of E_1S, corresponding to ovarian synthesis, range from 11 to 18 nmol/L and are affected by ovariectomy. On the contrary, the subsequent peak of liberation reaches more than 250 nmol/L and comes only from fetoplacental synthesis, descending drastically after fetal death (Pashen and Allen, 1979; Kindahl et al., 1982; Raeside et al., 1997; Satué et al., 2011, 2018).

This increase in estrogens temporarily coincides with the hypertrophy of fetal gonads, which together with local expression of the enzyme

17α-hydroxylase, lead to elevated umbilical levels of P5, T, and DHEA (Raeside, 1979; Hasegawa et al., 2001). At the same time, maternal plasma concentrations of DHEA and T increase after 100 days of gestation, obtaining maximum values at six months (Canisso et al., 2014; Satué et al., 2019), whose function is related to promoting greater perfusion in the fetal compartment and promoting uterine tonicity (Ginther, 1992; Ousey, 2011). Legacki et al. (2016) describe DHEA values that fluctuate between 1 and 3 ng/mL during the first two months of gestation and reach levels at around 17 ng/mL at 6 and 8 months, decreasing afterward.

In contrast, T concentrations found during this study were below detection limits for most of gestation. In any case, the absence of the enzyme 3β-HSD in fetal gonads shows that DHEA is the final product and that the rest of the androgens are synthesized in the placenta, where their expression is notably increased. Thus, this enzyme is responsible for the conversion of DHEA to A_4 and P5 to P4. As previously mentioned, the fetal adrenal glands contribute to the synthesis of steroid hormones during this period by producing P5. However, like gonads, they do not express 3β-HSD either, confirming that placenta is the main source P4 during the second half of gestation in the mare (Hasegawa et al., 2001; Arai et al., 2006). In contrast, the presence of the enzyme aromatase in the adrenal glands suggests the involvement of estrogens in the functionality and maturation of fetal organs as has been reported in piglets (Weng et al., 2007).

7.2.5 LATE-PREGNANCY PROGESTAGEN AND ESTROGEN MONITORING

The mitochondrial cytochrome P450 side-chain cleavage *enzyme*, necessary for the conversion of cholesterol into P5, is present in the glomerulosa and reticularis zone of the fetal adrenals from 150 days of gestation. However, its expression increases noticeably at the end of gestation, being also found in the fasciculata zone, in the placenta and in the uteroplacental tissues (Chavatte et al., 1997; Ousey, 2004). At the same time, fetal plasma levels of P5 and its uteroplacental diffusion are doubled and tripled between 200 and 300 days of gestation, obtaining concentrations of progestogens in maternal plasma that exceed 500 ng/mL, and that subsequently descend in the days prior to birth (Ousey et al., 2003; Ousey, 2006; Fowden et al., 2008). The increase of progestagens during this period is associated with the development of the mammary gland and its decrease coincides with the fetal synthesis of cortisol. However, one of the main metabolites of P4, the 5α-DHP, returns to umbilical circulation after synthesis in the endometrium, excreting only 30% of its production to maternal circulation. Thus, it has been suggested that it could play a relevant role within fetoplacental tissues (Hamon et al., 1991; Ousey et al., 2003). In fact, levels of progestogens and estrogens in maternal plasma are considered as indicators of FPU function, as will be described in the next section.

Although total estrogen levels decrease in term gestation, E_2 increases dramatically in the hours before parturition and plays a fundamental role. Specifically, during the last three weeks of gestation, this steroid presents a pattern of constant secretion with higher levels at night and lower levels before sunset. In the days prior to delivery, differences are accentuated and myoelectric activity at the uterine level increases, suggesting the involvement of E_2 in myometrial activation (O'Donnell et al., 2003; McGlothlin et al., 2004; Fowden et al., 2008). In fact, estrogens promote PGs synthesis and increase endometrial sensitivity to oxytocin, stimulating myometrial contractile activity during delivery (Ousey, 2004). Pashen and Allen (1979) reported that females with experimentally gonadectomized fetuses, which therefore do not release DHEA, have an immediate decrease in estrogen and that, although delivery occurs spontaneously, there is a significant decrease in the synthesis of $PGF_2\alpha$ and in myometrial contractibility. A higher probability of placental retention has been observed in these animals. In addition, gonadectomized fetuses had less weight and muscle development at birth than nongonadectomized fetuses.

A few days before parturition, the ripening of the hypothalamus–pituitary–adrenal (HPA) axis causes a change in the enzymatic routes. In this way, fetal adrenals change from mainly synthesizing P5 to producing cortisol in response to the stimulation of adrenocorticotropic hormone. Increased fetal cortisol is independent of changes in maternal corticoslemia and is not accompanied by changes in the expression of steroid receptors at the uterine level (Silver and Fowden, 1994). Thus, its function is related to preparing the fetus for extra-uterine life by stimulating different processes necessary for the maturation of organs such as the liver, thyroid gland, lungs, digestive system, bone marrow, and cardiovascular system (Ousey, 2006). In addition, cortisol activates the enzymes responsible for the synthesis of PGs which, without the presence of progestogens, increase continuously stimulating the onset of myometrial contractions. In addition, E_2 favors the uterine response to PGs and may also promote their synthesis (Kelleman and Act, 2013).

PGs play an important role during delivery by promoting myometrial contractibility ($PGF_2\alpha$), along with oxytocin, and cervical ripening and relaxation (PGE_2). Uteroplacental tissues are capable of synthesizing PGs and can be found in maternal plasma, fetal plasma, and allantoic fluid (Silver et al., 1979). However, its bioactivity is controlled by the enzyme 15-hydroxyprostaglandin dehydrogenase (PGDH), which converts the PGs into inactive metabolites, present in the maternal endometrium since approximately 150 days of pregnancy. In addition, the activity of this enzyme could be favored in the form of paracrine by P4 synthesized in the placenta (Han et al., 1995). On the other hand, the synthesis of PGs could be inhibited by P4, as described in pregnant sheep (Challis et al., 2000). Since the labile nature of PGs makes it difficult to measure one of these metabolites, 13,14-dihydro-15-keto-prostaglandin F-2α (PGFM) remained at low levels (<400 pg/mL) until day 200, then increased to peak pregnancy levels (>2000 pg/mL) by day 300 and remained at this value until parturition. PGFM uses one of its metabolites as an indicator of its circulating levels, with a term increase (2–4 ng/mL) being described, although it is during the second labor stage, when its value increases up to 50 times (Haluska and Currie, 1988; Vivrette et al. 2000) (Fig. 7.2).

Finally, relaxin is produced by the trophoblastic cells of the placenta (Klonisch and Hombach-Klonisch, 2000) and its activity is related to myometrial (Ousey, 2006), as well as of the cervix and pelvic ligaments relaxation (Bryant-Greenwood, 1982). Maternal plasma levels increase at the end of gestation (4–7 ng/mL) and during the second labor stage (11 ng/mL). After the expulsion of the placenta, it returns to basal values below the detection limit at 36 h (Stewart et al., 1982a), remaining elevated in cases of placental retention. However, important variations associated with breed have been described, a fact that does not seem to be related to the placental size or sex of the offspring (Stewart et al. 1992). The functional significance of these differences in terms of actions of relaxin is unknown.

7.3 ABNORMAL ENDOCRINE PATTERNS ALONG PREGNANCY IN THE MARE

Early detection of committed pregnancies can allow timely interventions and reduce foal losses. This section reviews the abnormal hormonal patterns and analyzes the available evidence that supports or refutes the clinical benefits of the most commonly used treatments in such cases (Table 7.1).

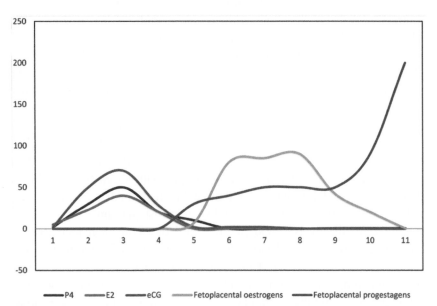

FIGURE 7.2   Normal hormonal P4, E_2, ecG, fetoplacental estrogens, and progestagen patterns in pregnant mares.

7.3.1   *PROGESTAGENS*

7.3.1.1   *PROGESTERONE*

Pregnancy loss is often divided in two categories: early pregnancy loss (EPL) or embryonic death (first 42 days) and fetal losses (after 42 days). The most common endocrine disorder incriminated in EPL in practice is luteal insufficiency. Luteal insufficiency implicates primarily of stimuli that trigger $PGF_2\alpha$ release, since primary luteal insufficiency does not appear to be a clinically significant problem in mares (Allen, 2001b; Morris and Allen, 2002). Around of 60% of EPL occurs during the first 42 days postovulation, when pregnancy maintenance is notably dependent on P4 produced by the primary CL, since essential developmental events including maternal recognition of pregnancy, embryogenesis, and initial organogenesis, disintegration of the blastocyst capsule, endometrial cup

TABLE 7.1 Clinical Interpretation of Pregnancy Hormones in the Mare.

Hormone	Normal values	Interpretation
P4	Adequate to support pregnancy to 120 days >4.0 ng/mL Mid-pregnancy to term: <1 ng/mL	Inadequate to support pregnancy: <2.0 ng/mL
eCG	40–140 days > 10 IU/mL 50–120 days > 100 IU/mL 150–200 days: undetectable	Risk of loss pregnancy: <10 IU/mL
T estrogens E_1S	>110 days > 200 ng/mL 150–300 days > 1000 ng/mL 45 days or greater > 10.0 ng/mL 80 days or greater > 60.0 ng/mL	Severely compromised or death fetus < 500 ng/mL Stress or fetal weakness 500–800 ng/mL Placentitis or fetal compromise < 10.0 ng/mL
Progestagens Pregnanes	90–325 days, 4–15 ng/mL 326–330 days, 6–20 ng/mL 331 days to term: 20–40 ng/mL \5αDHP: from 1.5 in 1st week to 38 ng/mL at term 20α5P: from 5 ng/mL to 69 ng/mL at 200 days, and 300 ng/mL at term βα-diol, 3β5P, P5ββ, and ββ-diol: 484 ng/mL, 100 ng/mL, 10 ng/mL, and 100 ng/mL at term, respectively Allopregnanolone: 16 ng/mL at mild and 20 ng/mL at term	Fetal compromise or placentitis: <4 ng/mL Placentitis P5, P4, 3β5P, P5ββ, ββ-diol, βα-diol, DHP, 20α5P, 20αDHP, and 20β-hydroxyprogesterone
Relaxin	>80 days of pregnancy: 45–85 ng/mL Last 7 weeks: 63.0 ng/mL	Placentitis: 33.0–53.0 ng/mL Hydrops: 33.2 ng/mL Oligohydrallantois: 42.3 ng/mL

formation, and the onset of definitive (chorio-allantoic) placenta formation take place (Stout, 2012). Though the cause may be unknown, may be due to illness, injury, colic, laminitis, or other situations that cause maternal stress (Canisso et al., 2013; Sieme et al., 2015). In addition, luteal insufficiency may be due to poor luteinization in mares with postmating endometritis particularly associated with premature luteal regression induced by cloprostenol (Bergfelt and Adams, 2007). If the CL does not produce enough P4 or is destroyed, pregnancy loss occurs. It is hypothesized that luteal insufficiency is related to deficient GnRH or gonadotrophin secretion, which may have luteotropic effects, since exogenous supplementation with GnRH analogous reduce pregnancy loss at 30 days postovulation (Newcombe, 2000a,b; Newcombe et al., 2001). Some individual case reports of luteal insufficiency which resulted in the birth of a healthy foal: one case without adjunctive hormone therapy (Newcombe, 2000a) and other case with supplementation of P4 during the first 150 days of pregnancy (Canisso et al., 2013) have been documented.

In early pregnancy, P4 concentrations above 4.0 ng/mL are considered adequate to support pregnancy. However, when levels are below 2.0 ng/mL, P4 supplementation is considered (Ousey, 2006). For this reason, serum P4 may be helpful in the decision to supplement mares with this hormone. Canisso et al. (2012) reported a case of a pregnant mare in which serum P4 concentrations had decreased below baseline by 15 days postovulation. The embryo was markedly smaller than average for the gestational age and the pregnancy was successfully rescued with the administration of P4.

Several types of P4 products have been used in an attempt to maintain pregnancies in mares. Altrenogest (allyltrenbolone, 17a-allyl-17b-hydroxy-estra-4,9,11-trien-3-one) is a synthetic progestin widely used in equine reproduction. After oral administration altrenogest is readily absorbed, reaching peak levels after 3–6 h (Machnik et al., 2007). Altrenogest acts by binding to the P4 receptors but has little effect on endogenous plasma total progestagen concentrations (Jackson et al., 1986). Specifically, altrenogest is not metabolized to 5α-pregnanes in the horse (Ousey et al., 2002). For this reason, the only scientific evidence that altrenogest prevents loss pregnancy in mares is during the first trimester, when it prevented abortion induced by repeated administration of $PGF_2\alpha$ (cloprostenol) (Daels et al., 1995). P4 may exert its effects by interfering with PG production stimulated by proinflammatory cytokines. Daels et al. (1996b) demonstrated that the rise in endogenous $PGF_2\alpha$ concentrations was inhibited by altrenogest treatment. Indeed, when early pregnant mares (21–35 days postovulation) were exposed to *Salmonella typhimurium* endotoxin all mares supplemented with altrenogest until day 70 remained pregnant, whereas six out of seven mares aborted when altrenogest therapy was discontinued on day 50 (Daels et al. 1991a).

Mares with suspected luteal insufficiency can be supplemented with altrenogest (0.044 mg/kg per os once or twice daily) or P4 (150 mg/day IM) starting on day 3 after ovulation and continuing until 100–120 days of pregnancy. Long-acting injectable formulations of P4 and altrenogest are available in some countries (Vanderwall et al., 2007). Administration of the GnRH analog, buserelin (40 μg), 10 or 11 days after ovulation has been reported to improve luteal function and reduce EPL in some studies (Pycock and Newcombe, 1996). Panzani et al. (2009) showed that the use of altrenogest improved recipient pregnancy rates compared with untreated controls. A recent clinical study showed a positive effect of altrenogest supplementation on embryonic growth rates between 35 and 45 days after ovulation in Warmblood mares older than 8 years (Willmann et al., 2011). P4 may need to be supplemented generally in early pregnant mares showing estrus signs, with a history of repeated EPL in case of endotoxemia and of stressful events. In mares under P4 supplementation, continuation of pregnancy has to be monitored regularly, since many will lose their pregnancy despite supplementation of P4 and this will prevent those mares returning to estrus (Sieme et al., 2015). In addition, altrenogest can be used to save pregnancy after inadvertent PG injection, provided altrenogest administration is begun within 18 h after PG injection (Daels et al. 1996b).

It has been reported, that administration of a singular dose of 20–40 μg buserelin between day 9 and 10 after ovulation increase the embryo numbers in multiple ovulating and pregnancy rates up to 5–10% (Newcombe et al., 2001; Kanitz et al., 2007; Newcombe and Peters, 2014). Buserelin does not increase circulating P4 levels or preventing the luteolysis, acting independently of CL in the mare (Stout et al., 2002). These effects prevent EPL that operate between day 9–10 and day 13–14 of pregnancy.

In a recent study, Köhne et al. (2014) reported that human chorionic gonadotropin (hCG) administration for induction of ovulation in mares increased progestin concentration in plasma of early pregnancy as well as the embryo size at the time of the start of placentation. Periovulatory treatment of mares with hCG may thus be a valuable tool to enhance conceptus growth during early pregnancy. These later authors showed that in contrast to direct progestin supplementation with altrenogest, hCG-treatment-stimulated endogenous P4 secretion. However, Biermann et al. (2014) report that hCG treatment of mares on day 5 or day 11 postovulation influenced peripheral P4 concentrations due to secondary luteal tissue but did not alter ovarian and uterine blood flow or increase pregnancy rates.

Three pathological profiles of P4 may be described in late gestation (Daels et al., 1991b):

Sudden decrease: This pattern is related with an acute condition, such as colic, uterine torsion, mare stress, and indicates high probability of fetal death.

Rapid increase: A rapid P4 level increase prior to the mare entering the normal window of parturition (prior to 320 days of pregnancy) indicates the possibility of placental pathology (placentitis) and often results in preterm labor of an immature foal.

Lack of P4 peak: A lack of P4 prior to delivery occurs with poisoning with fescue grass or tall fescue. Because of variations in P4 levels among mares, it is necessary to determine the individual baseline for each mare. The recommended frequency of blood sampling varies from as frequently as three times a day to as little as once every 2–3 days because only regular testing provides reliable information on placental and fetal condition (Daels et al. 1991b; Conley, 2016). Due during mid- and late-pregnancy progestagens are produced solely by the FPU, it is possible that a progestagen other than P4 (or synthetic P4) may be more effective at preventing preterm birth in the mare. Nevertheless, to date, P4 supplementation remains a part of the standard therapy protocol in placentitis cases (Ousey, 2006).

7.3.1.2 PROGESTAGENS

Several pathological conditions such as placentitis, placental separation, or fetus, alteration in umbilical blood flow attributable to a cord pathologic condition stimulates inflammatory and immune responses leading disrupt the endocrine capacity of the FPU and alterations in endocrine profile in plasma maternal attributed to disturbances to the normal synthetic pathway for these pregnanes. Fetoplacental function can be monitored by measuring total progestins in three or more samples of maternal plasma obtained at 48–72-h intervals (LeBlanc, 2008) in spontaneous and experimental placentitis (Douglas, 2004; Morris et al. 2007; Conley, 2016; Shikichi et al., 2017). Three patterns of total pregnanes in cases of abnormal pregnancy have been established (Ousey et al., 2002; Ousey, 2006):

First pattern: The total progestagen concentrations declining rapidly (over a few hours or days) or are already close to zero. Progestagens in maternal plasma have revealed that all the metabolites of P5 and P4 are less than 95%, consistent with failure of the fetus and fetoplacental tissues to produce and metabolize progestagens (LeBlanc et al., 2004). This pattern is associated with fetal death or imminent fetal expulsion due to uterine torsion, colic, maternal stress, or acute cases of experimentally induced placentitis when the mares abort rapidly (within 7 days of infection) (Santschi et al., 1991; Mizushima, 2005; Morris et al. 2007).

Another potential cause is the death of a single fetus in a twin pregnancy. In this situation, the adjacent area between the placentas is already avillous (Jeffcott and Whitwell, 1973; Ousey et al., 2000), and when the placenta supporting the deceased fetus necrotizes, a substantial loss in pregnane metabolism occurs (Whitwell, 1980). As the fetus is responsible for production of P5, any case in of fetal demise will result in a loss of precursor and therefore a decline in measurable pregnanes in the mare's circulation.

Second pattern: Progestagen concentrations raised precociously to levels greater than 95% for healthy mares of a similar gestation age. Although higher concentrations are usually found only before spontaneous parturition at term, three different profiles associated with different placental problems have been documented (Ousey et al., 2000; LeBlanc et al., 2004):

First profile: This profile involves unusually high concentrations of nearly all the progestagens and has been observed most frequently in mares with chronic cases of placentitis, placental edema, and placentas with poorly developed or sparse microvilli (Ousey, 2006; Morris et al., 2007). This pattern indicates that the fetus and the uteroplacental tissues are metabolically active despite the presence of bacteria or their products (Ousey et al., 2000). In addition, Shikichi et al. (2017) demonstrated that mares with high concentration of progestins and low concentration of estrogens after day 241 of pregnancy were likely to deliver aborted/ dead foals with placentitis. These authors demonstrated elevated and low concentrations of protegins and estrogens in the maternal sera of all cases with placentitis in pregnant mares, respectively.

Second profile: The high progestagens contain elevated concentrations of P4, but concentrations of P5 and several metabolites are normal or low. This profile was found in two mares, one with extensive placental villous poverty (poor or sparsely developed microvilli) and other with placental edema. In these cases, it seems that the placenta was less capable of metabolizing P4 into 5αDHP and other progestagens (Ousey et al., 2000).

Third profile: Maternal progestagen may remain elevated for several weeks before delivery, and the foals, if born alive, often have normal or hyperadrenocortical function with raised plasma P5 concentrations, even when delivered before term (Rossdale et al., 1995). This profile has been associated with fetal stress which results in an increase in P5 production from the fetal adrenal that ultimately leads to an increase in total pregnanes (Rossdale et al., 1992). Though foals born to mares which display this pattern are often born prematurely, they tend to fare better than those born prematurely to mares which do not display this increase. This is thought to be due to the increased activation of the HPA axis (Gravett et al., 2000; Ousey, 2006).

Third pattern: Progestagens do not reveal the normal prepartum increase. This is most often seen in prolonged gestation caused by ingestion of tall fescue containing endophyte fungus (Ousey, 2006). This pattern is almost exclusively found in mares that are exposed to ergopeptine alkaloids from the endophyte fungus found on tall fescue grass (fescue toxicosis), although it has also been observed in apparently healthy mares with prolonged gestations (Brendemeuhl et al., 1995). Ergot alkaloids present in the fescue inhibit fetal CRH, inhibiting the normal function of the adrenal gland to produce the cortisol surge and associated changes in pregnane metabolism (Ousey, 2006). In mares with fescue toxicosis, prepartum total plasma progestagen concentrations remain low, their foals have low cortisol concentrations, indicating suppression of fetal adrenocortical activity and P5 production (Brendemeuhl et al., 1995).

Based on these three progestagen profiles, the data indicate that maternal plasma progestagen concentrations provide a measure not only of placental function but of fetal adrenocortical activity, and thus foal outcome. To monitor progestagen profiles of mares at risk of losing their pregnancies, it is recommended that, initially, three jugular blood samples were collected daily using an assay that has been well characterized for normal concentrations in late pregnancy. These samples should determine if profiles are increasing or decreasing. Thereafter, regular sampling will enable the clinician to monitor any changes in fetoplacental activity (Ousey et al., 2000).

In general, mares with high total progestagen concentrations are more likely to deliver live foals than those with low concentrations because there has been some degree of fetal HPA activity. Foals born after these chronic insults often show precocious fetal maturation even when born many weeks before term (Ousey and McGladdery, 2000). Although an increase in fetal cortisol is advantageous for fetal survival, exposure to high levels of glucocorticoids causes a reduction in fetal body weight at birth (Seckl, 2004).

Ousey et al. (2005) reported changes in 10 specific pregnanes as P5, P4, 3β5P, P5ββ, ββ-diol, βα-diol, DHP, 20α5P, 20α-DHP, and 20β-hydroxyprogesterone from healthy mares compared with mares with diverse placental abnormalities. Mares with pregnancy complications were grouped based upon diagnosis: placentitis, placental pathology without placentitis, and nonplacental problems. Results for the placentitis group showed increases in all measured pregnanes, including P4 and P5. This suggested an increase in precursors due to fetal stress and increased metabolites as a result. For the group with placental pathology but no placentitis (including placental edema and avillous placenta), an increase in total pregnanes was noted with P4, specifically, also increased. However, most of the individual pregnanes were either in a normal range or decreased. As this group had issues with the placenta, it appears as though the placental function was affected and its ability to metabolize pregnanes was reduced. For the group of mares with problems unrelated to the placenta (colic, uterine ruptura or torsion, laminitis, etc.), the majority had a decrease in total pregnanes. These mares also showed a decrease in most of the individual pregnanes. These fetuses were significantly compromised or dead; therefore, precursor was reduced, or nonexistent, with downstream metabolites reduced as well.

Recently, Wynn et al. (2018b) compared P4, 5α-DHP, allopregnanolone, 3β5P, 20α5P, βα-diol, and ββ-diol concentrations in plasma of mares with experimentally induced, ascending placentitis compared with gestationally age-matched control mares. In mares with chronic placentitis, concentrations of DHP and its metabolites (allopregnanolone, 3β5P, 20α5P, βα-diol) increased at 2–8 days prior to abortion compared with control mares. Of these pregnanes, 20α5P and βα-diol increased at 8 days prior to abortion and demonstrated the largest increase (3–4 times) in mares with chronic placentitis compared with control mares. P4 concentrations were at or below the limit of detection (0.5 ng/mL) for control mares and were increased at two days prior to abortion in mares with chronic placentitis but were not different from controls in mares with acute placentitis. In mares with acute placentitis, concentrations of DHP, allopregnanolone, 3β5P, 20α5P, and βα-diol decreased within 0–3 days prior to abortion. In mares with chronic placentitis, the patterns of increased pregnanes metabolized by the placenta were similar to changes in normal mares beyond day 300 of gestation and likely represent the effects of fetal stress and adrenal activation on pregnane metabolism by the fetus and placenta. Decreases in these same pregnanes in mares with acute cases likely reflect extreme fetal or placental compromise. These studies were useful to understand how differential issues during the pregnancy could present as different pregnane profiles.

Although it is advisable to determine the additional need for P4 between days 120 and 150 of gestation, it must be taken into account that progestogen levels can show cross-reactivities with P4 at the laboratory level. Also, P4 concentrations measured in blood are only 2–3 ng/mL during the second half of gestation, much lower than during the first trimester of pregnancy. For this reason, P4 should not be used for monitoring mid- and late-trimesters of pregnancy, since that other progestins maintain the pregnancy (Ousey, 2011). It is known that P4 maintains myometrial quiescence, but their effects can be questioned by (1) the number of progestagens that are quantitatively important in mares' plasma, (2) the information suggesting that 5αDHP or another progestagen may be biologically active in the pregnant uterus, and (3) the fact that progestagens did not prevent oxytocin-induced myometrial contractions *in vitro*. For this reason, both progestins and native P4 should be used in research or in practice for supplementation during pregnancy in mares (Daels et al., 1996a; Squires, 2008).

It is recommended that administration begin within a few days after ovulation and is often continued until day 120 of pregnancy. From day 35 onward, endometrial cups start to form and secrete eCG the latter resulting in formation of secondary CLs. This period of gestation is a good time to measure blood P4 levels in supplemented mares to decide if the treatment is still necessary. P4 levels in supplemented mares should be recontrolled at day 60–70. Despite the necessary requirement for an ovarian source of P4 to maintain pregnancy up to approximately day 100 in the mare (Hinrichs et al., 1987), there is a lack of scientific evidence supporting exogenous P4 supplementation as a means of improving pregnancy maintenance (Allen, 2001b; Squires, 2008; Vanderwall, 2008). Even though altrenogest will likely suppress endogenous P4 levels; it has been reported that administration of altrenogest in pregnant mares was associated with lower concentrations of endogenous P4 from day 14 to 18 and on day 21 compared with endogenous P4 levels in pregnant mares not administered altrenogest. This effect can be mediated by a reduction in pituitary LH release and a decrease in luteotropic support (De Luca et al., 2011).

Recent studies demonstrated that altrenogest, when given in combination with antimicrobials, pentoxifylline, and nonsteroidal anti-inflammatory (NSAIDs) drugs to mares with placentitis, decreased the incidence of abortion (Troedsson and Zent, 2003). In these cases, altrenogest counteract uterine contractility induced by inflammation of the fetal membranes. In the same way, in bacterial placentitis, a combination of trimethoprim sulfamethoxazole, pentoxifylline, and a double dose of altrenogest (0.088 mg/kg bwt per os s.i.d.) was successful in maintaining pregnancies to term (Bailey et al., 2010), while that untreated control mares aborted. When mares were treated with trimpethoprim sulfamethoxazole and pentoxifylline without altrenogest, only one live foal was born (Graczyk et al., 2006; Bailey et al., 2010). Despite of this, it is not clear what role, if any, altrenogest plays within this multitreatment approach. However, the mares can still abort while receiving altrenogest treatment in the last trimester of pregnancy.

If altrenogest acts in the same manner as P4 to regulate PG catabolism via PGDH in the placenta, this may provide one pathway by which altrenogest could regulate PG synthesis, and hence myometrial activity. Apparently, the upregulation of oxytocin and PG receptors is inhibited at that stage by the administration of P4, and without these receptors and the formation of gap junctions between the myometrial cells, uterine contraction cannot happen. The specific action and efficacy of P4 supplementation as a way to prevent abortion in late gestation still is subject to controversy (Ousey, 2006). Since the plasma P4 concentrations are increased in most of these placentitis mares, supplementation is questionable. Some authors believe that it might be contraindicated, since a supplement of P4 inhibits placental 3β-HSD, converting endogen P5 to P4 (Chavatte et al., 1995). A total blockage of 3β-HSD leads to parturition in most animals, but not in the mare (Chavatte et al. 1997). Most likely, other progestogens play a more determining role in preventing preterm birth in the mare (Ousey, 2006).

In relation to parturition, Neuhauser et al. (2008) showed that double dose of altrenogest given to healthy pony mares during late gestation induced prolongation of stage II of labor, and transient decrease in respiratory rate in newborn foals with higher plasma pH compared with foals born to untreated mares. These same authors also revealed that foals born to altrenogest-treated healthy mares showed a reduced neutrophil/lymphocyte ratio, which the authors attributed either to immunomodulatory effects of altrenogest or dysmaturity of the foals (Neuhauser et al. 2009).

7.3.2   ESTROGENS

In late gestation, total estrogen levels (including E_1S, E_2 and its metabolites, equilin, and equilenin) as well may be used for fetal and placental health monitoring. Although total estrogen concentration >1000 ng/mL between

150 and 280 days of gestation is considered to be normal, values <500 ng/mL have been associated with a severely compromised or death fetus and between 500 and 800 ng/mL indicate stress or fetal weakness. However, it is doubtful that total estrogen concentration can predict fetal death as the fetal gonads are unlikely to respond to fetal stress (Bucca, 2006; LeBlanc, 2010; Shikichi et al. 2017).

Since the production of estrogens requires both contribution by the fetus and placental, reduced concentrations in maternal circulation may indicate or predict a stressed or hypoxic fetus that is not producing the estrogen precursors (LeBlanc, 2010). Indeed, E_2 (Canisso et al., 2017) and E_1S (Kasman et al., 1988) concentrations decreased sharply in mares with placental dysfunction and after the induction of abortion. Indeed, while E_1S concentrations >100 ng/mL indicate the presence of a viable fetus, low levels <10 ng/mL indicate pregnancy loss or barren mare. If the fetus is severely compromised or die in uterus, maternal plasma E_1S are baseline because of the absence of the C19 precursors secreted by the fetal gonads. However, pregnancies compromised by equine herpesvirus-1 infection or severe colic can present normal or transiently decreased E_1S concentrations (Santschi et al., 1991). Compared with the adrenal glands, the gonads are unlikely to respond to fetal stress; consequently, so it is doubtful that total estrogen concentrations can predict fetal death. Frequent blood sampling of mares induced to abort with PG between 90 and 150 days of pregnancy indicated that E1S levels did not decline until within 5 h of abortion (Daels et al., 1995).

In cases of placentitis at gestational ages between 150 and 280 days, Douglas (2004) and Shikichi et al. (2017) showed hormonal alterations common as elevated progestogens and low estrogens in mares that aborted. Although the decline in E_2 associated with placental dysfunction is thought to reflect placental disease *per se*, Esteller-Vico et al. (2017) recommended the estrogen supplementation as a means to reduce the risk of abortion associated with placentitis in mares. Recently, Curcio et al. (2017) showed that in addition to basic treatment with trimethoprim-sulfa-methoxazole and flunixin meglumine, mares with experimentally induced ascending placentitis benefited from estradiol cypionate supplementation. Conversely, altrenogest did not appear to make a difference in outcomes.

After fetal death and stress or fetal weakness, androgens and estrogens levels drop rapidly. For better determination of the health state of fetus, due to metabolism of both steroids, it is recommended to monitor androgens and estrogens simultaneously (Conley, 2016).

7.3.3 RELAXIN

Relaxin is a useful biomarker to assess placental health and can be monitored in high-risk mares. Ryan et al. (2009) reported a positive relationship between circulating levels of relaxin and poor outcomes in high-risk pregnancies. Relaxin is detectable in blood after the 80th day of pregnancy (4–7 ng/mL) without any changes until the second stage of labor, when it increases rapidly up to 11 ng/mL (Stewart et al. 1982b).

Relaxin concentrations decrease below 4 ng/mL in mares with impaired placental function, in cases of placentitis, placental abruption, hydroallantois, and hidramnios (Stewart et al., 1992; Ryan et al., 2009). Low circulating levels of relaxin have been reported both in pony mares affected by fescue toxicosis associated with placental disease and agalactia and in thoroughbred mares, with other forms of placental disease or insufficiency (Ryan et al. 2009).

In the case of placental hydrops, the risk of spontaneous rupture of the fetal membranes increases significantly (Christensen et al., 2006). Relaxin has been explored as a potential marker of treatment success in placentitis due to its level decrease in cases of spontaneously occurring and experimentally induced pregnancy loss (Klein, 2016). However, using circulating relaxin levels is limited due to significant breed differences and lack of commercial tests for determining relaxin levels in blood samples (Rossdale, 1993; Klein, 2016).

7.3.4 PROSTAGLANDINS

Placentitis is characterized by the production of proinflammatory cytokines such as IL-6 and IL-8 and prostaglandins ($PGF_2\alpha$ and PGE_2) (LeBlanc et al., 2012; Lyle et al., 2006; Lyle, 2014). PG release increases uterine contractility and consequently increases the risk of premature delivery (McGlothlin et al., 2004). However, it is unlikely that these parameters can be used at the diagnostic level because they are rapidly metabolized and released within the uterus or fetus (Bucca, 2006; LeBlanc et al., 2002; LeBlanc, 2008).

Proinflammatory cytokines and the PGs of the FPU increment and both in response to inflammation and infection, inducing premature activation of the fetal HPA axis (Lyle et al., 2010) accelerating fetal maturation before parturition (McGlothlin et al., 2004; Canisso et al., 2015). The fetal adrenal produces both progestins and, once sufficiently mature, cortisol (Lyle et al., 2010). Fetal cortisol, in turn, enhances placental and uterine PGs production, further enhancing uterine contractility and resulting in fetal delivery. Since the maturation of the equine fetus occurs later in gestation (Ousey, 2006), this implies that placentitis or maternal disease could be devastating to the newborn foal. However, early fetal maturation likely counterbalances premature delivery and may help improve the chances for foal survival (McGlothlin et al., 2004; Canisso et al., 2015).

Daels et al. (1991b) addressed whether flunixin meglumine could prevent luteolysis and maintain pregnancy in mares that were administered endotoxin. Flunixin meglumine, an *NSAID* cyclo-oxygenase inhibitor interferes with the production of PG. When flunixin meglumine was administered to mares between days 21 and 44 of gestation 10 min before endotoxin administration, endogenous P4 production was maintained and none of the mares lost their pregnancy. In those mares in which flunixin meglumine was administered 1 h after endotoxic insult, systemic P4 fell <2 ng/mL for several days, and pregnancy was lost in one of three mares. When flunixin meglumine was administered 2 h after endotoxic insult, P4 fell <0.5 ng/mL, and all three pregnancies were lost. Likewise, the 12 pregnant mares administered only endotoxin had very low P4 concentrations, and all lost their pregnancies.

Daels et al. (1996b) examined the ability of P4 or altrenogest and flunixin meglumine administration to inhibit abortion induced by cloprostenol. Mares were either administered P4 300 mg (q 24 h, IM) or 44 mg altrenogest (q 24 h, PO; "double dose") beginning either 18 or 12 h, respectively, after the first cloprostenol injection. The P4 regimen was used in eight mares between 98 and 153 days of gestation, and, of these mares, only three aborted. When altrenogest was used in similar fashion in mares between 93 and 115 days of gestation, none of the mares aborted. In the contrary, when 500 mg flunixin (q 8 h, IV) was administered beginning 15 min before the first daily cloprostenol injection, all mares aborted. Thus, P4 or altrenogest supplementation but not flunixin administration blocked cloprostenol-induced abortion at these gestational ages. Taken together, these studies support the concept that progestin supplementation can maintain equine pregnancy when the mares were submitted to $PGF_2\alpha$ insults (Daels et al., 1991b, 1996b).

In addition, the administration of the PG synthetase inhibitor (meclofenamic acid) to pregnant mares after abdominal surgery diminishes the normal postsurgical rise in PGFM and facilitates fetal survival compared with that in untreated mares (Silver et al., 1979). In addition, Esteller-Vico et al. (2017) showed that estrogen suppression resulted in a decrease in circulating PGFM, which suggests that estrogens partially regulate PG production during pregnancy, since PGFM concentrations were lower but still increased during the last trimester of equine gestation in letrozole-treated mares.

7.4 CONCLUSIONS

The adequate interaction between ovary, placenta, and fetus guarantees the secretion of correct hormonal patterns necessary for successful pregnancy. Measurements of progestagen, estrogens, and relaxin among others, are useful to monitor the state of health of the placenta and fetal viability, since placental pathologies and/or compromised or death leads to alterations of these hormones. Diagnosis of hormones allows to temporalize and detect early pathological conditions to propose the suitable treatment for maintenance of pregnancy to produce viable foal. Substantial progress has been made in recent years in the identification of compromised pregnancy and their management.

KEYWORDS

- **endocrinology**
- **broodmare**
- **placenta**
- **pregnancy**
- **steroid hormones**

REFERENCES

Akison, L. K.; Boden, M. J.; Kennaway, D. J.; Russell, D. L.; Robker, R. L. Progesterone Receptor-Dependent Regulation of Genes in the Oviducts of Female Mice. *Physiol. Genomics* **2014**, *46* (16), 583–592.

Albrecht, B. A.; MacLeod, J. N.; Daels, P. F. Differential Transcription of Steroidogenic Enzymes in the Equine Primary Corpus Luteum During Diestrus and Early Pregnancy. *Biol. Reprod.* **1997,** *56* (4), 821–829.

Allen, W. R. Fetomaternal Interactions and Influences During Equine Pregnancy. *Reproduction* **2001a,** *121* (4), 513–527.

Allen, W. R. Luteal Deficiency and Embryo Mortality in the Mare. *Reprod. Domest. Anim.* **2001b,** *36,* 121–131.

Allen, W. R.; Gower, S.; Wilsher, S. Immunohistochemical Localization of Vascular Endothelial Growth Factor (VEGF) and Its Two Receptors (Flt-I and KDR) in the Endometrium and Placenta of the Mare During the Oestrous Cycle and Pregnancy. *Reprod. Domest, Anim.* **2007,** *42* (5), 516–526.

Allen, W. R.; Skidmore, J. A.; Stewart, F.; Antczak, D. F. Effects of Fetal Genotype and Uterine Environment on Placental Development in Equids. *J. Reprod. Fertil.* **1993,** *98* (1), 55–60.

Allen, W. R.; Wilsher, S.; Stewart, F.; Stewart, F.; Ousey, J.; Ousey, J.; Fowden, A. The Influence of Maternal Size on Placental, Fetal and Postnatal Growth in the Horse. II. Endocrinology of Pregnancy. *J. Endocrinol.* **2002,** *172* (2), 237–246.

Allen, W. R.; Wilsher, S. A Review of Implantation and Early Placentation in the Mare. *Placenta* **2009,** *30,* 1005–1015.

Alm, C. C.; Sullivan, J. J.; First, N. L. The Effect of a Corticosteroid (Dexamethasone), Progesterone, Oestrogen and Prostaglandin F_2 on Gestation Length in Normal and Ovariectomized Mares. *J. Reprod. Fertil. Suppl.* **1975,** *23,* 637–640.

Antczak, D. F.; de Mestre, A. M.; Wilsher, S.; Allen, W. R. The Equine Endometrial Cup Reaction: A Fetomaternal Signal of Significance. *Annu. Rev. Anim. Biosci.* **2013,** *1,* 419–442.

Arai, K. Y.; Tanaka, Y.; Taniyama, H.; Tsunoda, N.; Nambo, Y.; Nagamine, N.; Watanabe, G.; Taya, K. Expression of Inhibins, Activins, Insulin-Like Growth Factor-I and Steroidogenic Enzymes in the Equine Placenta. *Dom. Anim. Endocrinol.* **2006,** *31* (1), 19–34.

Aurich, C. Reproductive Cycles of Horses. *Anim. Reprod. Sci.* **2011,** *124,* 220–228.

Aurich, C.; Budik, S. Early Pregnancy in the Horse Revisited—Does Exception Prove the Rule? *J. Anim. Sci. Biotechnol.* **2015,** *6,* 50.

Bailey, C. S.; Macpherson, M. L.; Pozor, M. A.; Troedsson, M. H.; Benson, S. M.; Giguere, S.; Sanchez, L. C.; LeBlanc, M. M.; Vickroy, T. W. Treatment Efficacy of Trimethoprim Sulfamethoxazole, Pentoxifylline and Altrenogest in Experimentally Induced Equine Placentitis. *Theriogenology* **2010,** *74,* 402–412.

Bairagi, S.; Quinn, K. E.; Crane, A. R.; Ashley, R. L.; Borowicz, P. P.; Caton, J. S.; Redden, R. R.; Grazul-Bilska, A. T.; Reynolds, L. P. Maternal Environment and Placental Vascularization in Small Ruminants. *Theriogenology* **2016,** *86* (1), 288–305.

Baker, C. B.; Adams, M. H.; McDowell, K. J. Lack of Expression of Alpha or Omega Interferons by the Horse Conceptus. *J. Reprod. Fertil. Suppl.* **1991,** *44,* 439–443.

Bergfelt, D. R.; Adams, G. P. Ovulation and Corpus Luteum Development. In *Current Therapy in Equine Reproduction*; Samper, J. C., Pycock, J. F., McKinnon, A. O., Eds.; W. B. Saunders-Elsevier: Saint Louis, 2007; pp 1–13.

Biermann, J.; Klewitz, J.; Otzen, H.; Martinsson, G.; Burger, D.; Meinecke-Tillmann, S.; Sieme, H. The Effect of hCG, Administered in Diestrus, on Luteal, Ovarian and Uterine Blood Flow, Peripheral Progesterone Levels and Pregnancy Rates in Mares. *J. Equine Vet. Sci.* **2014,** *34,* 166.

Brendemeuhl, J. P.; Williams, M. A.; Boosinger, T. R.; Ruffin, D. C. Plasma Progestagen, Trioiodothyronine and Cortisol Concentrations in Postdate Gestation Foals Exposed in Utero to the Tall Fescue Endophyte *Acremonium coenophialum*. *Biol. Reprod. Monogr.* **1995**, *1*, 53–59.

Bryant-Greenwood, G. D. Relaxin as a New Hormone. *Endocr. Rev.* **1992**, *3* (1), 62–90.

Bucca, S. Diagnosis of the Compromised Equine Pregnancy. *Vet. Clin. North Am. Equine Pract.* **2006**, *22*, 749–761.

Canisso, I. F.; Ball, B.; Troedsson, M.; Klein, C.; Stanley, S. D. Diagnostic Markers for Experimentally Induced Ascending Placentitis in Mares. *J. Equine Vet. Sci.* **2012**, *32*, S73.

Canisso, I. F.; Ball, B. A.; Erol, E.; Squires, E. L.; Troedsson, M. H. T. In *Proceedings of the 61st Annual Convention of the American Association of Equine Practitioners*; Las Vegas, Nevada, USA, December 5–9, **2015**; pp 490–509.

Canisso, I. F.; Ball, B. A.; Esteller-Vico, A.; Squires, E. L.; Troedsson, M. H. Dehydro-epiandrosterone Sulfate and Testosterone Concentrations in Mares Carrying Normal Pregnancies. In *Proceedings of the Society for Theriogenology Annual Conference*; Portland, OR, USA, 2014.

Canisso, I. F.; Ball, B. A.; Esteller-Vico, A.; Williams, N. M.; Squires, E. L.; Troedsson, M. H. Changes in Maternal Androgens and Oestrogens in Mares with Experimentally Induced Ascending Placentitis. *Equine Vet. J.* **2017**, *49* (2), 244–249.

Canisso, I. F.; Beltaire, K. A.; Bedford-Guaus, S. J. Premature Luteal Regression in a Pregnant Mare and Subsequent Pregnancy Maintenance with the Use of Oral Altrenogest. *Equine Vet. J.* **2013**, *45*, 97–100.

Challis, J. R. G.; Cox, D. B.; Sloboda, D. M. Regulation of Corticosteroids in the Fetus: Control of Birth and Influence on Adult Disease. *Semin. Neonatol.* **1999**, *4*, 93–97.

Challis, J. R. G.; Matthews, S. G.; Gibb, W..; Lye, S. J. Endocrine and Paracrine Regulation of Birth at Term and Preterm. *Endocr. Rev.* **2000**, *21* (5), 514–550.

Chavatte, P.; Holtan, D.; Ousey, J. C.; Rossdale, P. D. Biosynthesis and Possible Biological Roles of Progestagens During Equine Pregnancy and in the Newborn Foal. *Equine Vet. J. Suppl.* **1997**, *24*, 89–95.

Chavatte, P. M.; Rossdale, P. D.; Tait, A. D. Modulation of 3 Beta-Hydroxysteroid Dehydrogenase (3 beta-HSD) Activity in the Equine Placenta by Pregnenolone and Progesterone Metabolites. *Equine Vet. J.* **1995**, *27*, 342–347.

Chavatte-Palmer, P.; Duchamp, G.; Palmer, E.; Ousey, J. C.; Rossdale, P. D.; Lombès, M. Progesterone, Oestrogen and Glucocorticoid Receptors in the Uterus and Mammary Glands of Mares from Mid- to-Late Gestation. *J. Reprod. Fertil. Suppl.* **2000**, *56*, 661–672.

Christensen, B. W.; Troedsson, M. H. T.; Murchie, T. A.; Pozor, M. A.; Macpherson, M. L.; Estrada, A. H.; Carrillo, N. A.; Mackay, R. J.; Roberts, G. D.; Langlois, J. Management of Hydrops Amnion in a Mare Resulting in Birth of a Live Foal. *J. Am. Vet. Med. Assoc.* **2006**, *228*, 1228–1233.

Conley, A. J. Review of the Reproductive Endocrinology of the Pregnant and Parturient Mare. *Theriogenology* **2016**, *86* (1), 355–365.

Cross, D. L.; Redmond, L. M.; Strickland, J. R. Equine Fescue Toxicosis: Signs and Solutions. *J. Anim. Sci.* **1995**, *73*, 899–908.

Curcio, B. R.; Canisso, I. F.; Pazinato, F. M.; Borba, L. A.; Feijo, L. S.; Muller, V.; Finger, I. S.; Toribio, R. E.; Nogueira, C. E. W. Estradiol Cypionate Aided Treatment for Experimentally Induced Ascending Placentitis in Mares. *Theriogenology* **2017,** *102,* 98–107.

Daels, P. F.; Chang, G. C.; Hansen, B..; Mohammed, H. O. Testosterone Secretion During Early Pregnancy in Mares. *Theriogenology* **1996a,** *45* (6), 1211–1219.

Daels, P. F.; Besognet, B.; Hansen, B.; Mohammed, H.; Odensvik, K.; Kindahl, H. Effect of Progesterone on Prostaglandin F_2 Alpha Secretion and Outcome of Pregnancy During Cloprostenol-Induced Abortion in Mares. *Am. J. Vet. Res.* **1996b,** *57,* 1331–1337.

Daels, P. F.; Albrecht, B. A.; Mohammed, H. O. Equine Chorionic Gonadotropin Regulates Luteal Steroidogenesis in Pregnant Mares. *Biol. Reprod.* **1998,** *59* (5), 1062–1068.

Daels, P. F.; DeMoraes, J. J.; Stabenfeldt, G. H.; Hughes, J. P.; Lasley, B. L. The Corpus Luteum: Source of Oestrogen During Early Pregnancy in the Mare. *J. Reprod. Fertil. Suppl.* **1991a,** *44,* 501–508.

Daels, P. F.; Stabenfeldt, G. H.; Hughes, J. P.; Odensvik, K.; Kindahl, H. Evaluation of Progesterone Deficiency as a Cause of Fetal Death in Mares with Experimentally Induced Endotoxemia. *Am. J. Vet. Res.* **1991b,** *52,* 282–288.

Daels, P. F.; Hussni, M.; Montavon, S. M. E.; Stabenfeldt, G. H.; Hughes, J. P.; Odensvik, K.; Kindahl, H. Endogenous Prostaglandin Secretion During Cloprostenol-Induced Abortion in Mares. *Anim. Reprod.* **1995,** *40,* 305–321.

Davies Morel, M. C. *Equine Reproductive Physiology, Breeding and Stud Management,* 3rd ed. Wallindorf, UK: New York, **2008.**

Davies Morel, M. C.; Newcombe, J. R.; Holland, S. J. Factors Affecting Gestation Length in the Thoroughbred Mare. *Anim. Reprod. Sci.* **2002,** *74* (3–4), 175–185.

De Falco, S. The Discovery of Placenta Growth Factor and Its Biological Activity. *Exp. Mol. Med.* **2012,** *44* (1), 1.

De Luca, C. A.; McCue, P. M.; Patten, M. L.; Squires, E. L. Effect of a Nonsurgical Embryo Transfer Procedure and/or Altrenogest Therapy on Endogenous Progesterone Concentration in Mares. *J. Equine Vet. Sci.* **2011,** *31,* 57–62.

Douglas, R. H. Endocrine Diagnostics in the Broodmare: What You Need to Know about Progestins and Estrogens. In *Annual Meeting for the Society for Theriogenology and American College of Theriogenologists*; Lexington, KY, August 4–7, **2004;** pp 106–115.

Esteller-Vico, A.; Ball, B. A.; Troedsson, M. H. T.; Squires, E. L. Endocrine Changes, Fetal Growth, and Uterine Artery Hemodynamics after Chronic Estrogen Suppression During the Last Trimester of Equine Pregnancy. *Biol. Reprod.* **2017,** *96,* 414–423.

Ferraz, L. E. S.; Vicente, W. R. R.; Ramos, P. R. R. Progesterone and Estradiol 17-β Concentration, and Ultrasonic Images of the Embryonic Vesicle During the Early Pregnancy in Thoroughbred Mares. *Arq. Bras. Med. Vet. Zootechnol.* **2001,** *53* (4), 1–7.

Flaminio, M. J.; Antczak, D. F. Inhibition of Lymphocyte Proliferation and Activation: A Mechanism Used by Equine Invasive Trophoblast to Escape the Maternal Immune Response. *Placenta* **2005,** *26* (2–3), 148–159.

Fowden, A. L.; Forhead, A. J.; Ousey, J. C. The Endocrinology of Equine Parturition. *Exp. Clin. Endocrinol. Diabetes* **2008,** *116,* 393–403.

Gastal, M. O.; Gastal, E. L.; Torres, C. A..; Ginther, O. J. Effect of PGE2 on Uterine Contractility and Tone in Mares. *Theriogenology* **1998,** *50* (7), 989–999.

Gerstenberg, C.; Allen, W. R.; Stewart, F. Factors Controlling Epidermal Growth Factor (EGF) Gene Expression in the Endometrium of the Mare. *Mol. Reprod. Dev.* **1999,** *53* (3), 255–265.

Ginther, O. J. Equine Pregnancy: Physical Interactions between the Uterus and Conceptus. In *Proceedings of the 44th Annual Convention of the American Association of Equine Practitioners*; Baltimore, Maryland, December 6–9, **1998**.

Ginther, O. J. Mobility of the Early Equine Conceptus. *Theriogenology* **1983**, *19* (4), 603–611.

Ginther, O. J. *Reproductive Biology of the Mare: Basic and Applied Aspects*, 2nd ed. Equiservices, Cross Plains: Wisconsin, **1992**.

Ginther, O. J.; Santos, V. G. Natural Rescue and Resurgence of the Equine Corpus Luteum. *J. Equine Vet. Sci.* **2015**, *35*, 1–6.

Graczyk, J.; Macpherson, M. L.; Pozor, M. A.; Troedsson, M. H. T.; Eichelberger, A. C.; LeBlanc, M. M.; Vickroy, T. W. Treatment Efficacy of Trimethoprim Sulfamethoxazole and Pentoxifylline in Equine Placentitis. *Anim. Reprod. Sci.* **2006**, *94*, 434–435.

Gravett, M. G.; Hitti, J.; Hess, D. L.; Eschenbach, D. A. Intrauterine Infection and Preterm Delivery: Evidence for Activation of the Fetal Hypothalamic-Pituitary-Adrenal Axis. *Am. J. Obstet. Gynecol.* **2000**, *182*, 1404–1413.

Haffner, J. C.; Fecteau, K. A.; Eiler, H.; Tserendorj, T.; Hoffman, R. M.; Oliver, J. W. Blood Steroid Concentrations in Domestic Mongolian Horses. *J. Vet. Diagn. Invest.* **2010**, *22* (4), 537–543.

Haluska, G. J.; Currie, W. B. Variation in Plasma Concentrations of Oestradiol-17 Beta and Their Relationship to Those of Progesterone, 13,14-Dihydro-15-keto-prostaglandin F-2 Alpha and Oxytocin across Pregnancy and at Parturition in Pony Mares. *J. Reprod. Fertil.* **1988**, *84* (2), 635–646.

Hamon, M.; Clarke, S. W.; Houghton, E.; Fowden, A. L.; Silver, M.; Rossdale, P. D.; Ousey, J. C.; Heap, R. B. Production of 5 Alpha-dihydroprogesterone During Late Pregnancy in the Mare. *J. Reprod. Fertil. Suppl.* **1991**, *44*, 529–535.

Han, X.; Rossdale, P. D.; Ousey, J.; Holdstock, N.; Allen, W. R.; Silver, M.; Fowden, A. L.; McGladdery, A. J.; Labrie, F.; Belanger, A. Localisation of 15-Hydroxy Prostaglandin Dehydrogenase (PGDH) and Steroidogenic Enzymes in the Equine Placenta. *Equine Vet. J.* **1995**, *27* (5), 334–339.

Hasegawa, T.; Sato, F.; Nambo, Y.; Ishida, N. Expression of Steroidogenic Enzyme Genes in the Equine Feto-placental Unit. *J. Equine Sci.* **2001**, *12* (1), 25–32.

Henderson, K..; Stewart, J. A Dipstick Immunoassay to Rapidly Measure Serum Oestrone Sulfate Concentrations in Horses. *Reprod. Fertil. Dev.* **2000**, *12* (3–4), 183–189.

Henderson, K. M.; Eayrs, K. Pregnancy Status Determination in Mares Using a Rapid Lateral Flow Test for Measuring Serum Oestrone Sulphate. *New Zealand Vet. J.* **2004**, *52* (4) 193–196.

Hinrichs, K.; Sertich, P. L.; Palmer, E.; Kenney, R. M. Establishment and Maintenance of Pregnancy after Embryo Transfer in Ovariectomized Mares Treated with Progesterone. *J. Reprod. Fert.* **1987**, *80*, 395–401.

Holtan, D. W.; Houghton, E.; Silver, M.; Fowden, A. L.; Ousey, J.; Rossdale, P. D. Plasma Progestagens in the Mare, Fetus and Newborn Foal. *J. Reprod. Fertil. Suppl.* **1991**, *44*, 517–528.

Holtan, D. W.; Squires, E. L.; Lapin, D. R.; Ginther, O. J. Effect of Ovariectomy on Pregnancy in Mares. *J. Reprod. Fertil. Suppl.* **1979**, *27*, 457–463.

Hyland, J. H.; MacLean, A. A.; Robertson-Smith, G. R.; Jeffcott, L. B.; Stewart, G. A. Attempted Conversion of Twin to Singleton Pregnancy in Two Mares with Associated Changes in Plasma Oestrone Sulphate Concentrations. *Aust. Vet. J.* **1985**, *62* (12), 406–409.

Jackson, S. A.; Squires, E. L.; Nett, T. M. The Effect of Exogenous Progestins in Endogenous Progesterone Secretion in Pregnant Mares. *Theriogenology* **1986**, *25*, 275–279.

Jeffcott, L. B.; Rossdale, P. D. A Critical Review of Current Methods for Induction of Parturition in the Mare. *Equine Vet. J.* **1977**, *9*, 208–215.

Jeffcott, L. B.; Whitwell, K. E. Twinning as a Cause of Foetal and Neonatal Loss in the Thoroughbred Mare. *J. Comp. Pathol.* **1973**, *83*, 91–106.

Kajihara, T.; Tanaka, K.; Oguro, T.; Tochigi, H.; Prechapanich, J.; Uchino, S.; Itakura, A.; Sucurovic, S.; Murakami, K.; Brosens, J. J.; Ishihara, O. Androgens Modulate the Morphological Characteristics of Human Endometrial Stromal Cells Decidualized *In Vitro*. *Reprod. Sci.* **2014**, *21* (3), 372–380.

Kanitz, W.; Schneider, F.; Hoppen, H. O.; Unger, C.; Nürnberg, G.; Becker, F. Pregnancy Rates, LH and Progesterone Concentrations in Mares Treated with a GnRH Agonist. *Anim. Reprod. Sci.* **2007**, *97*, 55–62.

Kasman, L. H.; Hughes, J. P.; Stabenfeldt, G. H.; Starr, M. D.; Lasley, B. L. Estrone Sulfate Concentrations as an Indicator of Fetal Demise in Horses. *Am. J. Vet. Res.* **1988**, *49* (2), 184–187.

Kelleman, A. A..; Act, D. Equine Pregnancy and Clinical Applied Physiology. In *Proceedings of the 59th Annual Convention of the American Association of Equine Practitioners*; Nashville, Tennessee, USA, December 7–11, **2013**.

Klein, C. The Role of Relaxin in Mare Reproductive Physiology: A Comparative Review with Other Species. *Theriogenology* **2016**, *86*, 451–456.

Klonisch, T.; Hombach-Klonisch, S. Review: Relaxin Expressed at the Feto-Maternal Interface. *Reprod. Dom. Anim.* **2000**, *35* (3–4), 149.

Köhne, M.; Ille, N.; Erber, R.; Aurich, C. Treatment with Human Chorionic Gonadotrophin before Ovulation Increases Progestin Concentration in Early Equine Pregnancies. *Anim. Reprod. Sci.* **2014**, *149*, 187–193.

LeBlanc, M. M. Ascending Placentitis in the Mare: An Update. *Reprod. Domest. Anim.* **2010**, *45*, 28–34.

LeBlanc, M. M. Common Peripartum Problems in the Mare. *J. Equine Vet. Sci.* **2008**, *28*, 709–715.

LeBlanc, M. M.; Giguere, S.; Brauer, K.; Paccamonti, D. L.; Horohov, D. W.; Lester, G. D.; O'Donnell, L. J.; Sheerin, B. R.; Pablo, L.; Rodgerson, D. H. Premature Delivery in Ascending Placentitis Is Associated with Increased Expression of Placental Cytokines and Allantoic Fluid Prostaglandins E2 and F$_2\alpha$. *Theriogenology* **2002**, *58*, 841–844.

LeBlanc, M. M.; Macpherson, M.; Sheerin, P. Ascending Placentitis: What We Know about Pathophysiology, Diagnosis and Treatment. *Proc. Am. Assoc. Equine Pract.* **2004**, *50*, 127–143.

LeBlanc, M. M.; Giguere, S.; Lester, G. D.; Bauer, K.; Paccamonti, L. Relationship between Infection, Inflammation and Premature Parturition in Mares with Experimentally Induced Placentitis. *Equine Vet. J. Suppl.* **2012**, *41*, 8–14.

Lefranc, A. C.; Allen, W. R. Influence of Breed and Oestrous Cycle on Endometrial Gland Surface Density in the Mare. *Equine Vet. J.* **2000**, *39* (6), 506–510.

Legacki, E. L.; Scholtz, E. L.; Ball, B. A.; Stanley, S. D.; Berger, T.; Conley, A. J. The Dynamic Steroid Landscape of Equine Pregnancy Mapped by Mass Spectrometry. *Reproduction* **2016**, *151* (4), 421–430.

Lennard, S. N.; Stewart, F.; Allen, W. R. Transforming Growth Factor Beta 1 Expression in the Endometrium of the Mare During Placentation. *Mol. Reprod. Dev.* **1995,** *42* (2), 131–140.

Lennard, S. N.; Gerstenberg, C.; Allen, W. R.; Stewart, F. Expression of Epidermal Growth Factor and Its Receptor in Equine Placental Tissues. *J. Reprod. Fertil.* **1998,** *112* (1), 49–57.

Lunn, P.; Vagnoni, K. E.; Ginther, O. J. The Equine Immune Response to Endometrial Cups. *J. Reprod. Immunol.* **1997,** *34* (3), 203–216.

Lyle, S. K. Immunology of Infective Preterm Delivery in the Mare. *Equine Vet. J.* **2014,** *46,* 661–668.

Lyle, S. K.; Paccamonti, D. L.; Hubert, J. D.; Schlafer, D. H.; Causey, R. C.; Eilts, B. E.; Johnson, J. R. Laparoscopic Placement of an Indwelling Allantoic Catheter in the Mare: Biochemical, Cytologic, Histologic, and Microbiologic Findings. *Anim. Reprod. Sci.* **2006,** *94,* 428–431.

Lyle, S. K.; Hague, M.; Lopez, M. J.; Beehan, D. P.; Staempfil, S.; Len, J. A.; Eilts, B. E.; Paccamonti, D. L. *In Vitro* Production of Cortisol by Equine Fetal Adrenal Cells in Response to ACTH and IL-1b. *Anim. Reprod. Sci.* **2010,** *121,* 322.

Machnik, M.; Hegger, I.; Kietzmann, M.; Thevis, M.; Guddat, S.; Schänzer, W. Pharmacokinetics of Altrenogest in Horses. *J. Vet. Pharmacol. Therap.* **2007,** *30,* 86–90.

McGlothlin, J. A.; Lester, G. D.; Hansen, P. J.; Thomas, M.; Pablo, L.; Hawkins, D. L.; LeBlanc, M. M. Alteration in Uterine Contractility in Mares with Experimentally Induced Placentitis. *Reproduction* **2004,** *127* (1), 57–66.

Miller, W. L.; Auchus, R. J. The Molecular Biology, Biochemistry, and Physiology of Human Steroidogenesis and Its Disorders. *Endocr. Rev.* **2011,** *32* (1), 81–151.

Mizushima, C. Late-Term Abortion Associated with Umbilical Cord Torsion in the Mare: Case Report. *J. Equine Vet. Sci.* **2005,** 25, 162–163.

Morris, L. H. A.; Allen, W. R. Reproductive Efficiency of Intensively Managed Thoroughbred Mares in New Market. *Equine Vet. J.* **2002,** *34,* 51–60.

Morris, S.; Kelleman, A. A.; Stawicki, R. J.; Hansen, P. J.; Sheerin, P. C.; Sheerin, B. R. Paccamonti, D. L.; LeBlanc, M. M. Transrectal Ultrasonography and Plasma Progestin Profiles Identifies Feto-Placental Compromise in Mares with Experimentally Induced Placentitis. *Theriogenology* **2007,** *67,* 681–691.

Möstl, E. The Horse Feto-Placental Unit. *Exp. Clin. Endocrinol.* **1994,** *102* (3), 166–168.

Naber, M. E.; Shemesh, M.; Shore, L. S., Rios, C. Estrogen and Progesterone Levels in Pure Bred Arabian Horses During Pregnancy. *Israel J. Vet. Med.* **1999,** *54* (2), 33–35.

Nelis, H.; Vanden Bussche, J.; Wojciechowicz, B.; Franczak, A.; Vanhaecke, L.; Leemans, B.; Cornillie, P.; Peelman, L.; Van Soom, A.; Smits, K. Steroids in the Equine Oviduct: Synthesis, Local Concentrations and Receptor Expression. *Reprod. Fertil. Dev.* **2015,** *28* (9), 1390–1404.

Neuhauser, S.; Palm, F.; Ambuehl, F.; Aurich, C. Effects of Altrenogest Treatment of Mares in Late Pregnancy on Parturition and on Neonatal Viability of Their Foals. *Exp. Clin. Endocrinol. Diabetes* **2008,** *116,* 423–428.

Neuhauser, S.; Palm, F.; Ambuehl, F.; Möstl, E.; Schwendenwein, I.; Aurich, C. Effect of Altrenogest-Treatment of Mares in Late Gestation on Adrenocortical Function, Blood Count and Plasma Electrolytes in Their Foals. *Equine Vet. J.* **2009,** *41,* 572–577.

Newcombe, J. R. Embryonic Loss and Abnormalities of Early Pregnancy. *Equine Vet. Educ.* **2000a,** *12,* 88–101.

Newcombe, J. R. Spontaneous Oestrous Behaviour During Pregnancy Associated with Luteal Regression, Ovulation and Birth of a Live Foal in a Part Thoroughbred Mare. *Equine Vet. Educ.* **2000b,** *12,* 85–87.

Newcombe, J. R.; Martinez, T. A.; Peters, A. R. The Effect of the Gonadotropin-Releasing Hormone Analog, Buserelin, on Pregnancy Rates in Horse and Pony Mares. *Theriogenology* **2001,** *55,* 1619–1631.

Newcombe, J. R.; Peters, A. R. The Buserelin Enigma: How Does Treatment with this GnRH Analogue Decrease Embryo Mortality? *J. Vet. Sci. Technol.* **2014,** *5,* 151.

O'Donnell, L. J.; Sheerin, B. R.; Hendry, J. M.; Thatcher, M. J.; Thatcher, W. W.; LeBlanc, M. M. 24-Hour Secretion Patterns of Plasma Oestradiol 17Beta in Pony Mares in Late Gestation. *Reprod. Dom. Anim.* **2003,** *38* (3), 233–235.

Ousey, J. C. Peripartal Endocrinology in the Mare and Foetus. *Reprod. Domest. Anim.* **2004,** *39* (4), 222–231.

Ousey, J. C. Hormone Profiles and Treatments in the Late Pregnant Mare. *Vet. Clin. North Am. Equine Pract.* **2006,** *22* (3), 727–747.

Ousey, J. C. Endocrinology of Pregnancy. In *Equine Reproduction*; McKinnon, A. O., Squires, E. L., Vaala, W. E., Varner, D. D., Eds.; Wiley-Blackwell: Hoboken NJ, **2011**; pp 2222–2231.

Ousey, J.; McGladdery, A. Clinical Diagnosis and Treatment of Problems in the Late Pregnant Mare. *In Pract.* **2000,** *22,* 200–207.

Ousey, J. C.; Rossdale, P. D.; Dudan, F. E.; Houghton, E.; Grainger, L.; Fowden, A. L. The Effects of Intrafetal ACTH Administration on the Outcome of Pregnancy in the Mare. *Reprod. Fertil. Dev.* **1998,** *10,* 359–367.

Ousey, J. C.; Freestone, N.; Fowden, A. L.; Mason, W. T.; Rossdale, P. D. The Effects of Oxytocin and Progestagens on Myometrial Contractility in Vitro During Equine Pregnancy. *J. Reprod. Fertil. Suppl.* **2000,** *56,* 681–689.

Ousey, J. C.; Rossdale, P. D.; Palmer, L.; Houghton, E.; Grainger, L.; Fowden, A. L. Effects of Progesterone Administration to Mares During Late Gestation. *Theriogenology* **2002,** *58,* 793–795.

Ousey, J. C.; Forhead, A. J.; Rossdale, P. D.; Grainger, L.; Houghton, E.; Fowden, A. L. Ontogeny of Uteroplacental Progestagen Production in Pregnant Mares During the Second Half of Gestation. Biol. Reprod. **2003,** *69* (2), 540–548.

Ousey, J. C.; Houghton, E.; Grainger, L.; Rossdale, P. D.; Fowden, A. L. Progestagen Profiles During the Last Trimester of Gestation in Thoroughbred Mares with Normal or Compromised Pregnancies. *Theriogenology* **2005,** *63* (7), 1844–1856.

Panzani, D.; Crisci, A.; Rota, A.; Camillo, F. Effect of Day of Transfer and Treatment Administration on the Recipient on Pregnancy Rates after Equine Embryo Transfer. *Vet. Res. Commun.* **2009,** *33,* 113–116.

Parry-Weeks, L. C.; Holtan, D. W. Effect of Altrenogest on Pregnancy Maintenance in Unsynchronized Equine Embryo Recipients. *J. Reprod. Fertil. Suppl.* **1986,** *35,* 433–438.

Pashen, R. L.; Allen, W. R. The Role of the Fetal Gonads and Placenta in Steroid Production, Maintenance of Pregnancy and Parturition in the Mare. *J. Reprod. Fertil. Suppl.* **1979,** *27,* 499–509.

Pycock, J.; Newcombe, J. The Effect of the Gonadotrophin-Releasing Hormone Analog, Buserelin, Administered in Diestrus on Pregnancy Rates and Pregnancy Failure in Mares. *Theriogenology* **1996,** *46,* 1097–1101.

Raeside, J. I. Seasonal Changes in the Concentration of Estrogens and Testosterone in the Plasma of the Stallion. *Anim. Reprod. Sci.* **1979**, *1* (3), 205–212.

Raeside, J. I.; Christie, H. L.; Renaud, R. L.; Waelchli, R. O.; Betteridge, K. J. Estrogen Metabolism in the Equine Conceptus and Endometrium During Early Pregnancy in Relation to Estrogen Concentrations in Yolk-Sac Fluid. *Biol. Reprod.* **2004**, *71* (4), 1120–1127.

Raeside, J. I.; Christie, H. L.; Waelchli, R. O.; Betteridge, K. J. Biosynthesis of Oestrogen by the Early Equine Embryo Proper. *Reprod. Fertil. Dev.* **2012**, *24* (8), 1071–1078.

Raeside, J. I.; Renaud, R. L.; Christie, H. L. Postnatal Decline in Gonadal Secretion of Dehydroepiandrosterone and 3 Beta-hydroxyandrosta-5,7-dien-17-one in the Newborn Foal. *J. Endocrinol.* **1997**, *155* (2), 277–282.

Rambags, B. P.; van Tol, H. T.; van den Eng, M. M.; Colenbrander, B.; Stout, T. A. Expression of Progesterone and Oestrogen Receptors by Early Intrauterine Equine Conceptuses. *Theriogenology* **2008**, *69* (3), 366–375.

Ribatti, D. The Discovery of the Placental Growth Factor and Its Role in Angiogenesis: A Historical Review. *Angiogenesis* **2008**, *11* (3), 215–221.

Rossdale, P. D. Clinical View of Disturbances in Equine Fetal Maturation. *Equine Vet. J. Suppl.* **1993**, *25*, 3–7.

Rossdale, P. D.; Ousey, J. C.; Cottrill, C. M.; Chavatte, P.; Allen, W. R.; McGladdery, A. J. Effects of Placental Pathology on Maternal Plasma Progestagen and Mammary Secretion Calcium Concentrations and on Neonatal Adrenocortical Function in the Horse. *J. Reprod. Fertil. Suppl.* **1991**, *44*, 579–490.

Rossdale, P. D.; McGladdery, A. J.; Ousey, J. C.; Holdstock, N.; Grainger, L.; Houghton, E. Increase in Plasma Progestagen Concentrations in the Mare after Foetal Injection with CRH, ACTH or Betamethasone in Late Gestation. *Equine Vet. J.* **1992**, *24*, 347–350.

Rossdale, P. D.; Ousey, J. C.; McGladdery, A. J.; Prandi, S.; Holdstock, N.; Grainger, L.; Houghton, E. A Retrospective Study of Increased Plasma Progestagen Concentrations in Compromised Neonatal Foals. *Reprod. Fertil. Dev.* **1995**, *7*, 567–575.

Rowe, A. J.; Wulff, C.; Fraser, H. M. Localization of mRNA for Vascular Endothelial Growth Factor (VEGF), Angiopoietins and Their Receptors During the Peri-implantation Period and Early Pregnancy in Marmosets (*Callithrix jacchus*). *Reproduction* **2003**, *126* (2), 227–238.

Ryan, P. L.; Christiansen, D. L.; Hopper, R. M.; Bagnell, C. A.; Vaala, W. E.; LeBlanc, M. M. Evaluation of Systemic Relaxin Blood Profiles in Horses as a Means of Assessing Placental Function in High-Risk Pregnancies and Responsiveness to Therapeutic Strategies. *Ann. N.Y. Acad. Sci.* **2009**, *1160*, 169–178.

Santschi, E. M.; LeBlanc, M. M.; Weston, P. G. Progestagen, Oestrone Sulphate and Cortisol Concentrations in Pregnant Mares During Medical and Surgical Disease. *J. Reprod. Fertil. Suppl.* **1991**, *44*, 627–634.

Satué, K.; Domingo, R.; Redondo, J. I. Relationship between Progesterone, Oestrone Sulphate and Cortisol and the Components of Renin Angiotensin Aldosterone System in Spanish Purebred Broodmares During Pregnancy. *Theriogenology* **2011**, *76* (8), 1404–1415.

Satué, K.; Marcilla, M.; Medica, P.; Ferlazzo, A.; Fazio, E. Sequential Concentrations of Placental Growth Factor and Haptoglobin, and Their Relation to Oestrone Sulphate and Progesterone in Pregnant Spanish Purebred Mare. *Theriogenology* **2018**, *115*, 77–83.

Satué, K.; Marcilla, M.; Medica, P.; Ferlazzo, A.; Fazio, E. Testosterone, Androstenedione and Dehydroepiandrosterone Concentrations in Pregnant Spanish Purebred Mare. *Theriogenology* **2019**, *1* (123), 62–67.

Scholtz, E. L.; Krishnan, S.; Ball, B. A.; Corbin, C. J.; Moeller, B. C.; Stanley, S. D.; McDowell, K. J.; Hughes, A. L.; McDonnell, D. P.; Conley, A. J. Pregnancy without Progesterone in Horses Defines a Second Endogenous Biopotent Progesterone Receptor Agonist, 5α-Dihydroprogesterone. In *Proceedings of the National Academy of Sciences of the United States of America*, **2014**; pp 3365–3370.

Seckl, J. R. Prenatal Glucocorticoids and Long-Term Programming. *Eur. J. Endocrinol.* **2004**, *151*, 49–62.

Shikichi, M.; Iwata, K.; Ito, K.; Miyakoshi, D.; Murase, H.; Sato, F.; Korosue, K.; Nagata, S.; Nambo, Y. Abnormal Pregnancies Associated with Deviation in Progestin and Estrogen Profiles in Late Pregnant Mares: A Diagnostic Aid. *Theriogenology* **2017**, *98*, 75–81.

Sieme, J. L.; Sielhorst, J.; Martinsson, G.; Bollwein, H.; Thomas, S.; Burger, D. Improving the Formation and Function of the Corpus Luteum in the Mare. *Rev. Bras. Reprod. Anim.* **2015**, *39*, 117–120.

Silva, L. A.; Klein, C.; Ealy, A. D.; Sharp, D. C. Conceptus-Mediated Endometrial Vascular Changes during Early Pregnancy in Mares: An Anatomic, Histomorphometric, and Vascular Endothelial Growth Factor Receptor System Immunolocalization and Gene Expression Study. *Reproduction* **2011**, *142* (4), 593–603.

Silver, M.; Barnes, R. J.; Comline, R. S.; Fowden, A. L.; Clover, L.; Mitchell, M. D. Prostaglandins in Maternal and Fetal Plasma and in Allantoic Fluid During the Second Half of Gestation in the Mare. *J. Reprod. Fertil. Suppl.* **1979**, *27*, 531–539.

Silver, M.; Fowden, A. L. Prepartum Adrenocortical Maturation in the Fetal Foal. *J. Endocrinol* **1994**, *142*, 417–425.

Squires, E. L. Hormonal Manipulation of the Mare: A Review. *J. Equine Vet. Sci.* **2008**, *28*, 627–634.

Stewart, D. R.; Stabenfeldt, G. H.; Hughes, J. P. Relaxin Activity in Foaling Mares. *J. Reprod. Fertil. Suppl.* **1982a**, *32*, 603–609.

Stewart, D. R.; Stabenfeldt, G. H.; Hughes, J. P.; Meagher, D. M. Determination of the Source of Equine Relaxin. *Biol. Reprod.* **1982b**, *27*, 17–24.

Stewart, D. R.; Kindahl, H.; Stabenfeldt, G. H.; Hughes, J. P. Concentrations of 15-keto-13, 14-Dihydroprostaglandin F2 Alpha in the Mare During Spontaneous and Oxytocin Induced Foaling. *Equine Vet. J.* **1984**, *16*, 270–274.

Stewart, D. R.; Addiego, L. A.; Pascoe, D. R.; Haluska, G. J.; Pashen, R. Breed Differences in Circulating Equine Relaxin. *Biol. Reprod.* **1992**, *46* (4), 648–652.

Stewart, F.; Power, C. A.; Lennard, S. N.; Allen, W. R.; Amet, L.; Edwards, R. M. Identification of the Horse Epidermal Growth Factor (EGF) Coding Sequence and Its Use in Monitoring EGF Gene Expression in the Endometrium of the Pregnant Mare. *J. Mol. Endocrinol.* **1994**, *12* (3), 341–350.

Stewart, F.; Gerstenberg, C.; Allen, W. R. Factors Controlling Chorioallantoic Placentation in the Mare. *Pferdeheilkunde* **1999**, *15* (6), 611–613.

Stout, T. A. E. Prospects for improving the efficiency of Thoroughbred Breeding by Individual Tailoring of Stallion Mating Frequency. *Equine Vet. J.* **2012**, *44*, 504–505.

Stout, T. A. E.; Allen, W. R. Role of Prostaglandins in Intrauterine Migration of the Equine Conceptus. *Reproduction* **2001**, *121* (5), 771–775.

Stout, T. A. E.; Tremoleda, J. L.; Knaap, J.; Daels, P.; Kindahl, H.; Colenbrander, B. Mid-Diestrus GnRH-Analogue Administration Does Not Suppress the Luteolytic Mechanism in Mares. *Theriogenology* **2002**, *58*, 567–570.

Troedsson, M. H. T.; Zent, W. W. Clinical Ultrasonagraphic Evaluation of the Equine Placenta as a Method to Successfully Identify and Treat Mares with Placentitis. In *Proceedings of a Workshop on the Equine Placenta*; Kentucky Agricultural Experiment Station: Lexington, 2003; pp 66–67.

Troedsson, M. H. T.; Miller, L. M. J. Equine Placentitis. *Pferdeheilkunde* **2016**, *32*, 49–53.

Tsumagari, S.; Higashino, T.; Takagi, K.; Ohba, S.; Satoh, S.; Takeishi, M. Changes of Plasma Concentrations of Steroid Hormones, Prostaglandin F$_2$ Alpha-Metabolite and Pregnant Mare Serum Gonadotropin During Pregnancy in Thoroughbred Mares. *J. Vet. Med. Sci.* **1991**, *53* (5), 797–801.

van Niekerk, C. H.; Morgenthal, J. C. Fetal Loss and the Effect of Stress on Plasma Progestagen Levels in Pregnant Thoroughbred Mares. *J. Reprod. Fertil. Suppl.* **1982**, *32*, 453–457.

Vanderwall, D.; Marquardt, J.; Woods, G. Use of a Compounded Long-Acting Progesterone Formulation for Equine Pregnancy Maintenance. *J. Equine Vet. Sci.* **2007**, *27*, 62–66.

Vanderwall, D. K. Early Embryonic Loss in the Mare. *J. Equine Vet. Sci.* **2008**, *28*, 691–702.

Vivrette, S. L.; Kindahl, H.; Munro, C. J.; Roser, J. F.; Stabenfeldt, G. H. Oxytocin Release and Its Relationship to Dihydro-15-keto PGF$_2$ and Arginine Vasopressin Release During Parturition and to Suckling in Postpartum Mares. *J. Reprod. Fertil.* **2000**, *119* (2), 347–357.

Weng, Q.; Tanaka, Y.; Taniyama, H.; Tsunoda, N.; Nambo, Y.; Watanabe, G.; Taya, K. Immunolocalization of Steroidogenic Enzymes in Equine Fetal Adrenal Glands During Mid-Late Gestation. *J. Reprod. Dev.* **2007**, *53* (5), 1093–1098.

Whitwell, K. E. Investigations into Fetal and Neonatal Losses in the Horse. *Vet. Clin. North Am. Large Anim. Pract.* **1980**, *2*, 313–331.

Willmann, C.; Schuler, G.; Hoffmann, B.; Parvizi, N. Effects of Age and Altrenogest Treatment on Conceptus Development and Secretion of LH, Progesterone and eCG in Early-Pregnant Mares. *Theriogenology* **2011**, *75*, 421–428.

Wilsher, S.; Allen, W. R. Factors Influencing Equine Chorionic Gonadotrophin Production in the Mare. *Equine Vet. J.* **2011**, *43* (4), 430–438.

Wilsher, S.; Gower, S.; Allen, W. R. Immunohistochemical Localisation of Progesterone and Oestrogen Receptors at the Placental Interface in Mares During Early Pregnancy. *Anim. Reprod. Sci.* **2011**, *129* (3–4), 200–208.

Wynn, M. A. A.; Esteller-Vico, A.; Legacki, E. L.; Conley, A. J.; Loux, S. C.; Stanley, S. D.; Curry, T. E. Jr.; Squires, E. L.; Troedsson, M. H.; Ball, B. A. A. Comparison of Progesterone Assays for Determination of Peripheral Pregnane Concentrations in the Late Pregnant Mare. *Theriogenology* **2018a**, *106*, 127–133.

Wynn, M. A. A.; Ball, B. A.; May, J.; Esteller-Vico, A.; Canisso, I.; Squires, E.; Troedsson, M. Changes in Maternal Pregnane Concentrations in Mares with experimentally-Induced, Ascending Placentitis. *Theriogenology* **2018b**, *122*, 130–136.

CHAPTER 8

Equine Semen Preservation: Current and Future Trends

LYDIA GIL HUERTA[1*], CRISTINA ÁLVAREZ[2], and
VICTORIA LUÑO LÁZARO[1]

[1]*Department of Animal Pathology, Faculty of Veterinary Medicine,
Agroalimentary Institute of Aragón IA2, University of Zaragoza,
Center for Agrifood Research and Technology (CITA), Zaragoza,
C/Miguel Servet 133, 50013, Zaragoza, Spain*

[2]*Chief Veterinary Officer of the Veterinary Unit, Zaragoza, Spain*

Corresponding author. E-mail: lydiagil@unizar.es

ABSTRACT

Nowadays, stallion semen processing and preservation for artificial insemination (AI) is a widely used tool in modern horse reproduction. During the 20th century, AI had a strong development in most domestic animal species except in equine species, due to economic interests, traditional aspects and mistrust of horse owners. Semen conservation technologies based on temperature decrease to reduce or stop sperm metabolism are necessary to increase the lifespan of sperm and preserving sperm functionality and fertility. Currently, AI is performed mainly with fresh, chilled or frozen semen. Sperm refrigeration at 5°C has several advantages related to easy handling and shipping, low cost because it does not require special equipment and minor legal requirements for import and export. However, cryopreservation is the only viable method for spermatozoa storage during indefinite periods. The main problem of freezing semen is related to the low fertility rates obtained due to wide inter-individual sperm quality variability; therefore only some stallions produce suitable semen for cryopreservation. To solve these disadvantages, new methodologies have been studied during recent years with different results. Vitrification and lyophilization are promising stallion semen preservation techniques that require further study to be applied routinely during long-term periods.

8.1   INTRODUCTION

Equine sperm preservation methods have been linked to the development of artificial insemination (AI). The first reports of AI in horses were documented from Arabian texts, in which semen samples were obtained from recently covered mares of rival tribes and then utilized to inseminate their own mares. However, until the end of the 19th century, AI did not obtain promising results in mares due to researches carried out by Ivanow in Russia and Dr. Pearson at Pennsylvania University.

The decrease of equine population after the Second World War and the restrictive regulations regarding the use of AI in several equine breed organizations delayed the progress of this technique in horses. First, studies about stallion semen collection and handling were described by Mckenzie et al. (1939) and Berliner (1942) with suitable sperm quality results. The discovery of glycerol as cryoprotectant agent in 1949 by Polge et al., was the beginning of the development of preservation techniques of biological materials including equine sperm. Next year, Barker and Gandier (1957) obtained the first foal from cryopreserved epidydimal stallion sperm. During the 1970s and 1980s, the utilization of cooled semen on AI programs increased due to the development of a transport container (Equitainer) (Douglas-Hamilton et al., 1984), the use of Kenney extender (Kenney et al., 1975) and the acceptance of reproductive biotechnology by several breeders.

Several advantages show frozen-thawed sperm in comparison to cooled sperm, such as the scheduled use of stallions outside the competition period, easy international transport and the centralized processing of frozen semen by specialized laboratories, which decrease the variability of the seminal quality. Despite the current advances, cryopreserved semen shows some disadvantages, such as low fertility rates, control of the mare cycle, and a high cost along cryopreservation process (Brinsko and Varner, 1992; Samper and Morris, 1998; Loomis and Graham, 2008). Furthermore, it has been estimated that only 30–40% of stallions produce semen that is suitable for cryopreservation, and a large interindividual variation on sperm survival during the freezing and thawing procedures has been also reported (Loomis and Graham, 2008).

Nowadays, AI is the most common biotechnology utilized around the world in the horse industry and it has enabled the development of other technologies, such as sperm sexing, regulation of the estrous cycle, embryo transfer, cloning as well as improvement of semen preservation methods as sperm refrigeration or freezing and, currently, sperm vitrification and lyophilization.

8.2 SEMEN COLLECTION

Semen collection is an essential part of preservation protocols and AI programs. The quality of collected semen depends on numerous factors such as libido, season, age, or breed (Samper, 2000). Semen can be collected using different methods; condom, pharmacological induction, manual manipulation or by the use of artificial vagina, the tool most commonly used (Samper, 2000). There are several models of artificial vagina available commercially. The Colorado model is the most wide-spread at the beginning, but currently the most used is the Missouri model due to the improvements and efficiency.

The ejaculate is a liquid suspension composed of sperm and seminal plasma, which comprised a complex mixture of secretions (fructose, sorbitol, ascorbic acid, lactic acid, citric acid, proteins, enzymes, vitamins, and hormones). Seminal plasma-derived primarily from the epididymis and accessory sex glands of the male. It participates in the final sperm maturation, modifies spermatic membrane surface, besides acts as a vehicle for the ejaculated sperm and protects the spermatozoa during the female reproductive tract transport (Töpfer-Petersen et al., 2000). In stallion, the seminal plasma is normally separated from the semen during the cryopreservation process, since it has proved to be a harmful medium because decrease the percentage of sperm with progressive motility (Pickett et al., 1975; Jasko et al., 1992). The ejaculate should not be exposed to mechanical damage, light, cold, or heat and the equipment in contact with the sperm must be tempered, dry, clean, and free of toxic residues. After ejaculation, the semen will be kept at 30/32°C before the seminal evaluation and subsequent dilution (Brinsko and Varner, 1992).

Another effective way to recover genetic material in horses is to obtain it from the epididymis from castrated or slaughtered animals. This technique allows obtaining sperm from stallions of high genetic value that have suffered sudden death, major injuries, or castration. Different studies have demonstrated the efficiency of epididymal sperm recovery (Tiplady et al., 2002, Monteiro et al., 2011). In addition, several researchers suggest that sperm can be harvested immediately after orchiectomy or after 24 h of storage at 4°C–5°C without any difference in terms of viability (Bruemmer et al., 2006; Neild et al., 2006). Different methods have been used to collect epididymal sperm, including percutaneous epididymal sperm aspiration, the flotation method, the retrograde flush technique, or the standard flush technique of epididymis and ductus deferens (Cary et al., 2004; Bruemmer, 2006). This technique allows recovery of a high number of sperms compared with the collection by artificial vagina (Bruemmer, 2006). The motility of epididymal and ejaculated sperm in stallions has been found comparable and no differences were observed in terms of morphological defects and sperm viability (Weiss et al., 2008; Guimarães et al., 2012).

8.3   SEMEN PROCESSING

The semen quality is assessed immediately after collection. Andrological evaluation verifies the reproductive potential of a stallion in the buying and selling process, before the beginning of the reproductive season and before semen preservation or AI. The general parameters used for the analysis of semen quality include total volume, sperm concentration, motility, and normal morphology. Other tests, such as acrosome and membrane integrity, hypo-osmotic swelling test (HOST), mitochondrial activity, or the thermal resistance test can be used for assessment of semen quality (Love et al., 2018). However, some animals with apparently normal semen quality show very poor fertility rates; in these cases, a more exhaustive evaluation is necessary.

After the semen quality evaluation, equine ejaculate is usually centrifuged. In some countries, it is a standard practice prior to preparing sperm doses before AI. Centrifugation increases sperm concentration of the ejaculate and also removes the seminal plasma (Parlevliet and Colenbrander, 1999; Hoogewijs et al., 2010). However, it might generate negative effects on the conservation of equine sperm, decreasing the motility and viability of sperm (Martin et al., 1979), due to the physical damage on the cells and ROS production (Hoogewijs et al., 2010).

Contradictory results have been obtained in relation seminal plasma utilization on sperm preservation. Different studies showed that the removal of seminal plasma enhanced the survival spermatozoa (Parlevliet and Colenbrander, 1999; Aurich, 2005); however, the presence of a small amount of stallion seminal plasma (0.6–20%) increased sperm motility, plasma membrane integrity, and fertility (Jasko et al., 1992; Moore et al., 2006; Neuhauser et al., 2015). Beneficial effects may be related to antioxidant properties and the inhibitory effect on the binding of polymorphonuclear neutrophils on the female reproductive tract (Knop et al., 2005).

A special extender based on dense isotonic compounds is utilized during centrifugation. The most common mediums are citrate-ethylene acid (EDTA) (Cochran et al., 1984), Tyrode medium (Ljaz and Ducharme, 1995), and glucose-EDTA (Martin et al., 1979). The extender function is to maintain motility and protect the sperm during the centrifugation process and in a dilution ratio of 1:1 or 1:2. The centrifugation influences on equine sperm by the strength and time of centrifugation, the kind of extender, the presence or absence of the extender before centrifugation, and the concentration of seminal plasma (Pickett et al., 1975; Aurich, 2005). Different protocols have been used as shown in (Table 8.1).

TABLE 8.1   Different Stallion Sperm Centrifugation Protocols.

Centrifugation	References
1000g/5 min	Martin et al., 1979
600g/10 min	Palmer 1984
400g/12 min	Brinsko et al., 2011
400g/15 min	Cochran et al., 1984

8.4   SEMEN PRESERVATION TECHNIQUES

8.4.1   SPERM COOLING

The utilization of fresh semen avoids the damage by thermal shock derived from the conservation techniques at refrigeration or freezing temperatures. Nowadays, sperm quality is preserved just a few hours, therefore, the sperm conservation in refrigeration is the technique more used for semen storage and transportation. The cooling temperature reduces sperm metabolism sufficiently to maintain sperm viability, functionality, and fertility (Gibb and Aitken, 2016) for up to 96 h. Several studies have determined that AI with cooling semen shows a similar fertility rate in comparison with fresh semen (Jasko et al., 1992; Shore et al., 1998). In addition, the semen preserved in refrigeration at 5°C for 24 h maintains the same fertility rates as fresh semen (Aurich, 2005).

Semen preservation at low temperatures reduces sperm catabolism and cellular injury (Aurich, 2005). The metabolic rate restriction decreases the production of toxic metabolites (hydrogen peroxide, lipid aldehydes, or dioxide carbon), ATP and reactive oxygen species (ROS) (Vishwanath and Shannon, 1997; Gibb and Aitken, 2016). However, the cooling process involves a "cold-shock" that produces damage to the membrane, especially when the cooling rates are higher than 0.3°C/min (Aurich, 2005). This damage is characterized by abnormal patterns of movement, loss of motility during storage, acrosomal membrane damage, as well as a decrease of cellular metabolism due to the loss of enzymes and other intracellular components (Moran et al., 1992).

Several studies show that slow cooling rates (<0.3°C/min) maximize the motility and fertility of equine semen (Douglas-Hamilton et al., 1984; Varner et al., 1987), although equine semen can be refrigerated rapidly from 37°C to 20°C. Then, we should reduce to 0.1°C/min, preferably 0.05°C/min from 20°C to 5°C (Kayser et al., 1992). The time required for sperm cooling from 37°C to 4°C is between 2 and 4 h (Moran et al., 1992).

The extender most utilized in equine sperm refrigeration storage is INRA96®, a commercial media, made from purified fractions of milk that was developed by Batellier et al. in 1997. In this extender, the β-lactoglobulins and calcium phosphocaseins of milk were replaced by purified calcium phosphocaseins, which improve sperm membrane protection. In addition, it contains sugars and proteins that serve as an energy source and protect from thermal shock sperm, penicillin, and gentamicin to prevent bacterial growth and amphotericin B as a fungicide. The most common cooling extenders utilized are synthesized as given in Table 8.2 (Palmer, 1984; Aurich, 2004). The use of glucose (a source of energy), bicarbonate (buffer), and milk in the stallion cooling medium show the best results in progressive motility, viability, and fertility rates (Aurich, 2004). The inclusion of some antioxidants, such as taurine in INRA 82 and Kenney medium, improves motility and sperm viability (Ljaz and Ducharme, 1995). The addition of glutamine increases the fertility rates but not motility on equine chilled semen (Trimeche et al., 1999). Milk-based medium shows better semen analysis in comparison to egg yolk-based medium since the density of the milk does not interfere with the microscopic manipulations of semen. The gelatin of some extenders produces plasma membrane stabilization but interfere with microscopic evaluation (Pickett et al.,1975).

TABLE 8.2   Stallion Sperm Chilled Extenders.

Extender	References
Skim-milk-glucose Kenney I	Kenney et al., 1975
Skim-milk-glucose Kenney II	Kenney et al., 1975
E-Z Mixin	Province et al., 1985
INRA 82	Ljaz and Ducharme 1995
Skim-milk-gelatin	Ljaz and Ducharme 1995
INRA 96	Batellier et al., 1997

8.4.2   SPERM CRYOPRESERVATION

Cryopreservation is the only viable method for sperm storage during indefinite periods of time (Gibb and Aitken, 2016). However, freezing-thawing process produces several detrimental effects on the gametes such us loss on sperm viability and motility due to membrane damage caused by the production of ROS, interruption of the membrane functionality as result of separation of lipid bilayers, changes in water transport properties, and alteration in calcium channels (Hammerstedt et al., 1990; Kodoma et al., 1996; Watson, 2000). It also causes damage to the cytoskeleton, in the flagellum, in the acrosome with reduction of the acrosomal integrity, modifications in the head and in the subacrosomal space, in the DNA status, in the genes essential for fertilization and in normal embryonic development (Amann and Pickett, 1987; Valcarce et al., 2013). As a result of these alterations and modifications on sperm, the response to osmotic stress changes and the survival life in the female genital tract might reduce (Flesch and Gadella, 2000). The osmotic stress is due to the extracellular ice crystals development during the cooling process that produces a great increase in the osmolarity of the remaining liquids surround or inside the sperm (Amann and Pickett, 1987).

8.4.2.1   EXTENDERS

The special sensitivity of equine sperm to heat shock and the interest into increase sperm storage time have been possible in the development of methods to prevent cold-shock damage. Different extenders are added to ejaculate protecting the gametes from the effects of temperature changes. The main characteristics of a cooling medium are neutral pH or slightly acid, buffering power, isotonic osmotic pressure, an energy source for the metabolism of sperm, avoid or minimize the growth of microorganisms, stability against enzymatic degradation or oxidation, and protection against thermal shock using penetrating and nonpenetrating cryoprotectants (Aurich, 2005).

Egg yolk and skim milk are the most common protective nonpenetrating agents utilized against cold shock injury utilized on stallion sperm cryopreservation (Aurich, 2005). Milk is composed of caseins that are the proteins responsible for protecting the sperm during conservation (Lagares et al., 2012) and egg yolk exerts a protective effect due to its phospholipid components (Watson y Martin, 1974). However, several disadvantages are related to the utilization of these compounds, wide variability of composition, microbial contamination, and difficult manipulation (Aires et al., 2003). Different studies have determined other substances that might replace them, soy lecithin, pasteurized egg yolk, liposomes with high-density lipoproteins (LDL/HDL), or cyclodextrins saturated in cholesterol, with suitable results in the sperm samples after thawing (Marco-Jiménez et al., 2004; Papa et al., 2011; Pillet et al., 2011; Blommaert et al., 2016). On the other hand, different sugars have demonstrated the protective action on stallion sperm. Squires (2004) observed that raffinose and trehalose did not increase sperm motility or viability after the frozen-thawing process. However, methylcellulose improved stallion sperm quality.

Permeable cryoprotectants can pass across the membrane and rapidly enter and leave the cell reducing sperm osmotic stress (Alvarenga et al., 2005). Glycerol is one of the most widely used cryoprotectant for the stallion sperm cryopreservation (Gibb and Aitken, 2016). It is trivalent alcohol with low molecular weight and toxic effect because it produces disorders in the cytoplasm, in the permeability and stability of the plasma membrane, and in sperm metabolism (Amann and Pickett, 1987). This molecule passes across the sperm plasma membrane more slowly than other smaller molecular weight cryoprotective molecules, such as amides, dimethylsulfoxide, or ethylene glycol (Alvarenga et al., 2005). Dimethylformamide (or N, N-dimethylformamide, (CH_3) 2-N-CHO) is a nonpenetrating cryoprotectant of the group of amides that show the best results in relation to stallion sperm quality after cryopreservation (Gomes et al., 2002;

Alvarenga et al., 2005; Gibb et al., 2013). The amides improve motility, viability, and fertility parameters due to its ability to maintain the structural integrity of the plasma membrane and the organelles (Vidament et al., 2002). Alvarenga et al., (2005) described that the relatively lower viscosity and low molecular weight of the amides increase the permeability of these components across the sperm plasma membrane and decrease the osmotic damage to the equine sperm. The cryoprotective capacity is even more evident when the amides are used in horses that have shown low motility after freezing their semen with glycerol (Medeiros et al., 2002).

Amino acids protect mammalian cells against cold-shock damages. Koskinen et al. (1989) showed that betaine used at 2.5% increased the number of sperm with progressive motility in equine semen. The incorporation a range of 30–80 mM of glutamine and proline in the freezing medium increased motility parameters (Khlifaoui et al., 2005).

One reason related to the decrease of fertility rates during the cryopreservation process is the peroxidation of the lipids in the cell membrane. Lipid peroxidation is the oxidative degradation by ROS of lipids. Semen contains antioxidants that balance lipid peroxidation and prevents excessive formation of lipids peroxides (Griveau et al., 1995). High concentrations of superoxide dismutase have been found in equine seminal plasma (Mennella and Jones, 1980) and Kankofer et al. (2005) determined positive interaction between seminal plasma and milk-based extender increasing the antioxidant capacity. This hypothesis is supported by the fact that the addition of certain antioxidants, such as ascorbic acid (Aurich, 2005) or pyruvate (Bruemmer, 2006), improved sperm plasma membrane integrity, motility, and fertility of equine sperm. Detergents (Equex STM) have been added to the seminal freezing extenders. This compound increases the emulsion and dispersion of the egg yolk lipids and interact with the sperm plasma membrane. The presence of seminal plasma increases sperm resistance to cold-shock and the ability to survive during the freezing and thawing process. The individual differences of the seminal plasma composition could explain the variability between stallions for sperm tolerance to cryopreservation (Ramires Neto et al., 2014).

In the last 25 years, two extenders and their modifications have been most utilized in equine reproduction. Martin et al. (1979) together with Cochran et al. (1984) demonstrated that the lactose-egg-glycerol extender supplemented with EDTA and sodium bicarbonate maintained suitable percentages of motility and viability after thawing equine semen, achieving pregnancy rates of 63%. On the other hand, Palmer et al. (1984) proposed the alternative skimmed milk-egg yolk-glycerol extender with good sperm quality results after freezing. Currently, there is a wide variety of commercial extenders available that could be used for equine semen cryopreservation. Gent® (MinitubeIberica SL, Tarragona, Spain) and Botucrio® (BiotechBotu-catu, Sao Paulo, Brazil) are the most common commercial medium utilized (Macedo et al., 2017). INRA 96® (IMV Technologies, L'Aigle, France) is the most used in chilled doses, with the possibility of adding different permeable cryoprotectants agents for freezing (Álvarez et al., 2014).

8.4.2.2 CRYOPRESERVATION PROTOCOL

The first step in the cryopreservation protocol is the centrifugation of the semen sample in order to increase the concentration of semen and reduce the amount of seminal plasma (Hoogewijs et al., 2010). Previously, the ejaculate is usually diluted in semen/media ratio of 1:1 (Pickett et al., 1975; Martin et al., 1979; Cochran et al., 1984).

In relation to sperm concentration, Loomis et al. (1983) recommended that high concentrations are preferable, on the contrary to Heitland et al. (1995). Samper and Morris (1998) suggested that freezing at low sperm concentrations could provide high availability of nutrients and cryoprotec-tants per sperm. This fact would explain the high percentages of motile spermatozoa immediately after thawing when frozen at a concentration of 40×10^6 sperm/mL. Standard sperm concentrations ranges between $50/200 \times 10^6$ sperm/mL in equine semen. Several storage devices have been used, including vials or glass ampoules, straws of polypropylene, polyvinyl or plastic (generally with volumes between 0.5 and 1 cm³), macrotubes, containers of aluminum, pellets and plastic bags (Martin et al., 1979; Cochran et al., 1984). Nowadays, straws of 0.5 cm³ are the devices most utilized worldwide (Fig. 8.1).

Stallion sperm can be successfully frozen when the temperature drop ranges between 5°C and 45°C per min (Moore et al., 2006). In a study carried out by Salazar et al. (2011), he determined that a slow cooling curve prior to freezing improved the results with respect to rapid cooling.

Cryopreserved semen involves storage at extremely low temperatures in liquid nitrogen (–196°C). If the sperms are able to withstand the freeze-thaw cycles, sperm viability could be maintained indefinitely since the metabolic activity is considered null at this temperature (Brinsko et al., 2011).

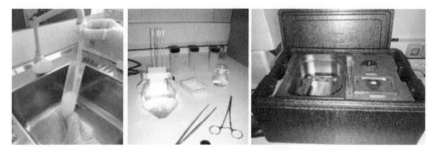

FIGURE 8.1   Steps and schematic design for sperm cryopreservation.

The success of freezing processes is also limited by the thawing process. In general, if the cooling rate is fast, the thawing should also be fast. Alternatively, if the cooling rate is slow, the process must be slow (Amann and Pickett, 1987). There are different thawing protocols, depending on the size of the container. If the sperms are frozen in macrotubes, they are normally thawed in the water at 50°C for 40 s (Martin et al., 1979). There are two protocols available in 0.5 mL straws: 37°C in water bath for 30 s (Cochran et al., 1984; Loomis et al., 1983) or 75°C for 7 s and immediately in another water bath at 37°C for 5 s (Cochran et al., 1984).

8.4.3   SPERM VITRIFICATION

In the last years, long-storage alternatives sperm preservation methods simplest and cost-effective have been proposed in several species. One of them is sperm vitrification. This method preserves the spermatozoa in a hypertonic medium by plunging the cells directly into liquid nitrogen (Rall y Fahy, 1985). The advantages of vitrification are related to the low cost of equipment, simplicity, and low exposure time at low temperatures. However, it produces adverse effects due to the use of hypertonic solutions and high concentrations of cryoprotectants (Lopera et al., 2007).

Vitrification is an ultrafast freezing method (from 37°C to–196°C in less than a second), based on the solidification of spermatozoa without the formation of ice crystals (Isachenko et al., 2004; Pradiee et al., 2015). This technique requires high concentrations of permeable cryoprotectants (Isachenko et al., 2008) that increase the viscosity of the medium and prevent the formation of intracellular ice during cooling (Rall and Fahy, 1985). It is the election method for preservation oocytes, embryos, and other tissues that require rapid cooling rates (Rall and Fahy, 1985).

However, the results obtained on sperm preservation are not satisfactory when compared with the results observed in oocytes or embryos applying the same protocols, due to the lack of tolerance of spermatozoa to the high concentration of cryoprotectants (Oldenhof et al., 2017). The kinetic of vitrification has been studied in order to improve vitrification results. It consists of the generation of small volumes of sperm solutions without any permeable cryoprotectant in LN2 (Isachenko et al., 2008), avoiding the formation of intracellular ice (Isachenko et al., 2004). Kinetic vitrification for sperm processing is different compared with the conventional term for vitrification associated with oocytes and embryos, where both the intracellular environment and the extracellular environment must be vitrified (Pradiee et al., 2015) (Fig. 8.2). There is no single protocol established, depending on of sensitivity of the sperm, extenders, cryoprotectants, and devitrification methods (Table 8.3). Recently, Álvarez et al. (2019) have determined that equine sperm vitrification is affected by sperm origin. Thus, vitrification with equine epididymal spermatozoa showed better quality results than equine ejaculates.

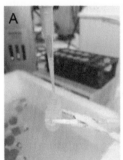
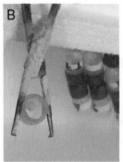
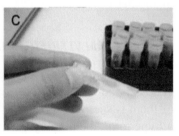

FIGURE 8.2   Stallion sperm vitrification process in cryotubes (A, B) and freeze-dried stallion sperm (C).

TABLE 8.3   Summary of the Principal Vitrification Protocols on Stallion Sperm.

Extender	Volume	Cryoprotectant	Desvitrification	References
Equipro	1.8 mL	8% egg yolk+DMF	37°C 5 min	Restrepo et al., 2012
INRA 96+BSA	25 µL	Sacarose and trehalose	65°C 5 s and 37°C 3 min	Pérez-Marín et al., 2018
INRA 96+BSA	30 µL	Sucrose	42°C 5 s	Hidalgo et al., 2018
INRA 96+BSA	0.25 mL	Sucrose	43°C 5 s	Consuegra et al., 2018

Perez-Marín et al. (2018) obtained better results in total and progressive motility with fresh and frozen ejaculate semen than vitrificated sperm with trehalose and sucrose (0.15 M). Another study conducted by Restrepo et al. (2012) found superior results of progressive motility with fresh semen and frozen semen than vitrificated semen. However, other studies determined better motility results when included sucrose and BSA in the vitrification medium with an equilibration period than the traditional freezing process (Consuegra et al., 2018; Hidalgo et al., 2018).

8.4.4 SPERM LYOPHILIZATION

Lyophilization is a preservation method in which frozen material is dried by sublimation of ice, thereby, involving a direct transition from a solid (ice) to a vapor (gas) phase. The main objective of the process is to remove water from the cells avoiding any chemical or biological reaction. It consists of three phases: sample freezing, sublimation (primary drying), and desorption (secondary drying) (Jennings, 2002).

The first attempts to lyophilize spermatozoa were made in rooster semen in 1949 (Polge et al., 1949) and then in human and bovine semen (Sherman, 1954; Bialy and Smith, 1957). Any of these studies did not demonstrate the fertility of freeze-dried sperm. In 1998, Wakayama and Yanagimachi reported the first offspring obtained from freeze-dried mouse sperm. This study demonstrated that although lyophilized sperm were dead, the DNA did not lose their ability to activate the oocyte with the subsequent embryonic development (Kusakabe et al., 2001).

One of the main advantages of this method is that nitrogen is no longer required for the storage and shipment, which can be stored at room temperature or 4°C. The storage and shipping costs are reduced. However, freeze-dried sperm lose their motility, even after rehydration (Kusakabe et al., 2001), therefore sperm are unable to fertilize oocytes by themselves *in vivo* as by *in vitro* (Fig. 1.2). It is necessary to use intracytoplasmic sperm injection (ICSI) to perform successful fertilization.

Several factors influence the lyophilization process and produce different sperm damage. One of them is the drying conditions during the lyophilization process (Hara et al., 2014). The interaction between temperature, vacuum pressure, and drying period regulates the kinetics and the degree of dehydration, which have a great impact on the sperm (Kawase et al., 2007). Lyophilized sperm preservation for a long period of time is essential to protect DNA from physical damage caused by the action of endogenous endonucleases during storage (Kaneko and Serikawa, 2012). Chelating agents, such as EDTA, are necessary. 1,2,2-diamino 2,2', 2", 2"-tetraacetic) or ethylene glycol-bis (2-aminoethyl ether)-N, N, N'N'-tetraacetic acid (EGTA) are incorporated in the lyophilization solution to prevent sperm DNA fragmentation (Kaneko and Nakagata, 2006). Olaciregui et al., (2016) determined that the presence of EGTA in the lyophilization media provided a protective effect on the DNA sperm than the presence of EDTA. Sugars have been studied as components of the lyophilization medium. Trehalose, a nonreducing disaccharide, plays an important role in the prevention of membrane alterations in cellular dehydration. The incorporation of trehalose to the lyophilization medium maintains the integrity of the DNA after the lyophilization process (McGinnis et al., 2005).

The pH of the lyophilization media is a factor to be taken into account. An alkaline pH (pH:8) contributes to the inactivation of DNA damage. Kaneko and Serikawa (2012) showed that lyophilized sperm in a medium with an alkaline pH maintained the DNA integrity as well as their capacity for embryonic development. Another factor that may influence sperm preservation is the conditions of conservation. Currently, it is considered that 4°C is the optimum temperature to preserve lyophilized semen samples for long periods of time (Kaneko and Serikawa, 2012).

The rehydration process restores the lyophilized cell to the original formulation. It is a critical step in the process since when reintroducing water into the cells, all the chemical and biological reactions are reactive. The lyophilized sperm are normally rehydrated by adding ultra-pure water, in an equal volume as the original (Gil et al., 2014). Finally, another important factor is the technique of ICSI. After the lyophilization process, the sperm lose motility, so the ICSI technique is necessary to fertilize the oocytes. The development of the ICSI is the key to success in obtaining offspring from lyophilized semen, as published for the first time by Wakayama and Yanagimachi (1998) and Choi et al. (2011) because they obtained the first foal born alive.

In small and farm animal species, satisfactory results have not been obtained, except in the equine species (Choi et al., 2011). In this case, lyophilized stallion semen and sperm extract suspension were utilized from different males. Five pregnancies were obtained an only two foals born. One of them was originated from lyophilized sperm and the other was from the stallion that provides the sperm extract. The lyophilized sperm and sperm processed by multiple unprotected freezing and thawing cycles (such as sperm extract) can originate viable foals. To our knowledge, this is the first report on the production of live offspring by ICSI with lyophilized sperm in a nonlaboratory animal species.

Lyophilization is a promising semen preservation technique that requires further study to be applied routinely during long-term conservation periods. This technique would be a suitable alternative biobanking option for high genetic values animals.

KEYWORDS

- **stallion**
- **semen preservation**
- **cryopreservation**
- **vitrification**
- **lyophilization**

REFERENCES

Aires, V. A.; Hinsch, K.; Mueller-Schloesser, F.; Bogner, K.; Mueller-Schloesser, S. *In Vitro* and *in Vivo* Comparison of Egg Yolk-Based and Soybean Lecithin-Based Extenders for Cryopreservation of Bovine Semen. *Theriogenology* **2003,** *60,* 269–279.

Álvarez, C.; Gil, L.; González, N.; Olaciregui, M.; Luño, V. Equine Sperm Post-Thaw Evaluation After the Addition of Different Cryoprotectants Added to INRA 96® Extender. *Cryobiology* **2014,** *69,* 144–148.

Álvarez, C.; González N.; Luño, V., Gil, L. Ejaculated compared to epididymal stallion sperm vitrification. Animal Reproduction Science **2019,** 211, 106205.

Alvarenga, M. A.; Papa, F. O.; Landim-Alvarenga, F. C.; Medeiros, A. S. L. Amides as Cryoprotectants for Freezing Stallion Semen: A Review. *Anim. Reprod. Sci.* **2005,** *89,* 105–113.

Amann, R. P.; Pickett, B. W. Principles of Cryopreservation and A Review of Cryopreservation of Stallion Spermatozoa. *J. Equine. Vet. Sci.* **1987,** *7* (3), 145–173.

Aurich, C. Factors Affecting the Plasma Membrane Function of Cooled-Stored Stallion Spermatozoa. *Anim. Reprod. Sci.* **2005,** *89,* 65.

Brinsko, S. P.; Varner, D. D. Artificial Insemination and Preservation of Semen. *Vet. Clin. Noth. Equine Pract.* **1992,** *8* (1), 205–218.

Brinsko, S. P.; Blanchard, T.; Varner, D. D.; Schumacher, J.; Love, C. H.; Hinrichs, K. *Manual of Equine Reproduction*, 3rd ed; Maryland Heights: Mosby, 2011.

Barker, C. A.; Gandier, J. C. Pregnancy in a Mare Resulting from Frozen Epididymal Spermatozoa. *Can. J. Comp. Med. Vet. Sci.* **1957,** *21* (2), 47–51.

Batellier, F.; Magistrini, M.; Fauguant, J.; Palmer, E. Effect of Milk Fractions on Survival of Equine Spermatozoa. *Theriogenology* **1997**, *48* (3), 391–410.

Berliner, V. R. Dilutors for Stallion and Jack Semen. *J. Anim. Sci.* **1942**, *1*, 314–319.

Bialy, G.; Smith, V. R. Freeze-drying of Bovine Spermatozoa. *J. Dairy Sci.* **1957**, *40*, 739–745.

Blommaert, D.; Franck, T.; Donnay, I.; Lejeune; J. P.; Detilleux, J.; Serteyn, D. Substitution of Egg Yolk by a Cyclodextrin–Cholesterol Complex Allows a Reduction of the Glycerol Concentration into the Freezing Medium of Equine Sperm. *Cryobiology* **2016**, *72* (1), 27–32.

Brinsko, S. P.; Varner, D. D. Artificial Insemination and Preservation of Semen. *Vet. Clin. North Am. Equine Pract.* **1992**, *8*, 205–218.

Bruemmer, J. E. Collection and Freezing of Epididymal Stallion Sperm. *Vet. Clin. North Am. Equine Pract.* **2006**, *22* (3), 677–682.

Cary, J. A.; Madill, S.; Farnsworth, K.; Hayna, J. T.; Duoos, L.; Fahning, M. L. A Comparison of Electroejaculation and Epididymal Sperm Collection Techniques in Stallions. *Can. Vet. J.* **2004**, *45*, 35–41.

Choi, Y. H.; Varner, D. D.; Love, C. C.; Hartman, D. L.; Hinrichs, K. Production of Live Foals Via Intracytoplasmic Injection of Lyophilized Sperm and Sperm Extract in the Horse. *Reproduction* **2011**, *142*, 529–538.

Cochran, J. D.; Amann, R. P.; Froman, D. P.; Pickett, B. W. Effects of Centrifugation, Glycerol Level, Cooling to 5°C, Freezing Rate on the Post-Thaw Motility of Equine Spermatozoa. *Theriogenology* **1984**, *22* (1), 25–38.

Consuegra, C.; Crespo, F.; Dorado, J.; Ortiz, I.; Diaz-Jimenez, M.; Pereira, B.; Hidalgo, M. Comparison of different sucrose-based extenders for stallion sperm vitrification straws. *Reprod. Domest. Anim.* **2018**, *53* (2), 59–61.

Douglas-Hamilton, D. H.; Osol, R.; Osol, G.; Driscoll, D.; Noble, H. A Field Study of Fertility of Transported Equine Semen. *Theriogenology* **1984**, *22*, 291–304.

Flesch, F.M.; Gadella, B. M. Dynamics of the Mammalian Sperm Plasma Membrane in the Process of Fertilization. *Biochim. Biophys. Acta.* **2000**, *1469*, 197–235.

Gibb, Z.; Morris, L. H.; Maxwell, W. M.; Grupen, C. G. Dimethyl Fomamide Improves the Postthaw Characteristics of Sex-Sorted and Nonsorted Stallion Sperm. *Theriogenology* **2013**, *79* (7), 1027–1033.

Gibb, Z.; Aitken, R. J. The Impact of Sperm Metabolism During *In Vitro* Storage: The Stallion as a model. *BioMed Res. Int.* **2016**, *9380608*, 8.

Gil, L.; Olaciregui, M.; Luño, V.; Malo, C.; Gonzalez, N.; Martínez, F. Current Status of Freeze-Drying Technology to Preserve Domestic Animal's Sperm. *Reprod. Domest. Anim.* **2014**, *49* (4),72–81.

Gomes, G. M.; Jacob, J. C. F.; Medeiros, A. S.; Papa, F. O.; Alvarenga, M. A. Improvement of Stallion Spermatozoa Preservation with Alternative Cryoprotectants for the Mangalarga Marchador Breed. *Theriogenology* **2002**, *58* (2), 277–279.

Griveau, J. F.; Dumont, E.; Renard, P.; Callegari, J. P.; Le Lannou, D. Reactive Oxygen Species, Lipid Peroxidation and Enzymatic Defense Systems in Human Spermatozoa. *J. Reprod. Fertil.* **1995**, *103* (1), 17–26.

Guimarães, T.; Lopes, G.; Ferreira, P.; Leal, I.; Rocha, A. Characteristics of Stallion Epididymal Spermatozoa at Collection and Effect of Two Refrigeration Protocols on the Quality of the Frozen/Thawed Sperm Cells. *Anim. Reprod. Sci.* **2012**, *136*, 85–89.

Hammesterdt, R.; Graham, J.; Nolan, J. P. Cryopreservation of Mammalian Sperm: What We Ask Them to Survive. *J. Androl.* **1990**, *11* (1), 73–88.

Hara, H.; Tagiri, M.; Hwang, I. S.; Takahashi, M.; Hirabayasi, M. Adverse Effect of Cake Collapse on the Functional Integrity of Freeze-Dried Bull Spermatozoa. *Cryobiology* **2014**, *68*, 354–360.

Heitland, A. V.; Jasko, K. J.; Squires, E. L.; Graham, J. K.; Pickett, B. W.; Hamilton, C. Factors Affecting Motion Characteristics of Frozen-Thawed Stallion Spermatozoa. *Equine Vet. J.* **1996**, *28*, 47–53.

Hidalgo, M.; Consuegra, C.; Dorado, J.; Diaz-Jiménez, M.; Ortiz, I.; Pereira, B.; Sánchez, R.; Crespo, F. Concentrations of Non-Permeable Cryoprotectants and Equilibration Temperatures are Key Factors for Stallion Sperm Vitrification Success. *Anim. Reprod. Sci.* **2018**, *196*, 91–98.

Hoogewijs, M.; Rjsselaere, T.; De Vliegher, S.; Vanhaesebrouck, E.; De Schauwer, C.; Govaere, J.; Thys, M.; Hoflack, G.; Van Soom, A.; De Kruif, A. Influence of Different Centrifugation Protocols on Equine Semen Preservation. *Theriogenology* **2010**, *74* (1), 118–126.

Isachenko, V.; Isachenko, E.; Katkov, I. I.; Montag, M.; Dessole, S.; Nawroth, F.; Van Der Ven, H. Cryoprotectant-free Cryopreservation of Human Spermatozoa by Vitrification and Freezing in Vapor: Effect on Motility, DNA Integrity, and Fertilization Ability. *Biol. Reprod.* **2004**, *71*, 1167–1173.

Isachenko, E.; Isachenko, V.; Weiss, J.M.; Kreienberg, R.; Katkov, I. I.; Schulz, M.; Lulat, A. G.; Risopatron, M. J.; Sanchez, R. Acrosomal Status and Mitochondrial Activity of Human Spermatozoa Vitrified with Sucrose. *Reproduction* **2008**, 136, 167–173.

Jasko, D. J.; Hathaway, J. A.; Schaltenbrand, V. L.; Simper, W. D.; Squires, E. L. Effect of Seminal Plasma and Egg Yolk on Motion Characteristics of Cooled Stallion Spermatozoa. *Theriogenology* **1992**, *37*, 1241–1252.

Jennings, T. A. Lyophilization. In: *Introduction and Basic Principles*; Ed.; Interpharm CRC, New York, 2002.

Kaneko, T.; Serikawa, T. Long-term Preservation of Freeze-dried Mouse Spermatozoa. *Cryobiology* **2002**, *64*, 211–214.

Kaneko, T.; Nakagata, N. Improvement in the Long-term Stability of Freeze-Dried Mouse Spermatozoa by Adding of a Chelating Agent. *Cryobiology* **2006**, *53*, 279–282.

Kankofer, M.; Kolm, G.; Aurich, J.; Aurich, C. Activity of Glutathione Peroxidase, Superoxide Dismutase and Catalase and Lipid Peroxidation Intensity in Stallion Semen During Storage at 5 Degrees C. *Theriogenology* **2005**, *63* (5), 1354–1365.

Kayser, J. P.; Amann, R. P.; Shideler, R. K.; Squires, E. L.; Jasko, D. J.; Pickett, B. W. Effects of Linear Cooling Rate on Motion Characteristics of Stallion Spermatozoa. *Theriogenology* **1992**, *38* (4), 601–614.

Kawase, Y.; Hani, T.; Kamada, N.; Jishage, K.; Suzuki, H. Effect of Pressure at Primary Drying of Freeze-drying Mouse Sperm Reproduction Ability and Preservation Potential. *Reproduction* **2007**, *133*, 841–846.

Kenney, R. M.; Bergman, R. V.; Cooper, W. L. Minimal Contamination Techniques and Preliminary Findings, Proceedings of the Annual Conference of American Association of Equine Practitioners, Boston, USA, **1975**.

Khlifaoui, M.; Battut, I.; Bruyas, J. F.; Chatagnon, G.; Trimeche, A.; Tainturier, D. Effects of Glutamine on Post-Thaw Motility of Stallion Spermatozoa: An Approach of the Mechanism of Action at Spermatozoa Level. *Theriogenology* **2005**, *63* (1), 138–149.

Knop, K.; Hoffmann, N.; Rath, D.; Sieme, H. Effects of Cushioned Centrifugation Technique on Sperm Recovery and Sperm Quality in Stallions with Good and Poor Semen Freezability. *Anim. Reprod. Sci.* **2005**, *89* (1–4), 294–297.

Kodama, H., Kuribayashi, Y.; Gagnon, C. Effect of Sperm Lipid Peroxidation on Fertilization. *J. Androl.* **1996**, *17* (2), 151–157.

Koskinen, E.; Junnila, M.; Katila, T.; Soini, H. A Preliminary Study on the Use of Betaine as a Cryoprotective Agent in Deep Freezing of Stallion Semen. *J. Vet. Med.* **1989**, *39*, 110–111.

Kusakabe, H.; Szczygiel, M. A.; Whittingham, D. G.; Yanagimachi, R. Maintenance of Genetic Integrity in Frozen and Freeze-Dried Mouse Spermatozoa. *Proc. Natl. Acad. Sci. USA.* **2001**, *98*, 13501–13506.

Lagares, M. A.; Martins, H. S.; Carvalho, I. A.; Oliverira, C. A.; Souza, M. R.; Penna, C. F.; Cruz, B. C.; Stahlberg, R.; Henry, M. R. Caseinates Protects Stallions Perm During Semen Cooling and Freezing. *Cryo. Letters.* **2012**, *33* (3), 214–219.

Ljaz, A.; Ducharme, D. Effects of Various Extenders and Taurine on Survival of Stallion Sperm Cooled to 5 Degrees C. *Theriogenology* **1995**, *44* (7), 1039–1050.

Loomis, P. R.; Amann, R. P.; Squires, E. L.; Pickett, B. W. Fertility of Unfrozen and Frozen Stallion Spermatozoa Extended in EDTA-Lactose-Egg Yolk and Packaged in Straws. *J. Anim. Sci.* **1983**, 56, 693–697.

Loomis, P. R.; Graham, J. K. Commercial Semen Freezing: Individual Male Variation in Cryosurvival and the Response of Stallion Sperm to Customized Freezing Protocols. *Anim. Reprod. Sci.* **2008**, *105*, 119–128.

Lopera, V.; Méndez, I.; Peña, M.; Góngora, A. Vitrificación de ovocitos bovinos inmaduros por el método de la pajilla abierta y estirada (Open pulled Straw - OPS). *RCCP.* **2007**, *20*, 532–540.

Love, C. C. Sperm Quality Assays: How Good are They? The Horse Perspective. *Anim. Reprod. Sci.* **2018**, **194**, 63–70.

Macedo, S.; Bliebernicht, M.; Carvalheira, J.; Costa, A.; Ribeiro, F.; Rocha A. Effects of Two Freezing Methods and two Cryopreservation Media on Post-Thaw Quality of Stallion Spermatozoa. *Reprod. Dom. Anim.* **2017**, *53* (2), 519–524.

Marco-Jiménez, F.; Puchades, S.; Moce, E. Use of Powdered Egg Yolk *vs.* Fresh Egg Yolk for the Cryopreservation of Ovine Semen. *Reprod. Dom. Anim.* **2004**, *441*, 438–441.

Martin, J. C.; Klug, E.; Gunzel, A. R. Centrifugation of Stallion Semen and its Storage in Large Volume Straws. *J. Reprod. Fertil.* **1979**, *27*, 47–51.

McGinnis, L. K.; Zhu, L.; Lawitts, J. A.; Bhowmick, S.; Toner, M.; Biggers, J. D. Mouse Sperm Desiccated and Stored in Trehalose Medium Without Freezing. *Biol. Reprod.* **2005**, *73*, 627–633.

McKenzie, F. F.; Lasley, J. F.; Phillips, R. W. The Storage of Horse and Swine Semen. *Am. Soc. Anim. Prod.* **1939**, *1*, 222–225.

Medeiros, A. S. L.; Gomes, G. M.; Carmo, M. T.; Papa, F. O.; Alvarenga, M. A. Cryopreservation of Stallion Sperm Using Different Amides. *Theriogenology* **2002**, 58, 273–276.

Mennella, M. R.; Jones, R. Properties of Spermatozoa Superoxide Dismutase and Lack of Involvement of Superoxides in Metal-Ion-Catalysed Lipid Peroxidation and Reactions in Semen. *Biochem. J.* **1980**, *191* (2), 289–297.

Monteiro, G. A.; Papa, F. O.; Zahn, F. S.; Dellaqua, J. A.; Melo, C. M.; Maziero, R. R. D.; Guasti, P. N. Cryopreservation and Fertility of Ejaculated and Epididymal Stallion Sperm. *Anim. Reprod. Sci.* **2011**, *127* (3–4), 197–201.

Moore, A.; Squires, E.; Bruemmmer, J.; Graham, J. Effect of Cooling Rate and Cryoprotectant on the Cryosurvival of Equine Spermatozoa. *J. Equine Vet. Sci.* **2006**, *26* (5), 215–218.

Moran, D.; Jasko, D.; Squires, E.; Amann R. P. Determination of Temperature and Cooling Rate Which Induce Cold Shock in Stallion Spermatozoa. *Theriogenology* **1992**, *38*, 999–1012.

Neild, D.; Miragaya, M.; Chaves, G.; Pinto, M.; Alonso, A.; Gambarotta, M.; Losinno, L.; Aguero, A. Cryopreservation of Cauda Epididymis Spermatozoa from Slaughterhouse Testicles 24 h After Ground Transportation. *Anim. Reprod. Sci.* **2006**, *94*, 92–95.

Neuhauser, S.; Dörfel, S.; Handler J. Dose-dependent Effect of Homologous Seminal Plasma on Motility and Kinematics Characteristics of Post-Thaw Stallions Epididymal Spermatozoa. *Andrology* **2015**, *3* (3), 536–543.

Olaciregui, M.; Luño, V.; Martí, J. I.; Aramayona, J.; Gil, L. Freeze-dried Stallion Spermatozoa: Evaluation of two Chelating Agents and Comparative Analysis of Three Sperm DNA Damage Assays. *Andrologia* **2016**, *48* (9), 900–906.

Oldenhof, H.; Bigalk, J.; Hettel, C.; De Oliveira Barros, L.; Sydykov, B.; Bajcsy, A. C.; Sieme, H.; Wolkers, W. F. Stallion Sperm Cryopreservation Using Various Permeating Agents: Interplay Between Concentration and Cooling Rate. *Biopreserv. Biobank.* **2017**, *15*, 422–431.

Palmer, E. Factors Affecting Stallion Semen Survival and Fertility. Proceedings 10th International Congress of Animal Reproduction and Artificial Insemination. Urbana-Champaign, Illinois, USA, **1984**.

Papa, F. O.; Barcelos, G.; Marini, C.; Alvarenga, M. A.; Vita, B.; Trinque, C.; Pouli-Filho, J. N.; Dell'Aqua, J. A. Replacing Egg Yolk with Soybean Lecithin in the Cryopreservation of Stallion Semen. *Anim. Reprod. Sci.* **2011**, *129*,173–179.

Parlevliet, J. M.; Colenbrander, B. Prediction of First Season Stallion Fertility of 3-year-ols Dutch Warmbloods with Prebreeding Assessment of Percentage of Morphologically Normal Live Sperm. *Equine Vet. J.* **1999**, *31* (3), 248–251.

Pérez-Marín, C. C; Requena, F. D.; Arando, A.; Ortiz-Villalón, S.; Requena, F.; Agüera, E. I. Effect of Trehalose- and Sucrose-based Extenders on Equine Sperm Quality After Vitrification: Preliminary Results. *Criobiology* **2018**, *80*, 62–69.

Pickett, B. W.; Sullivan, J. J.; Seidel, G. E. Effect of Centrifugation and Seminal Plasma on Motility and Fertility of Stallion and Bull Spermatozoa. *Fertil. Steril.* **1975**, *26*, 167–174.

Pillet, E.; Duchamp, G.; Batellier, F.; Beaumal, V.; Anton, M.; Desherces, S.; Magistrini, M. Egg Yolk Plasma Can Replace Egg Yolk in Stallion Freezing Extenders. *Theriogenology* **2011**, *75* (1), 105–114.

Polge, C.; Smith, A. U.; Parks, A. S. Revival of Spermatozoa After Vitrification and Dehydration at Low Temperatures. *Nature* **1949**, *164*, 666.

Pradiee, J.; Esteso, M. C.; Lopez-Sebastián, A.; Toledano-Díaz, A.; Castaño, C.; Carrizosa, J. A.; Urrutia, B.; Santiago-Moreno, J. Successful Ultrarapid Cryopreservation of Wild Iberian ibex (Capra pyrenaica) Spermatozoa. *Theriogenology* **2015**, *84*, 1513–1522.

Province, C. A.; Squires, E. L.; Pickett, B. W.; Amann R. P. Cooling Rates, Storage Temperatures and Fertility of Extended Equine Spermatozoa. *Theriogenology* **1985**, *23*, 925–933.

Rall, W. F.; Fahy, G. M. Ice-free Cryopreservation of Mouse Embryos at -196 Degrees C by Vitrification. *Nature* **1985**, *313*, 573–575.

Ramires-Neto, C.; Monteiro, G. A.; Sancler-Silva, Y. R. F.; Maziero, D. D. R.; Lisboa, F. P.; Freitas-Dell'Aqua, C. P.; Alvarenga, M. A.; Papa, F. 0. Influence of Addition of Motility

Stimulators in Cryopreservation of Sperm from Subfertile Stallions. *J. Equine Vet. Sci.* **2014,** *34* (1), 98.

Restrepo, G.; Duque, J. E.; Montoya, J. D. Effect of Two Protocols of Cryopreservation on Fertilizing Capacity of Stallion (Equus caballus) Semen. *Rev. Fac. Nal. Agr. Medellín.* **2012,** *65* (2): 6711–6718.

Salazar, J. L.; Teague, S.; Love, C. C.; Brinsko, S.; Blanchard, T.; Varner, D. Effect of Cryopreservation Protocol on Post-thraw Characteristics of Stallion Sperm. *Theriogenology* **2011,** *76* (3), 409–418.

Samper, J. C.; Morris, C. A. Current Methods for Stallion Semen Cryopreservation: A Survey. *Theriogenology* **1998,** *49,* 895–903.

Samper, J. C. *Equine Breeding Management and Artificial Insemination;* Saunders: Philadelphia, **2000.**

Sherman, J. K. Freezing and Freeze-drying of Human Spermatozoa. *Fertil. Steril.* **1954,** *5,* 357–371.

Shore, M. D.; Macpherson, M. L.; Combes, G. B.; Varner, D. D.; Blanchard, T. L. Fertility Comparison Between Breeding at 24 Hours or at 24 and 48 Hours After Collection with Cooled Equine Semen. *Theriogenology* **1998,** *50* (5), 693–698.

Squires, E. L.; Keith, S. L.; Graham, J. K. Evaluation of Alternative Cryoprotectants for Preserving Stallion Spermatozoa. *Theriogenology* **2004,** *62,* 1056–1065.

Tiplady, C. A.; Morris, L. H. A.; Allen, W. R. Stallion Epididymal Spermatozoa: Pre-freeze and Post-thaw Motility and Viability After Three Treatments. *Theriogenology* **2002,** *58,* 225–228.

Töpfer-Petersen, E.; Petrounkina, A. M.; Ekhlasi-Hundrieser, M. Oocyte–sperm Interactions. *Anim. Reprod. Sci.* **2002,** *60,* 653–662.

Trimeche, A.; Yvon, J. M.; Vidament, M.; Palmer, E.; Magistrini, M. Effects of Glutamine, Proline, Histidine and Betaine on Post-taw Motility of Stallion Spermatozoa. *Theriogenology* **1999,** *52* (1), 181–191.

Valcarce, D. G.; Cartón-García, F.; Riesco, M. F.; Harráez, M. P.; Robles, V. Analysis of DNA Damage After Human Sperm Cryopreservation in Genes Crucial for Fertilization and Early Embryo Development. *Andrology* **2013,** *1* (5), 723–730.

Varner, D.D.; Blanchard, T.; Love, C.; Garcia, M.; Kenney, R. Effects of Semen Fractionation and Dilution Ratio on Equine Spermatozoal Motility Parameters. *Theriogenology* **1987,** *28* (5), 709–723.

Vidament, M.; Daire, J. M.; Yvon, J. M.; Doligez, P.; Bruneau, B.; Magistrini, M.; Ecot, P. Motility and Fertility of Stallion Semen Frozen with Glycerol and/or Dimethyl Formamide. *Theriogenology* **2002,** *58,* 1–3.

Vishwanath, R.; Shannon, P. Do Sperm Cells Age? A Review of the Physiological Changes in Sperm During Storage at Ambient Temperature. *Reprod. Fert. Dev.* **1997,** *9,* 321–331.

Wakayama, T.; Yanagimachi, R. Development of Normal Mice from Oocytes Injected with Freeze-Dried Spermatozoa. *Nat. Biotechnol.* **1998,** *16,* 639–641.

Watson, P. F.; Martin, I. C. The Influence of Some Fractions of Egg Yolk on the Survival of Ram Spermatozoa at 5°C. *Aust. J. Biol. Sci.* **1974,** *28,* 145–152.

Watson, P. F. The Causes of Reduced Fertility with Cryopreserved Semen. *Anim. Reprod. Sci.* **2000,** *60–61,* 481–492.

Weiss, R. R.; Muradas, P. R.; Graneman, L. C.; Meira, C. Freezing Sperm from Cauda Epididymis of Castrated Stallions. *Anim. Reprod. Sci.* **2008,** *107* (3), 356.

CHAPTER 9

The Journey of the Porcine Spermatozoa from Its Origin to the Fertilization Site: The Road *In Vivo* vs. *In Vitro*

CRISTINA SORIANO-ÚBEDA*, FRANCISCO ALBERTO GARCÍA-VÁZQUEZ, and CARMEN MATÁS

Department of Physiology, Faculty of Veterinary Science, International Excellence Campus for Higher Education and Research "Campus Mare Nostrum", University of Murcia, Murcia, Spain Institute for Biomedical Research of Murcia (IMIB-Arrixaca), Murcia, Spain

Corresponding author. E-mail: cmsu1@um.es

ABSTRACT

Assisted reproduction techniques (ARTs) are of great interest in both research and animal production. The porcine species is especially important due to its anatomical, physiological, and genetic similarities with the human species which makes the pig of special relevance as a biomedical model. In this sense, all the critical points during animal production must be controlled. *In vitro* production of embryos (IVP) is no exception. Fertilization is a complex biological process in which innumerable factors are directly and/or indirectly involved. For healthy animals, the efficiency of *in vitro* fertilization (IVF) and IVP is lower than *in vivo*. However, in some mammalian species such as bovine and murine a high yield has been achieved but, in porcine species, it is still suboptimal. With a focus on the special requirements of pig reproduction, different studies have been conducted over the last several decades to improve IVP efficiency by using a variety of methods to prepare and co-culture gametes and develop normal embryos. The knowledge of the differences between the *in vitro* and *in vivo* environments in which fertilization occurs plays a key role, and the *in vitro* simulation of *in vivo* conditions is postulated as the best strategy to improve ARTs. This chapter summarizes the spermatozoa physiology and functionality from their origin in the testicle to the fertilization site in the oviductal ampulla and exposes the main strategies currently used in porcine IVP.

9.1 INTRODUCTION

Assisted reproduction techniques (ARTs) have helped to understand many of physico-chemical events around reproductive physiology in animals, with a remarkable increase in mammals and profound implications for human beings. Researchers have been looking for ways to expand the knowledge about the genetic influence in reproduction, the hormonal reproductive cycle regulation, superovulation and embryo collection, culture, freezing and transfer. The achievements have allowed the development of various techniques that have been gaining much interest in recent years in mammals, such as *in vitro* fertilization (IVF). In the particular case of porcine species, reproductive technologies have been directed toward both swine production and research. The economic interest of this species has produced the development of numerous systems for production of pigs for human food that are continuously undergoing changes to reduce costs and increase production efficiency (Day, 2000). Moreover, although not classically thought of as an obvious model organism, the pig has recently become relevant in research due to its anatomy, genetics and physiology are closer to human, at least more than other classic animal models as mice. Several notable advancements have been achieved in the use of this species as a biomedical model in the genetic technology and have motivated the interest in the possible use of swine as donors of specific proteins and even organs for the improvement of human health (Watson et al., 2016; Mourad and Gianello, 2017). At the same time, the scientific interest on swine reproduction has undergone significant progress in basic science and ARTs. Particular emphasis has been made in the development of different protocols for IVF and *in vitro* production and culture of viable embryos in pigs. For these purpose, numerous studies have been carried out related to the sperm capacitation process signalling, the molecules involved in the gametes interaction and fertilization and in early embryo development, both *in vivo* and *in vitro* (reviewed by Romar et al., 2016).

However, while these techniques have achieved a good efficiency in some mammalian species such as bovine or murine, the results obtained in porcine species are so far not comparable to *in vivo* output. The study of spermatozoa physiology and functionality, from their origin in the testicle to the fertilization site, and also of the oocyte and its interaction with the spermatozoon gains special importance in the purpose to increase the efficiency of the processes of *in vitro* sperm capacitation (the ability of spermatozoa to fertilize oocytes) and fertilization.

Up to now, the journey of the sperm to the egg and fertilization *in vivo* is still poorly understood, but what seems clear is that all the processes and physico-chemical events that the spermatozoon undergoes from its origin in the testis to the fertilization site are a coordinated system in which each step is important for the success of the spread of genetics. Increasing this knowledge can be key in order to improve the current techniques of assisted reproduction. Below, what is currently understood about some of the most important *in vivo* events in these processes is detailed.

9.2 THE SPERMATOZOA IN THE MALE GENITAL TRACT

9.2.1 *SPERMATOZOA IN THE TESTICLE AND EPIDIDYMIS: ORIGIN, MATURATION AND STORAGE*

The spermatozoa originate in the germinal epithelium of the seminiferous tubules of the testis during spermatogenesis in which the male produces spermatozoa from spermatogonial stem cells by consecutive mitotic and meiotic divisions. The immature spermatozoa leave the rete testis by passing through the efferent ducts, they enter a unique tubule, the epididymis, in which the final stages of spermatozoa differentiation occur (Joseph et al., 2009).

During the transit through the epididymis, there are progressive and sequential modifications of maturing male gametes that have been demonstrated to be essential for the acquisition of motility and fertility (Wolf, 1981).

The morphological, biochemical and physiological changes as they move along the epididymis basically are: (i) changes in motility pattern, (ii) modifications in the metabolism and the distribution of tail organelles, (iii) chromatin restructuring, (iv) acrosome shape remodeling, (v) water reabsorption and an increased concentration of cells, (vi) cytoplasmic droplet migration and detachment, and (vii) modifications in the spermatozoa plasma membrane. A specific composition in proteins (Syntin et al., 1996) and other organic molecules and ions (Cooper, 1986; Rodriguez-Martinez et al., 1990; Setchell et al., 1993) in each epididymal region allows the maturation of spermatozoa. The proteins are incorporated to the spermatozoa through specific exosomes of the epididymis to which proteins are associated, called epididymosomes. These little membranous particles selectively transfer the proteins to spermatozoa during the epididymal transit playing a major role in the production of fully functional gamete (Sullivan et al., 2005). After that, a high proportion of mature spermatozoa are stored in the cauda in a state of quiescence until ejaculation (Briz et al., 1995).

The epididymal influences on spermatozoa maturation and storage have two clear objectives: (i) promoting the ability of spermatozoa to respond appropriately to conditions within the female genital tract so they can fertilize the oocyte, and (ii) preventing this response within the male tract itself (Cooper, 1986). This state of inactivity also is associated with low extracellular pH in the cauda epididymis (pH ~6.2) resulting from a low bicarbonate (HCO_3^-) concentration of ~3–4 mmol/L (Okamura et al., 1985; Rodriguez-Martinez et al., 1990).

9.2.2 SPERMATOZOA IN THE EJACULATE

During ejaculation in the boar, spermatozoa emitted together with cauda epididymal fluid are poured into the urethra and are sequentially exposed and resuspended in different mixtures of accessory sex gland secretions. The fluid portion of this suspension, which is called the seminal plasma (SP), nourishes, transports and protects spermatozoa and modulates the uterine immunological response during their journey through the female genital tract (Schuberth et al., 2008). The SP regulates spermatozoa motility and acquisition of the ability of spermatozoa to fertilize oocytes (sperm capacitation), modulates the recognition and interaction between gametes, maintains spermatozoa fertility, buffers the extracellular media, maintains the osmolarity and is a source of energy for spermatozoa metabolism (Mann and Lutwak-Mann, 1981). The molecular changes that SP provokes in the spermatozoa enhance their lifespan and fertilizing capacity but cannot be totally responsible for it. The action of SP antioxidants, secreted by the male reproductive tract, protect spermatozoa from the toxic effect of reactive oxygen species (ROS) after ejaculation (Koziorowsk-Gilum et al., 2011).

Once spermatozoa are ejaculated and in contact with the SP, they display one type of physiological motility called 'activated' motility. They become motile and undergo an increase in metabolic activity due to the release from the suppressive conditions in the epididymis. During the ejaculation, spermatozoa are suddenly immersed in a HCO_3^--rich fluid, particularly in the sperm-richest fraction (Okamura et al., 1985; Rodriguez-Martinez et al., 1990) and the pH of the media surrounding the spermatozoa also increases to between 7.3 and 7.8 (Garner and Hafez, 2000).

The main ion transporters for spermatozoa pH_i regulation can be arranged into two groups: membrane H^+ transporters and HCO_3^- transporters. The first group (Fig. 9.1) involves the membrane Na^+/H^+ exchangers (sNHE) (Orlowski and Grinstein, 2011) and H^+ channels (H_v) (Lishko et al., 2010). The second group consists of membrane proteins that carry HCO_3^- across the plasma membrane, such as solute carriers 4 and 26 families (SLC4 and SLC26) and the cystic fibrosis transmembrane conductance regulator (CFTR) (Liu et al., 2012) that acts as an ion channel. Moreover, the CO_2/HCO_3^- is equilibrated by membrane associated carbonic anhydrases (CAs) that catalyzes the reversible conversion of cytosolic CO_2 to HCO_3^- and H^+ release ($CO_2 + H_2O \leftrightarrow H_2CO_3 \leftrightarrow HCO_3^- + H^+$) (reviewed by Nishigaki et al., 2014). Upon ejaculation, HCO_3^- is the unique activator that makes the quiescent spermatozoa motile (Okamura et al., 1985; Tajima et al., 1987). The SP activates certain channels in the spermatozoa plasma membrane during ejaculation that causes them to pass from immobile and inactive in the epididymis to mobile and active in SP. However, although the SP activates sperm motility, it does not activate other pathways related to sperm capacitation and contains specific 'decapacitating' factors that prevent the premature capacitation of spermatozoa in the ejaculate.

For the sperm capacitation process to occur normally, it is necessary to have SP removal and plasma membrane decoating of the decapacitating factors that are inhibiting or blocking that process. These SP factors will be lost *in vivo* along the spermatozoa journey through the female genital tract.

9.3 THE SPERMATOZOA IN THE FEMALE GENITAL TRACT: CERVIX AND UTERINE HORNS

Spermatozoa transport from the place where semen is deposited to the fertilization site is a complex process in which spermatozoa are progressively exposed to a dynamic and hostile environment and a strict selection process. Billions of spermatozoa are deposited into the cervix during mating or common AI in porcine, but only a limited number reach the

UTJ and the large majority of those do not pass through it (Hunter and Nichol, 1988). It involves numerous interactions between semen and the female genital tract that ensures that a sufficient number of fertilization-competent spermatozoa colonize the oviduct.

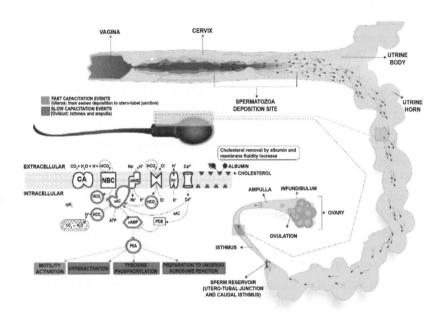

FIGURE 9.1 Sperm molecular basis of the spermatozoa capacitation pathway with special attention to bicarbonate (HCO$_3^-$). Fast and slow capacitation events depending on HCO$_3^-$ uptake. The fast capacitation events (represented in green) take place as soon as spermatozoa are capacitated and deposited in the uterus: HCO$_3^-$ uptake and subsequent intracellular pH alkalinization (pH$_i$) and motility activation (fast capacitation events). The slow capacitation events (represented in red) occur once spermatozoa achieve the oviduct (from isthmus to ampulla): hyperactivation, tyrosine phosphorylation (Tyr-P) and preparation to undergo acrosome reaction (AR) develop in a sequential and parallel way. Both fast and slow events depend on the HCO$_3^-$ and Ca^{2+} concentrations in the medium, but the slow ones also depend on the presence of albumin as membrane cholesterol acceptor. Membrane HCO$_3^-$ transporters: Na$^+$/HCO$_3^-$ co-transporters (NBC) and Cl$^-$/HCO$_3^-$ anion exchangers. Membrane H$^+$ transporters: Na$^+$/H$^+$ exchangers (sNHE), H$^+$ channels (H$_v$). The CO$_2$/HCO$_3^-$ is equilibrated by membrane associated carbonic anhydrases (CAs) that catalyzes the reversible conversion of cytosolic CO$_2$ to HCO$_3^-$ and H+ release (CO$_2$ + H$_2$O $\leftrightarrow$ H$_2$CO$_3$ $\leftrightarrow$ HCO$_3^-$ + H$^+$). After changes in sperm membrane fluidity and lipid scrambling HCO$_3^-$-dependent pathway is activated (Visconti et al., 1995). In the presence of albumin, HCO$_3^-$ leads to the activation of the soluble adenylyl cyclase (sAC) of the sperm membrane, which catalyzes cAMP metabolism and regulate the protein kinase A substrates phosphorylation (PKAs-P) (Visconti, 2009) on which fast and slow events depend.

9.3.1 SEMEN DEPOSITION AND SPERMATOZOA TRANSPORT

During natural mating or AI in porcine, billions of spermatozoa are deposited in the uterus but only a few thousand reach the oviducts (First et al., 1968; Sumransap et al., 2007) (Fig. 9.2). The fact that these processes happen in the uterus suggests that spermatozoa are subjected to strict selection during their transport towards the oviduct. Nevertheless, and under normal circumstances, spermatozoa are able to reach the oviduct within 1 h after semen deposition (Hunter, 1981).

The displacement of spermatozoa through the female genital tract to the site of fertilization seems to be a combination of passive and active transport. In the 'passive transport', the action of the uterus is essential to spermatozoa moving forward. The vigorous contractile activity of the myometrium directed forward and backward favors, on one hand, the advance of spermatozoa through the uterine horns towards the oviduct, and on the other hand, contractile activity eliminating part of the spermatozoa in the backflow (García-Vázquez et al., 2015). Reproductive hormones modulate contractions in the myometrium, which are inhibited by progesterone (P4) and reaches maximum activity during estrus by the action of estrogens, oxytocin, and prostaglandins (Langendijk et al., 2005). The rate of spermatozoa transport along the uterus is much faster if spermatozoa swim efficiently in the uterine fluid (UF), which is commonly called 'active transport'. This kind of transport is especially important to maintain the spermatozoa in suspension in the UF. Rapid transport of spermatozoa through the uterus can enhance spermatozoa survival by helping them to evade the local immune reaction. Gaddum-Rosse (1981) observed that immotile spermatozoa were unable to reach the last portion of the uterine horns, the utero-tubal junction (UTJ). The UTJ, the second great anatomical barrier of the uterus for the spermatozoa, is extremely narrow and tortuous and only a few thousand manage to pass through it and enter the oviduct.

9.3.2 SPERMATOZOA INTERACTION WITH UTERINE ENVIRONMENT

The epithelial uterine cells act creating an immunological barrier for spermatozoa and biological agents like viruses and bacteria. In the estrus stage of the cycle there is a massive migration of leukocytes (mainly PMN) to the sub-epithelial stroma (reviewed by Taylor et al., 2009). The presence of semen constituents, whether during coitus or AI, enhances the immunological reaction, trying to eliminate the foreign material including any bacteria (Schuberth et al., 2008), and produces an ideal environment for embryo implantation (Rozeboom et al., 1998). The PMNs collaborate in spermatozoa selection in the uterus due to their phagocytic action on non-motile or damaged spermatozoa (Tomlinson et al., 1992; Matthijs et al., 2003). One of the mechanisms to avoid the selective action of backflow and neutrophil attack is spermatozoa adhesion to the uterine epithelial cells (UEC) apical membrane (Taylor et al., 2008). The communication with the UECs is maintained mainly by spermadhesin-, lectin- or lectin-like protein-mediated interactions (Töpfer-Petersen et al., 1998; Bergmann et al., 2012). Only viable, membrane-intact and motile spermatozoa attach to the UECs (Rath et al., 2008) and it is probable that spermatozoa selection also depends on a specific morphology (reviewed by García-Vázquez et al., 2016).

Transport of spermatozoa into the uterus influences capacitation because spermatozoa are separated from the 'decapacitating factors' and other inhibitors and protectors present in the SP such as spermadhesins (Dostàlovà et al., 1995; Garner and Hafez, 2000) and spermatozoa are significantly diluted in luminal secretions and are susceptible to the changes of characteristics or composition of UF. The acidity or excessive alkalinity immobilizes spermatozoa, but moderately alkaline fluid enhances their motility (Garner and Hafez, 2000). In general terms, at the time of ovulation porcine cervical mucus is most alkaline (pH ~8.4, Hafez and Hafez, 2000), in which only some of the spermatozoa survive, which contributes to the selection of spermatozoa that are resistant to pH changes.

After the passage throughout all selective barriers aforementioned, the number of spermatozoa that reach the lower oviduct has been considerably reduced.

9.4   THE SPERMATOZOA IN THE FEMALE GENITAL TRACT: THE OVIDUCT

The mammalian oviduct provides a suitable environment for spermatozoa transport, storage and capacitation, oocyte pick-up, transport, maturation and fertilization, and early embryo development (Hunter and Rodriguez-Martinez, 2004). In some species of mammals including pigs and cows, oocytes are rapidly fertilized after ovulation; however, spermatozoa do not always colonize the oviduct at the same time as ovulation occurs. Spermatozoa need to survive and keep their fertility potential while waiting for ovulation within a certain time window. For this purpose, a storage site for spermatozoa is formed in the caudal isthmus, the sperm reservoir (SR), which has been described to be functional in pigs up to 30 h from onset of estrous (Rodríguez-Martínez et al., 2005). The SR ensures that a suitably low number of viable and potentially fertile spermatozoa are available to reach the fertilization site. Spermatozoa remain attached to the oviductal (isthmus) epithelial cells (OECs) in the SR and remain in a state of quiescence. After ovulation, spermatozoa are progressively released from OECs, their motility pattern changes (termed hyperactivation) and their plasma membrane is destabilized as part of the sperm capacitation process. In porcine, unlike other mammalian species where fertilization takes place in the oviductal ampulla, spermatozoa reach the AIJ where they interact with the ZP of the oocytes and undergo the AR to fertilize them. Finally, spermatozoa penetrate the zona pellucida and fuse with the oolemma (Yanagimachi, 1994a). During all these events in the oviduct, the specific characteristics and composition of the oviductal fluid (OF) in the periovulatory stage are essential to ensure proper sperm capacitation and gamete interaction.

9.4.1 SPERMATOZOA-OVIDUCT ADHESION AND RELEASE FROM THE 'SPERM RESERVOIR'

Only a small part of the inseminated spermatozoa achieves the caudal part of the oviduct, and transiently adhere to the ciliated OECs forming the SR (Fig. 9.2). The SR provides a selective barrier in the oviduct more specific than that of the uterus and allow the survival of spermatozoa with certain qualities and extension of their lifespan. The spermatozoa remain bound to OECs for up to 36–40 h before ovulation with no reduction in their fertilizing ability (Tienthai, 2015) and they are the most competent for fertilization based on their functionality (reviewed by Holt and Fazeli, 2010). The SR formation has been described as a crucial phase for fertilizing potential before gametes interact, which ensures that a suitable number of viable and potentially fertile spermatozoa are available (Hunter, 1984). The more probable significance of the SR establishment is to sequentially release the attached spermatozoa after ovulation to allow only a small quantity of them to reach the oocyte at any given time and therefore reduce the possibility of polyspermy (Hunter, 1973).

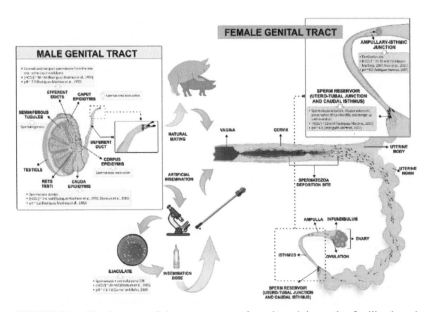

FIGURE 9.2 The journey of the spermatozoa from its origin to the fertilization site. Functions, bicarbonate (HCO_3^-) concentration and pH in each section of the male and female genital tract. The spermatozoon must travel first from its production site in the seminiferous tubules of the testis, to the maturation site along the epididymis (caput and corpus) and to its site of storage in the epididymis (cauda), where they encounter an acidic environment with ~3–4 mmol/L of HCO_3^- and pH ~6.2. During ejaculation, spermatozoa are emitted together with the seminal plasma (SP) formed by the cauda epididymal fluid and accessory sex glands secretions. SP contains ~20 mmol/L of HCO_3^- and pH 7.3–7.8. During natural mating, the ejaculate is deposited into the anterior cervix. From ejaculate, insemination doses can also be obtained for artificial insemination that can be deposited in anterior cervix or uterine body using the appropriate insemination catheter. Spermatozoa move through the uterus by passive transport favored by myometrial contractions and also active transport by sperm swimming. Billions of spermatozoa are deposited into the female reproductive tract but only a limited number reach de utero-tubal junction (UTJ) and the large majority of those do not even pass through it. In the UTJ and caudal isthmus, spermatozoa attach to the oviductal epithelial cells (OECs) forming the sperm reservoir (SR). The SR selects the spermatozoa, extends their lifespan, preserves their functionality and storages them up until ovulation. The HCO_3^- concentration in SR is low (~10 mmol/L) and pH slightly acid (pH 6.5) to allow spermatozoa quiescence. Once ovulation occurs, an increase of HCO_3^- concentration (~25–90 mmol/L) and pH (~8.0) takes place that triggers the hyperactivation of spermatozoa that allows its release from the SR. The spermatozoa enter into the oviductal lumen in which they complete the capacitation process: the transport to the fertilization site in ampullary-isthmic junction (AIJ), the preparation to undergo the acrosome reaction (AR) to go through the egg vestments and the contact with the oocytes and penetration.

The microenvironment of the SR favors the adhesion of competent spermatozoa that seems to be mediated by molecules exposed on the spermatozoa surface, such as lectin-like proteins of the rostral region of the spermatozoa head. The OECs have the ability to select viable and uncapacitated spermatozoa and protect them during a certain time window from being damaged and capacitated until the ovulated egg arrives (Töpfer-Petersen et al., 2002). However, not all spermatozoa are able to bind and take part in the SR.

It has been reported in *in vitro* studies that OECs binds sperm in a selective manner. For example, OECs only bind mature (Petrunkina et al., 2001), viable (Fazeli et al., 1999; Yeste et al., 2009), morphologically normal (Fazeli et al., 1999; Waberski et al., 2006; Yeste et al., 2012), uncapacitated (Fazeli et al., 1999; Petrunkina et al., 2001; Yeste et al., 2009; López-Úbeda et al., 2017) and fertile spermatozoa (Holt and Fazeli, 2010; López-Úbeda et al., 2017), with non-fragmented chromatin (Ardón et al., 2008), good osmoregulatory abilities (Petrunkina et al., 2007) and that express certain surface proteins such as spermadhesin AQN1 (Talevi and Gualtieri, 2010). All these strict requisites enable the selection of a higher quality spermatozoa population with greater fertilizing potential, and is the basis of the spermatozoa competition that has been speculated by several authors in porcine and other mammalian species (Gualtieri and Talevi, 2003; López-Úbeda et al., 2017;).

It has even been suggested that the action of the lowest isthmus on spermatozoa is more to delay the capacitation progress than promote it (Smith, 1998; Rodriguez-Martinez et al., 2001). In the SR, spermatozoa are quiescent, and capacitation is delayed until specific and partially unknown signals around the time of ovulation that induce the spermatozoa release. Spermatozoa release could be a combination of periovulatory signals secreted by the oviduct itself or stimulated by *cumulus*-oocyte complexes (COCs), follicular fluid (FF) and the presence of spermatozoa in the oviduct (reviewed by Georgiou et al., 2007; Brüssow et al., 2008; Hunter, 2008), in combination with the P4 levels in the periovulatory stage (Bureau et al., 2002). Other oviductal factors such as Ca^{2+} concentration in OF are also important to produce the state of hyperactivation in spermatozoa that allows the bound spermatozoa to be released from OECs (Flesch and Gadella, 2000; Gadella and Harrison, 2000; Petrunkina et al., 2001). The power of the increased bend amplitude of the sperm tail during hyperactivation can overcome spermatozoa-epithelial binding, and it has been demonstrated that only hyperactivated spermatozoa are able to detach from OECs (Suarez et al., 1992). And also, the modifications in the spermatozoa surface (Suarez, 2016) and action of determined molecules, as heparin, are essential to produce spermatozoa detachment from OECs (Ardon et al., 2016).

9.4.2   THE SPERM CAPACITATION PROCESS IN THE OVIDUCT

Sperm capacitation is a complex and lengthy physiological process that involves a combination of sequential and parallel molecular changes that affect both the spermatozoa head and tail (Suarez, 2007). It is a critical point to the acquisition of the ability of the spermatozoa to fertilize the oocyte.

Sperm capacitation includes many changes in sperm, such as alterations in plasma membrane fluidity, protein tyrosine phosphorylation (Tyr-P), and a change in motility pattern (hyperactive motility) and the ability to undergo the AR. Some of these changes take place as the spermatozoa are ejaculated but others require a longer period and develop along the female genital tract, specifically in the oviduct. What seems clear is that all these processes are triggered by HCO_3^- and regulated by protein kinase A (PKA) in the soluble adenylyl cyclase (sAC)/adenosine 3':5'-cyclic monophosphate (cAMP) pathway (Visconti et al., 1995; Visconti, 2009) (Fig. 9.1).

One of the first events of capacitation is the activation of spermatozoa motility by the action of HCO_3^- that stimulates the flagellum (García Herreros et al., 2005), which involves HCO_3^- uptake from the extracellular medium, producing a slight alkalinization of the spermatozoa cytosol. The later events of capacitation take place in the oviduct, that involves first a remodeling of plasma membrane architecture and cholesterol-efflux due to the action of albumin and high-density lipoproteins present in the OF, which increases membrane fluidity. The consequence of this increase in membrane fluidity is membrane depolarization, which causes an increase in spermatozoa Ca^{2+} permeability (Wennemuth et al., 2003). The spermatozoa motility pattern also changes drastically (hyperactivation) and the spermatozoon acquires the ability to fertilize the oocyte (Visconti, 2009).

Spermatozoa are firstly inactive in the SR and then activated and free in the oviductal lumen moving towards the ovulated oocyte, ready for ZP binding, undergoing the AR, and fertilizing the oocyte.

9.4.3 FERTILIZATION

Fertilization is the process in which two haploid gametes (spermatozoon and oocyte) unite to form a genetically distinct individual. It comprises a series of sequential and coordinated phases that result in a diploid zygote. In porcine, fertilization takes places in the AIJ (Hunter, 1974) and begins when the capacitated spermatozoa in the immediate vicinity of oocyte pass through the *cumulus oophorus* and interact with the glycoproteins of the ZP of the oocyte (Yanagimachi, 1994b; Kim et al., 2008). Spermatozoa-ZP recognition and binding is mediated by carbohydrate interactions that can be divided into two phases:

i) Primary binding: the capacitated spermatozoon recognizes the ZP mainly by apical surface spermadhesins and proacrosin and binds to the ZP glycoproteins in a specific manner (Töpfer-Petersen et al., 1985; Töpfer-Petersen and Henschen, 1987; Harris et al., 1994; Töpfer-Petersen et al., 1998; 2008). This interaction triggers the initiation of the AR, in which acrosomal enzymes are discharged into the ZP (Yanagimachi, 1994b). The hyperactivated spermatozoon then uses the impulse of flagellar beating to pass through the ZP.

ii) Secondary binding: the acrosome reacted spermatozoa expose a set of intraacrosomal proteins with high affinity for ZP. Spermatozoa become firmer attached to the ZP and definitely crosses it (Bleil et al., 1988).

After spermatozoa penetration of the egg vestments, the acrosome-reacted sperm goes through the perivitelline space and adheres its equatorial region and fuses with the egg plasma membrane, the oolemma (sperm-egg fusion). The cortical reaction then takes place, which results in changes to the structure of the ZP and its proteins (Wolf, 1981). This converts the ZP into a 'hardened' state, which helps to block polyspermy. This particular phenomenon is of special interest in porcine because this species has a high incidence of polyspermy under *in vitro* conditions (Funahashi et al., 2000). The spermatozoon next penetrates the oocyte and introduces its nucleus into the ooplasm (Yanagimachi, 1994b). Despite the continuous advance in the knowledge of the physiology of gametes as well as their interaction, there are still many aspects to be clarified to efficiently extrapolate the *in vivo* environment in the oviduct to the *in vitro* conditions in the laboratory. Many strategies and protocols have been carried out so far; however, the efficiency obtaining quality embryos *in vitro* remains lower than that of them *in vivo* counterparts.

9.5 *IN VIVO VS. IN VITRO* SPERM CAPACITATION AND FERTILIZATION

The rapid advance of ARTs in mammals has led to reliable and standardized protocols of obtaining zygotes and embryos in the laboratory with a relatively reasonable success rate. Establishment of *in vitro* systems has been assisted and encouraged by the ready availability of protocols for preparation of gametes, chemically-defined culture media, disposable plastic dishes and tubes, and computer-controlled incubators set to a predetermine gas concentration, humidity and temperature (Hunter and Rodriguez-Martinez, 2002). However, conditions applied fruitfully *in vitro* may not be closely representative of those found *in vivo*, and levels of success *in vitro* seldom match those found *in vivo* (reviewed by Hunter and Rodriguez-Martinez, 2002).

The population of spermatozoa selected or capacitated *in vitro* probably is different from the small proportion of competent spermatozoa that would reach the site of fertilization *in vivo* close to the time of ovulation. As an example, a droplet of culture medium containing spermatozoa and COCs represents, strictly speaking, a post-ovulatory milieu, but is probably much different from the preparatory milieu to which gametes are exposed *in vivo* (Rodríguez-Martínez et al., 2005). The current conditions in porcine IVF are still far from optimal since none has managed to reduce the unacceptably high incidence of polyspermy in this species. *In vitro* techniques have resulted in pregnancies and live offspring through embryo transfer in multiple mammalian species. For decades, research in this field has increased the knowledge in basic science about physiology of gametes and their interaction, even in the complex uterine environment. However, while good performance of these techniques has been achieved in some mammalian species such as bovine or murine, the results obtained in porcine so far are not comparable to the *in vivo* output. In pigs, differences between *in vivo* and *in vitro* environment in which sperm capacitation and fertilization take place could be a determinant of the low success in obtaining potentially viable zygotes. A summary of the main differences between *in vivo* and *in vivo* sperm capacitation and fertilization are shown in Table 9.1.

TABLE 9.1 Differences Between *In Vivo* and *In Vitro* Sperm Capacitation and Fertilization in Mammals, with Special Attention to Porcine Species.

Parameter/Factor	*In vivo* (*)	*In vitro* (†)	Reference
Source of spermatozoa	Ejaculate	Epididymis or ejaculate	* Yanagimachi, 1994b † Matás et al., 2010
Spermatozoa selection and capacitation	Backflow, phagocytosis by neutrophils and formation of sperm reservoir (SR)	Washes with albumin or through colloids and sperm pelleting, filtration with Sephadex gel or glass wool	* García-Vázquez et al., 2015; Holt and Fazeli, 2010; Taylor et al., 2008; Matthijs et al., 2003; † Matás et al., 2011; Holt et al., 2010; Matás et al., 2003
Sperm capacitation site	During the transport through the female reproductive tract	Plastic tubes and dishes in computer-controlled incubators set to predetermine gas phase, humidity and temperature	* Yanagimachi, 1994a † Hunter and Rodriguez-Martinez, 2002
Sperm capacitation media	Uterine and oviductal fluids (UF and OF)	Chemically defined media	* Rodriguez-Martinez, 2007. † Rath et al., 1999; Abeydeera and Day, 1997; Mattioli et al., 1988
Spermatozoa response to capacitation	Progressive and sequential. Heterogeneity among spermatozoa subpopulations	High proportion of partially-reacted spermatozoa	* Suarez, 2007 † reviewed by Funahashi, 2003
Timing of sperm capacitation	2–3 h depending on the place of deposition	Initiated in max. 60 s. The latter signs occur after 60 min incubation	* Harrison, 1996; Hunter and Dziuk, 1968 † Rath et al., 1999; Harrison, 2004
Source of matured oocytes	Follicle (ovulated oocytes)	Follicle (ovulated oocytes) or *in vitro* matured oocytes in plastic dishes	* Yanagimachi, 1994a † Hunter and Rodriguez-Martinez, 2002

TABLE 9.1 (Continued)

Parameter/Factor	In vivo (*)	In vitro (†)	Reference
Cumulus oophorus	Present	Present or absent	* Yanagimachi, 1994a † Coy et al., 1993c
Oocytes and zygotes ZP thickness	Thick	Thin	* Funahashi et al., 2001; Wang et al., 1998 † Funahashi et al., 2001
Spermatozoa and oocytes coincubation time	-	From 15 s to 18 h	† Almiñana et al., 2008; Coy et al., 2008b; Matás et al., 2003; Coy et al., 1993a
Spermatozoa concentration for insemination	From 30–60 million (AI) to hundreds of millions (natural mating) spermatozoa/ml	From tens of thousands to millions spermatozoa/ml	* Waberski et al., 2008 † Ballester et al., 2014; Almiñana et al., 2008; Coy et al., 1993b
Capacitating and fertilizing environment	Dynamic	Static	* Rodriguez-Martinez, 2007 † Nagai, 1994
Fertilization site	Ampullary-isthmic junction (AIJ)	4-wells multidish, microdrops, caps of tubes, straws, microchannels, microfluidic sorters, 3-D OECs cultures	* Yanagimachi, 1994a † Ferraz et al., 2017; Sano et al., 2010; Clark et al., 2005; Li et al., 2003; Funahashi and Nagai, 2000
Fertilization media	Periovulatory oviductal fluid (OF)	TCM-199, TALP, BO, TBM	* Yanagimachi, 1994b † Coy and Romar, 2002; Coy et al., 2002
Regulation and synchronization of environment	Oviductal and follicular factors	Technical and human factors	* Hunter, 1990 † Hunter and Rodriguez-Martinez, 2002

TABLE 9.1 *(Continued)*

Parameter/Factor	In vivo (*)	In vitro (†)	Reference
Environmental HCO$_3^-$ concentration	~10 mmol/L in isthmus and 25–90 mmol/L in AIJ	25 mmol/L	* Rodriguez-Martinez, 2007; Rodriguez-Martinez et al., 1990 † Parrish, 2014; Yoshioka et al., 2008; Bedu-Addo et al., 2007; Coy et al., 2002; Rath et al., 1999; Quinn, 1995
Environmental pH	~8.0	7.4–8.0	* Rodriguez-Martinez, 2007 † Matás et al., 2010; Abeydeera and Day, 1997; Coy et al., 1993b; Soriano-Úbeda et al., 2017
Biofluids presence	Uterine or oviductal fluids (UF or OF)	Uterine, oviductal or follicular fluids (UF, OF or FF) incorporated to the media	* Leese et al., 2001; Nichol et al., 1992; Leese, 1988 † Cánovas et al., 2017; Coy and Avilés, 2010; Coy et al., 2008b; Coy et al., 2002; Kim et al., 1997; Kim et al., 1996; Funahashi and Day, 1993; Nagai and Moor, 1990

Spermatozoa fertility usually refers to the ability of spermatozoa to fertilize oocytes, either *in vivo* or *in vitro*. In most mammalian species including porcine, spermatozoa acquire fertilization ability once the reach the corpus epididymis or proximal segment of the cauda epididymis (Yanagimachi, 1994a). In *in vivo* conditions, both in natural mating and in AI, spermatozoa entering the uterus are ejaculated spermatozoa; that is, spermatozoa that have had contact with the SP. There are also studies in porcine in which sows were inseminated with epididymal spermatozoa (fresh or frozen-thawed) but fertilization and conception rates and litter size after AI were much lower than those obtained with ejaculated spermatozoa (Holtz and Smidt, 1976; Okazaki et al., 2012). *in vitro*, two sources of spermatozoa can be used—ejaculated or epididymal—depending on the objective and the technical constraints. In fact, there are numerous studies in which both ejaculated and epididymal spermatozoa have been used and compared (Matás et al., 2010). The fertility and response to treatments usually is variable in ejaculated spermatozoa both within and between individual boars and ejaculates, probably due to the variable effects of SP components on the different subpopulations of spermatozoa. In this sense, epididymal spermatozoa tend to be more 'stable' in their response to selection or capacitation treatments (Matás et al., 2010). It has been reported that epididymal spermatozoa *in vitro* can reach capacitation and fertilize oocytes much easier than ejaculated spermatozoa (Yanagimachi, 1994b), but this depends on the specific treatments used for sperm selection and capacitation.

Over years, different types of *in vitro* spermatozoa selection techniques have been developed with the main objective to eliminate the SP and decapacitating factors, residues of diluents used for spermatozoa preservation, or certain contaminating particles. Many of these selection methods involve the centrifugation (washing with albumin or through colloids and sperm pelleting) or the use of a non-physiological composition of selection media (for example, spermatozoa filtration with Sephadex gel or glass wool) that select spermatozoa by their physical characteristics, but some of these procedures can produce cellular damage (Holt et al., 2010; Matás et al., 2011).

Once spermatozoa are released from SR and enter the oviductal lumen, they are exposed to the specific and dynamic milieu of the oviduct, which due to its particular temperature, oxygen and pH provides a suitable environment to promote sperm capacitation and fertilization (De Lamirande et al., 1997). *in vivo*, sperm capacitation occurs during the transport through the female reproductive tract, is progressive and sequential due to the dynamic environments encountered by the spermatozoa from the site of semen deposition to the site of fertilization in terms of biofluid composition, pH, temperature, percentage of oxygen, etc. The diversity and heterogeneity in responsiveness among spermatozoa subpopulations allow different grades of sperm capacitation in each uterine section. The specific composition of UF and OF in the periovulatory stage is still partially unknown, which makes it difficult to mimic *in vitro*. *In vitro* sperm capacitation is conducted in plastic tubes or dishes, in static systems, in chemically defined media of differing complexity but limited and fixed composition and physical characteristics, probably much different from that encountered in UF and OF. One of the main consequences of these static systems is that under *in vitro* conditions most of spermatozoa are capacitated simultaneously (Rodriguez-Martinez, 2007). *In vitro* capacitation can occur by incubating spermatozoa at physiological temperature of 38.5°C, in the presence of HCO_3^- and Ca^{2+}, with albumin as a protein source, and with energy substrate molecules such as glucose, pyruvate and lactate, in a balanced salt solution in which slightly alkaline pH is maintained, normally at 7.4 (Harrison, 1996; Visconti and Kopf, 1998; Watson and Green, 2000).

It is difficult to specify the exact timing of the events that take place during the sperm capacitation process. Under *in vivo* conditions, sperm capacitation could last 2 or 3 hours, depending on the place of semen deposition (Hunter and Dziuk, 1968; Harrison, 1996). What seems clear is that OF modulates the rate of sperm capacitation events *in vivo*, and probably also when it is added to an *in vitro* system. Once spermatozoa are sequentially exposed to UF and OF, these fluids should be able to regulate the rate of the process (Rodriguez-Martinez, 2007). However, it has been described that *in vitro* capacitation is initiated within a few seconds or minutes after spermatozoa come into contact with a HCO_3^--enriched capacitating medium because HCO_3^- rapidly stimulates sAC (maximum within 60 s) that triggers PKA-dependent protein phosphorylation cascade (Harrison, 2004; Visconti, 2009). One of the first signals of that is the activation of spermatozoa motility, but also a scrambling of plasma membrane phospholipids that produces an increase in plasma membrane fluidity (Harrison and Miller, 2000). Significantly later, the membrane fluidity increases again but by the action of the presence of albumin in the incubation medium, which removes or redistributes the cholesterol in the spermatozoa plasma membrane (Flesch et al., 2001). Another late effect (>60 min) of HCO_3^- in *in vitro* sperm capacitation is the activation of tyrosine kinases and the subsequent Tyr-P (Visconti, 2009).

The process of fertilization *in vivo* is precisely and strictly regulated and synchronized. In the oviduct, oviductal and follicular factors coordinate gamete interaction and function (Hunter, 1990). Only few capacitated spermatozoa reach the COCs and undergo the AR during passage through the *cumulus* (Mattioli et al., 1998) or ZP (Cummins and Yanagimachi, 1982). However, *in vitro* sperm capacitation and fertilization provides a static system controlled by technical (incubators, thermostats, gas infusion pumps, etc.) and human factors (time of manipulation of gametes, maintenance of asepsis, contamination, abrupt fluctuations of temperature, etc.) (Hunter and Rodriguez-Martinez, 2002) that are far from resembling the dynamic system to which gametes are exposed *in vivo* (Nagai, 1994; Visconti, 2009). In IVF, there is no single medium commonly used by researches, but what seems clear is the importance of Ca^{2+} availability in the medium and its uptake by oocytes and spermatozoa. Currently, conditions used for IVF differ enormously from those *in vivo* but all the *in vivo* parameters should first be determined to be efficiently mimicked and applied *in vitro*. The strict control by the female reproductive tract of spermatozoa functions and capacitation state enables, in physiological conditions in the oviduct, monospermic penetration of oocytes in porcine of around 95% of total fertilizations (reviewed by Funahashi, 2003). The strategies employed by the uterus to reduce the number of spermatozoa that reach the site of fertilization, select the most suitable spermatozoa for fertilization and modulate their state of activation-quiescence-capacitation are still largely unknown. As previously described, the mechanisms that control the number of porcine spermatozoa that are fertilization competent are well developed *in vivo* and effectively reduce polyspermy, but the complexity of these mechanisms make it difficult to reproduce *in vitro* (reviewed by Funahashi, 2003). Thus, it seems nearly impossible to obtain the high rate of monospermy in pigs *in vitro* that has been achieved in other mammals. In fact, it has been proposed that polyspermy is the bottleneck to improvements in porcine IVF and this has been related to the induction of partial AR of boar spermatozoa in IVF media and thus to the use of a highly non-physiological number of spermatozoa which are simultaneously capacitated and ready to fertilize. The percentage of polyspermy *in vitro* is directly related to the number of spermatozoa used, but, unfortunately, simply reducing the number of spermatozoa per oocyte not only does not address the problem of polyspermy but decreases the penetration rate. The current conditions of preparation of the gametes prior to porcine IVF are still far from optimal since none of them has managed to reduce the unacceptably high incidence of polyspermy in this species. One strategy is to modulate the *in vitro* sperm capacitation to impede the simultaneous presence of massive numbers of capacitated spermatozoa around the oocytes at the time of fertilization.

On the other hand, polyspermy has been also related to the significant differences in organization and ultrastructure of ZP proteins in pig between *in vitro* and *in vivo* matured and fertilized oocytes (Coy et al., 2008a). ZP of ovulated oocytes has a rather thick mesh-like fibrillar network structure whereas in *in vitro* matured oocytes the ZP is more compacted and smoother. After the contact with spermatozoa, *in vitro* matured oocytes undergo a delayed or incomplete zona reaction far from the complete polyspermy-blocking reaction that takes place *in vivo* in the oviduct (Funahashi, 2003). Polyspermic penetration in porcine oocytes also occurs *in vivo*; however, there are physiological mechanisms, many of them unknown, that modulate this incidence. Additional macromolecules have been reported in the ZP of ovulated pig oocytes (Hedrick et al., 1987), such as oestrogen-dependent oviductal glycoproteins, which are secreted into the oviductal lumen (Brown and Cheng, 1986; Coy et al., 2008a). With the current media used in the IVF laboratories, it has not yet been possible to reproduce this phenomenon. During final maturation, the ZP of *in vivo* matured oocytes adds oviductal glycoproteins, which allows the change of conformation in the inner ZP necessary to undergo an appropriate ZP reaction when fertilized. Changes in ovulated oocytes that are conferred by OF seem to produce ZP resistance to digestion by pronase (Wang et al., 1998); this ZP resistance can be increased in *in vitro* matured oocytes by exposing them to OF (Coy et al., 2008a).

Despite the development of different spermatozoa-oocyte co-incubation times (Coy et al., 1993a; Matás et al., 2003; Almiñana et al., 2008; Coy et al., 2008b), spermatozoa concentration for insemination (Coy et al., 1993b; Almiñana et al., 2008; Ballester et al., 2014), presence of the *cumulus oophorus* (Coy et al., 1993c), sperm capacitation methods (Matás et al., 2003) and innovative IVF protocols in which gametes are physically separated (Funahashi and Nagai, 2000; Li et al., 2003; Clark et al., 2005; Sano et al., 2010), polyspermy in porcine IVF is not yet solved. Moreover, there are numerous studies attempting to improve IVF by developing defined capacitation and fertilization media for pigs (Mattioli et al., 1988; Abeydeera and Day, 1997; Rath et al., 1999) and comparing their efficiency, such as TCM-199, Tyrode's albumin lactate pyruvate (TALP), Brackett-Oliphant solution (BO) or Tris-buffered medium (TBM) (reviewed by Coy et al., 2002; Coy and Romar, 2002). Other variables studied have been the spermatozoa concentration used for insemination, coincubation time, source of spermatozoa or volume of coculture medium, but there is a lack of conclusive results and standardized protocols in porcine (reviewed by Coy and Romar, 2002).

   Therefore, more studies are needed to deepen the knowledge of the oviductal microenvironment in which porcine capacitation and fertilization take place *in vivo* to try to mimic them *in vitro*. At present, the main objectives of the research carried out in our laboratories are aimed at improving media and conditions of culture, the incorporation of biofluids and the development of IVF devices in which gamete functionality is more similar to physiological conditions (Cánovas et al., 2017; Soriano-Úbeda et al., 2017). Some of these factors, still to be optimized, such as HCO_3^- concentration, pH, use of biofluids and IVF devices that allow much more physiological contact between gametes, are reviewed below.

9.5.1   BICARBONATE (HCO_3^-) CONCENTRATION

HCO_3^- has been identified *in vitro* as a key capacitating agent that promotes lipid rearrangement-disorder in the spermatozoa plasma membrane that initiates the capacitation. It acts by activating the sAC/cAMP-dependent pathway (Visconti et al., 1995). Sperm capacitation in the isthmus is initiated under a concentration of HCO_3^- around 10 mmol/L (Rodriguez-Martinez et al., 1990) and spermatozoa are progressively exposed to higher HCO_3^- as they ascend to the fertilization site. *in vivo*, the number of capacitated spermatozoa at one particular time and place of the oviduct would be low. The capacitated state is transient and irreversible *in vivo*. So, there should be a continuous replacement of capacitated, short-lived spermatozoa leading to low spermatozoa number per area at one time, ensuring the availability of capacitated spermatozoa for an extended period between spermatozoa deposition and ovulation (Rodriguez-Martinez, 2007). However, far from these dynamic environments that spermatozoa go through and the progressive and sequential events in capacitation of spermatozoa subpopulations *in vivo*, currently most of the *in vitro* capacitation and fertilization protocols result in the majority of spermatozoa being capacitated and available to fertilize at the same time. The most common media for *in vitro* sperm capacitation and IVF contains a fix concentration of 25 mmol/L of HCO_3^-, whatever the origin of the spermatozoa (epididymal or ejaculated) and the treatments received (dilution in an extender, refrigeration, selection process) (Quinn, 1995; Rath et al., 1999; Coy et al., 2002; Bedu-Addo et al., 2007; Yoshioka et al., 2008; Parrish, 2014). HCO_3^-, as a key effector in sperm capacitation, needs to be adjusted in the medium in an attempt to produce more physiological sperm capacitation and combat the problem of polyspermy. For that purpose, some authors proposed reduction of HCO_3^- concentration in the media for porcine *in vitro* sperm capacitation and fertilization to 15 mmol/L. This concentration activates the porcine sperm capacitation but with slower progression, which seems to be related with increased rates of monospermy in the IVF (Soriano-Úbeda et al., 2019).

9.5.2 pH

In addition to be a capacitating effector, HCO_3^- acts to buffer the reproductive environments in which gametes are found. One of the consequences of the exposure of spermatozoa to HCO_3^- is the alkalinization of the intracellular fluid, which in the oviduct activates spermatozoa motility and triggers the cascade of molecular events of capacitation (Visconti, 2009).

The pH in the oviductal lumen, due to the production of HCO_3^- in the OECs, greatly increases in the periovulatory stage, reaching around pH 8.0 at the site of fertilization at the time of the encounter between gametes (Rodriguez-Martinez, 2007). However, media commonly used for *in vitro* sperm capacitation and IVF have a fixed pH of 7.4 (Coy et al., 1993a,b,c; Abeydeera and Day, 1997; Matás et al., 2010). It is known that most of biological processes in organisms are regulated by pH (Lodish et al., 2000), and mammalian capacitation, fertilization and polyspermy blocking could be some of them. For this reason, one of the plausible strategies to improve IVF output is increasing the pH of the medium (although maintaining its concentration of HCO_3^-) to 8.0 to be more like the physiological pH at the place of fertilization (Soriano-Úbeda et al., 2017).

9.5.3 BIOFLUIDS

As discussed, under *in vitro* conditions, the pattern of sperm capacitation and fertilization is not similar to the situation *in vivo*. The media used in laboratories is not similar to OF and there is not a single medium commonly used in all laboratories that allows standardization of IVF in porcine (Coy et al., 2002). Chemically defined media are currently used for these techniques, with more or less complex composition based in salts, sugars, proteins such as albumin and other components. However, the media composition has not been able to equate with OF, as it is still unknown. In order to increase the performance of IVF in pigs, several protocols have been developed that include OF in the medium (Coy et al., 2010; Cánovas et al., 2017) although the lack of knowledge of OF composition remains a handicap in achieving consistency.

The effect of OF on sperm has been described to prolong survival and delay destabilization processes at the plasmalemma, even during capacitation, and resulting hyperactivation (reviewed by Rodriguez-Martinez et al., 2016). Briefly, OF seems to modulate spermatozoa functionality and capacitation process. Moreover, the intraluminal periovulatory OF is the optimal medium to transport gametes allowing the interaction between them and also to promote early embryonic development (Yanagimachi, 1994b). Periovulatory OF is formed by specific OECs secretions and by transudation of blood serum, but OF differs from serum in terms of ionic composition, osmolarity, pH and macromolecular content (Leese, 1988; Nichol et al., 1992). Regional differences also exist in the composition of OF and this seems to be related with the process of gamete preparation for fertilization (Leese et al., 2001). There are also differences in OF composition by the mere fact of gametes presence (Georgiou et al., 2007).

Incubation of spermatozoa with undefined oviductal components before or during IVF as has been done for OECs, has demonstrated that OF or FF improve IVF (Kim et al., 1997; Funahashi and Day, 1993; Nagai and Moor, 1990). In addition, specific oviductal components such as glycoproteins (Kouba et al., 2000; Coy et al., 2008a; Algarra et al., 2016), GAGs such as HA (Suzuki et al., 2000) or proteins such as osteopontin (Hao et al., 2006) have shown beneficial effects. *In vitro*, the preincubation of porcine oocytes in OF from early-luteal phase increased ZP hardening and pronase digestion time, which has been linked with higher monospermy rate (Kim et al., 1996; Coy et al., 2002; Coy et al., 2008a; Coy and Avilés, 2010). It has been described that the inclusion of OF in IVF systems reduces polyspermy, probably by preventing the spermatozoa AR (Kim et al., 1997), regulating the capacitation rate and making it slower before ovulation and faster after it (Rodriguez-Martinez et al., 1998; Coy et al., 2010; Avilés, 2011).

Other difference between *in vivo* and *in vitro* interactions between porcine gametes is that many IVF protocols remove the *cumulus* cells that surround the oocyte. In these cases, the secretory products of *cumulus* cells derived from their metabolism are absent in many of the current IVF systems. In pigs, the presence of *cumulus* cells has been shown to improve fertility and monospermy ratios (Coy et al., 1993c). In bovine, granulosa cells obtained from the follicular wall increase the fertilization rate and decrease polyspermy (Fukui and Ono, 1989). The FF, which is a product of the follicular wall, is also important in the oviductal milieu as during ovulation it is poured into the oviduct and forms part of the OF. In porcine, the effect of including FF in the pre-fertilization media for spermatozoa incubation has been studied and during IVF results in a reduction of polyspermy and number of spermatozoa bound to the ZP (Funahashi and Day, 1993). Some substances existing in the FF and OF and also produced by *cumulus* cells play a significant role in sperm capacitation and survival, as hyaluronic acid (HA). HA from OF and FF can modulate sperm capacitation and promote sperm survival (Rodriguez-Martinez, 2007), and HA from *cumulus* cells promote the AR close to the oocyte (Suzuki et al., 2002).

There is a large gap in knowledge of the exact composition of biofluids, but what seems clear is that despite the use of chemically defined culture media has not been able to match the results of biofluids *in vivo* or the addition of biofluids to IVF systems. More studies are needed to analyze in depth the composition of biofluids with the objective to establish a chemically defined culture medium or system for sperm capacitation and IVF that more closely resembles the physiological environment.

9.5.4 *IN VITRO FERTILIZATION (IVF) DEVICES*

The most used systems for IVF in porcine have been 4-well dishes and microdrops, but with the objective to mimic the strict spermatozoa selection process that takes place in the female genital tract and to allow the establishment of competition between spermatozoa, several methods and devices have been developed: IVF by climbing-over-a-wall (Funahashi and

Nagai, 2000; Soriano-Úbeda et al., 2017), using biomimetic microfluidic technology (Clark et al., 2005), IVF in straws (Li et al., 2003), applying modified swim-up for spermatozoa selection (Park et al., 2009), using a microfluidic spermatozoa sorter (Sano et al., 2010) or 3-D OECs culture systems for IVF and embryo production (reviewed by Ferraz et al., 2017). Most of these methods reduce the number of spermatozoa that contact the oocytes, allowing a certain selection of spermatozoa population and expression of their heterogeneity in terms of motility, capacitation state and fertility. Many of them can include biofluids that can be replaced over time to mimic the dynamic oviductal environment in terms of composition of proteins, hormones and other molecules, and they even have different compartments for male and female gametes and/or OECs. Normally, there are methods or devices in which gametes, female and male, are physically distant from each other and spermatozoa must cross an artificial obstacle to reach the oocytes, more similar to the situation *in vivo*. However, none of them has managed to eliminate the problem of polyspermy under *in vitro* conditions in the pig. Many studies are currently underway to develop new devices in which spermatozoa are guided to the oocytes through the so-called 'taxis': chemo-, rheo- and thermotaxis. In each one of them, spermatozoa are attracted by a different stimulus gradient: chemical, fluid flow or temperature, respectively (revised by Pérez-Cerezales et al., 2015).

9.6 CONCLUDING REMARKS

From the studies reviewed, major research progress has been made in reproductive physiology and technology in swine. However, attempts to improve *in vitro* reproduction in pigs have not been enough. Lack of knowledge of many factors involved in *in vitro* sperm capacitation and fertilization and its regulation could contribute to the abnormally high incidence of polyspermy in this species. The use of simple *in vitro* systems of pre-treatment of gametes and IVF have been well demonstrated to be valid to analyze the complex processes of fertilization and evaluate several sperm, oocyte and embryo parameters. However, they suffer from serious limitation for the *in vitro* production of embryos due to fact that the available capacitation media produce a large percentage of capacitated spermatozoa that ready for fertilize at the same time. The direction in which we must advance is to allow oocytes to express their natural ability to block polyspermy, with more studies on the physiology of gametes, as well as with the development of new strategies for modulation of sperm capacitation. To do this, it would seem logical to first adjust the known parameters involved in *in vitro* sperm capacitation and fertilization processes that are far from their counterparts *in vivo* and that could firmly establish the basis of these techniques in the porcine species.

ACKNOWLEDGMENTS

The authors would like to thank the Spanish Ministry of Economy and Competitiveness (MINECO), the European Regional Development Fund (FEDER), Grants AGL2012-40180-C03-01-02 and AGL2015-66341-R) for the support and Dr. Lawrence Reynolds and Jordana Portugal Sena Lopes for their critical revision and assistance with the language.

KEYWORDS

- **porcine**
- **spermatozoa**
- **capacitation**
- **bicarbonate**
- **pH**
- **oviductal fluid**
- ***in vitro* fertilization**

REFERENCES

Abeydeera, L. R.; and Day, B. N. Fertilization and Subsequent Development *in Vitro* of Pig Oocytes Inseminated in a Modified Tris-Buffered Medium with Frozen-Thawed Ejaculated Spermatozoa. *Biol. Reprod.* **1997,** *57*(4), 729–734.

Algarra, B.; Han, L.; Soriano-Úbeda, C.; Avilés, M.; Coy, P.; Jovine, L.; Jimenez-Movilla, M. The C-Terminal Region of OVGP1 Remodels the Zona Pellucida and Modifies Fertility Parameters. *Sci. Rep.* **2016,** *6*, 32556.

Almiñana, C.; Gil, M. A.; Cuello, C.; Parrilla, I.; Roca, J.; Vazquez, J. M.; Martinez, E. A. Effects of Ultrashort Gamete Co-Incubation Time on Porcine *In Vitro* Fertilization. *Anim. Reprod. Sci.* **2008,** *106* (3), 393–401.

Ardón, F.; Helms, D.; Sahin, E.; Bollwein, H.; Töpfer-Petersen, E.; Waberski, D. Chromatin-Unstable Boar Spermatozoa have Little Chance of Reaching Oocytes *In Vivo. Reproduction.* **2008,** *135* (4), 461–470.

Ardon, F.; Markello, R D.; Hu, L.; Deutsch, Z. I.; Tung, C. K.; Wu, M.; Suarez, S. S. Dynamics of bovine sperm interaction with epithelium differ between oviductal isthmus and ampulla. *Biol. Reprod.* **2016,** *95* (4), 90–1.

Avilés, K. Estudio de la funcionalidad espermática, interacción de gametos y análisis proteico en espermatozoides epididimarios y eyaculados en la especie porcina. PhD Dissertation, University of Murcia, Murcia, Spain, **2011.**

Ballester, L.; Romero-Aguirregomezcorta, J.; Soriano-Úbeda, C.; Matás, C.; Romar, R.; Coy, P. Timing of Oviductal Fluid Collection, Steroid Concentrations, and Sperm Preservation Method Affect Porcine *In Vitro* Fertilization Efficiency. *Fertil. Steril.* **2014,** *102* (6), 1762–1768.

Bedu-Addo, K.; Barratt, C. L. R.; Kirkman-Brown, J. C.; Publicover, S. J. Patterns of $[Ca^{2+}]_i$ Mobilization and Cell Response in Human Spermatozoa Exposed to Progesterone. *Dev. Biol.* **2007,** *302* (1), 324–332.

Bergmann, A.; Taylor, U.; Rath, D. Sperm Binding to Porcine Uterine Epithelial Cells Might be Lectin Mediated. *Reprod. Fertil. Dev.* **2012,** *25* (1), 152–152.

Bleil, J. D.; Greve, J. M.; Wassarman, P. M. Identification of a Secondary Sperm Receptor in the Mouse Egg Zona Pellucida: Role in Maintenance of Binding of Acrosome-Reacted Sperm to Eggs. *Dev. Biol.* **1988,** *128*, 376–385.

Briz, M. D.; Bonet, S.; Pinart, B.; Egozcue, J.; Camps, R. Comparative Study of Boar Sperm Coming from the Caput, Corpus, and Cauda Regions of the Epididymis. *J. Androl.* **1995,** *16* (2), 175–188.

Brown, C. R.; Cheng, W. K. Changes in Composition of the Porcine Zona Pellucida During Development of the Oocyte to the 2- to 4-Cell Embryo. *J. Embryol. Exp. Morphol.* **1986,** *92* (1), 183–191.

Brüssow, K. -P.; Rátky, J.; Rodriguez-Martinez, H. Fertilization and Early Embryonic Development in the Porcine Fallopian Tube. *Reprod. Domest. Anim.* **2008,** *43* (s2), 245–51.

Bureau, M.; Bailey, J. L.; Sirard, M. -A. Binding Regulation of Porcine Spermatozoa to Oviductal Vesicles *In Vitro. J. Androl.* **2002,** *23* (2), 188–193.

Cánovas, S.; Ivanova, E.; Romar, R.; García-Martínez, S.; Soriano-Úbeda, C.; García-Vázquez, F.A.; Saadeh, H.; Andrews, S.; Kelsey, G.; Coy, P. DNA Methylation and Gene Expression Changes Derived from Assisted Reproductive Technologies can be Decreased by Reproductive Fluids. *Elife.* **2017,** *6*, 1–24.

Clark, S. G.; Haubert, K.; Beebe, D. J.; Ferguson, C. E.; Wheeler, M. B. Reduction of Polyspermic Penetration Using Biomimetic Microfluidic Technology During *In Vitro* Fertilization. *Lab Chip.* **2005,** *5* (11), 1229–1232.

Cooper, T.G. *The Epididymis, Sperm Maturation and Fertilization.* Springer-Verlag: Berlin, **1986.**

Coy, P.; Romar, R. In Vitro Production of Pig Embryos: a Point of View. *Reprod. Fertil. Dev.* **2002,** *14* (5), 275–286.

Coy, P.; Avilés, M. What Controls Polyspermy in Mammals, the Oviduct or the Oocyte? *Biol. Rev.* **2010,** *85* (3), 593–605.

Coy, P.; Martínez, E.; Ruiz, S.; Vázquez, J. M.; Roca, J.; Matás, C.; Pellicer, M. T. *In Vitro* Fertilization of Pig Oocytes After Different Coincubation Intervals. *Theriogenology.* **1993a,** *39* (5), 1201–1208.

Coy, P.; Martínez, E.; Ruiz, S.; Vázquez, J. M.; Roca, J.; Matas, C. Sperm Concentration Influences Fertilization and Male Pronuclear Formation *In Vitro* in Pigs. *Theriogenology.* **1993b,** *40* (3), 539–546.

Coy, P.; Martínez, E.; Ruiz, S.; Vázquez, J. M.; Roca, J.; Gadea, J. Environment and Medium Volume Influence *In Vitro* Fertilisation of Pig Oocytes. *Zygote.* **1993c,** *1* (3), 209–13.

Coy, P.; Gadea, J.; Romar, R.; Matás, C.; García, E. Effect of *In Vitro* Fertilization Medium on the Acrosome Reaction, Cortical Reaction, Zona Pellucida Hardening and *In Vitro* Development In Pigs. *Reproduction.* **2002,** *124* (2), 279–288.

Coy, P.; Cánovas, S.; Mondéjar, I.; Saavedra, M. D.; Romar, R.; Grullón, L.; Matás, C.; Avilés, M. Oviduct-Specific Glycoprotein and Heparin Modulate Sperm-Zona Pellucida Interaction During Fertilization and Contribute to the Control of Polyspermy. *Proc. Natl. Acad. Sci.* **2008a,** *105* (41), 15809–15814. *The Journey of the Porcine Spermatozoa from Its Origin* 275.

Coy, P.; Grullon, L.; Canovas, S.; Romar, R.; Matas, C.; Aviles, M. Hardening of the Zona Pellucida of Unfertilized Eggs can Reduce Polyspermic Fertilization in the Pig and Cow. *Reproduction.* **2008b,** *135* (1), 19–27.

Coy, P.; Lloyd, R.; Romar, R.; Satake, N.; Matas, C.; Gadea, J.; Holt, W. V. Effects of Porcine Pre-Ovulatory Oviductal Fluid on Boar Sperm Function. *Theriogenology.* **2010,** *74* (4), 632–642.

Cummins, J. M.; Yanagimachi, R. Sper-Egg Ratios and the Site of the Acrosome Reaction During *In Vivo* Fertilization in the Hamster. *Gamete Res.* **1982,** *5* (3), 239–256.

Day, B. N. Reproductive Biotechnologies: Current Status in Porcine Reproduction. *Anim. Reprod. Sci.* **2002,** *60–61,* 161–172.

De Lamirande, E.; Leclerc, P.; Gagnon, C. Capacitation as a Regulatory Event that Primes Spermatozoa for the Acrosome Reaction and Fertilization. *Mol. Hum. Reprod.* **1997,** *3* (3), 175–194.

Dostàlovà, Z.; Töpfer-Petersen, E.; Calvete, J. J. Interaction of Non-Aggregated Boar AWN-1 and AQN-3 with Phospholipid Matrices. A Model for Coating of Spermadhesins to the Sperm Surface. *Biol. Chem. Hoppe. Seyler.* **1995,** *376* (4), 237–242.

Fazeli, A.; Duncan, A. E.; Watson, P. F.; Holt, W. V. Sperm-Oviduct Interaction: Induction of Capacitation and Preferential Binding of Uncapacitated Spermatozoa to Oviductal Epithelial Cells in Porcine Species. *Biol. Reprod.* **1999,** *60* (4), 879–886.

Ferraz, M. A. M. M.; Henning, H. H. W.; Stout, T. A. E.; Vos, P. L. A. M.; Gadella, B. M. Designing 3-Dimensional *In Vitro* Oviduct Culture Systems to Study Mammalian Fertilization and Embryo Production. *Ann. Biomed. Eng.* **2017,** *45* (7), 1731–1744.

First, N. L.; Short, R. E.; Peters, J. B.; Stratman, F. W. Transport and Loss of Boar Spermatozoa in the Reproductive Tract of the Sow. *J. Anim. Sci.* **1968,** *27* (4), 1037–1040.

Flesch, F. M.; Brouwers, J. F.; Nievelstein, P. F.; Verkleij, A. J.; van Golde, L. M.; Colenbrander, B.; Gadella, B. M. Bicarbonate Stimulated Phospholipid Scrambling Induces Cholesterol Redistribution and Enables Cholesterol Depletion in the Sperm Plasma Membrane. *J. Cell Sci.* **2001,** *114* (19), 3543–3555.

Flesch, F. M.; Gadella, B. M. Dynamics of the Mammalian Sperm Plasma Membrane in the Process of Fertilization. *Biochim. Biophys. Acta - Rev. Biomembr.* **2000,** *1469* (3), 197–235.

Fukui, Y.; Ono, H. Effects of Sera, Hormones and Granulosa Cells Added to Culture Medium for *In Vitro* Maturation, Fertilization, Cleavage and Development of Bovine Oocytes. *J. Reprod. Fertil.* **1989,** *86* (2), 501–506.

Funahashi, H. Polyspermic Penetration in Porcine IVM-IVF Systems. *Reprod. Fertil. Dev.* **2003,** *15* (3), 167–177.

Funahashi, H.; Day, B. Effects of Follicular Fluid at Fertilization *In Vitro* on Sperm Penetration in Pig Oocytes. *J. Reprod. Fertil.* **1993,** *99* (1), 97–103

Funahashi, H.; Nagai, T. Sperm Selection by a Climbing-Over-A-Wall IVF Method Reduces the Incidence of Polyspermic Penetration of Porcine. *J. Reprod. Dev.* **2000,** *46* (5), 319–324.

Funahashi, H.; Ekwall, H.; Rodriguez-Martinez, H. Zona Reaction in Porcine Oocytes Fertilized *In Vivo* and *In Vitro* as Seen with Scanning Electron Microscopy. *Biol. Reprod.* **2000,** *63* (5), 1437–1442.

Funahashi, H.; Ekwall, H.; Kikuchi, K.; Rodriguez-Martinez, H. Transmission Electron Microscopy Studies of the Zona Reaction in Pig Oocytes Fertilized *In Vivo* and *In Vitro*. *Reproduction.* **2001,** *122* (3), 443–452.

Gaddum-Rosse, P. Some Observations on Sperm Transport Through the Uterotubal Junction of the Rat. *Am. J. Anat.* **1981,** *160* (3), 333–341.

Gadella, B. M.; Harrison, R. A. P. The Capacitating Agent Bicarbonate Induces Protein Kinase A-Dependent Changes in Phospholipid Transbilayer Behavior in the Sperm Plasma Membrane. *Development.* **2000,** *127* (11), 2407–2420.

García Herreros, M.; Aparicio, I. M.; Núñez, I.; García-Marín, L. J.; Gil, M. C.; Peña Vega, F. J. Boar Sperm Velocity and Motility Patterns Under Capacitating and Non-Capacitating Incubation Conditions. *Theriogenology.* **2005,** *63* (3), 795–805.

García-Vázquez, F. A.; Hernández-Caravaca, I.; Matás, C.; Soriano-Úbeda, C.; Abril-Sánchez, S.; Izquierdo-Rico, M. J. Morphological Study of Boar Sperm During Their Passage Through the Female Genital Tract. *J. Reprod. Dev.* **2015,** *61* (5), 407–413.

García-Vázquez, F. A.; Gadea, J.; Matás, C.; Holt, W. V. Importance of Sperm Morphology During Sperm Transport and Fertilization in Mammals. *Asian J. Androl.* **2016,** *18* (6), 844–850.

Garner, D. L.; Hafez, E. S. E. Spermatozoa and Seminal Plasma. In *Reproduction in Farm Animals*. Lippincott Williams and Wilkins: Baltimore, pp. 96–109, 2000.

Georgiou, A. S.; Snijders, A. P. L.; Sostaric, E.; Aflatoonian, R.; Vazquez, J. L.; Vazquez, J. M.; Roca, J.; Martinez, E. A.; Wright, P. C.; Fazeli, A. Modulation of the Oviductal Environment by Gametes. *J. Proteome Res.* **2007,** *6* (12), 4656–4666.

Gualtieri, R.; Talevi, R. Selection of Highly Fertilization-Competent Bovine Spermatozoa Through Adhesion to the Fallopian Tube Epithelium *In Vitro*. *Reproduction.* **2003,** *125* (2), 251–258.

Hafez, E. S. E.; Hafez, B. Transport and survival of gametes. In *Reproduction in Farm Animals*. Lippincott Williams and Wilkins: Baltimore, pp. 82–95, **2000**.

Hao, Y.; Mathialagan, N.; Walters, E.; Mao, J.; Lai, L.; Becker, D.; Li, W.; Critser, J.; Prather, R. S. Osteopontin Reduces Polyspermy During *In Vitro* Fertilization of Porcine Oocytes. *Biol. Reprod.* **2006,** *75* (5), 726–733.

Harris, J.; Hilber, D.; Fontenot, G.; Hsu, K.; Yurewicz, E.; Sacco, A. Cloning and Characterization of Zona Pellucida Genes and cDNAs from a Variety of Mammalian Species: the ZPA, ZPB and ZPC Gene Families. *DNA Seq. - J. Seq. Mapp.* **1994,** *4* (6), 361–393.

Harrison, R. A. P. Capacitation Mechanisms, and the Role of Capacitation as seen in Eutherian Mammals. *Reprod. Fertil. Dev.* **1996,** *8* (4), 581–594.

Harrison, R. A. P. Rapid PKA-Catalysed Phosphorylation of Boar Sperm Proteins Induced by the Capacitating Agent Bicarbonate. *Mol. Reprod. Dev.* **2004,** *67* (3), 337–352.

Harrison, R. A. P.; Miller, N. G. A. cAMP-Dependent Protein Kinase Control of Plasma Membrane Lipid Architecture in Boar Sperm. *Mol. Reprod. Dev.* **2000,** *55* (2), 220–228.

Hedrick, J. L.; Wardrip, N. J.; Berger, T. Differences in the Macromolecular Composition of the Zona Pellucida Isolated from Pig Oocytes, Eggs, and Zygotes. *J. Exp. Zool.* **1987,** *241* (2), 257–262.

Holt, W. V.; Fazeli, A. The Oviduct as a Complex Mediator of Mammalian Sperm Function and Selection. *Mol. Reprod. Dev.* **2010,** *77* (11), 934–943.

Holt, W. V.; Hernandez, M.; Warrell, L.; Satake, N. The Long and the Short of Sperm Selection *In Vitro* and *In Vivo*: Swim-Up Techniques Select for the Longer and Faster Swimming Mammalian Sperm. *J. Evol. Biol.* **2010,** *23* (3), 598–608.

Holtz, W.; Smidt, D. The Fertilizing Capacity of Epididymal Spermatozoa in the Pig. *J. Reprod. Fertil.* **1976,** 46(1), 227–229.

Hunter, R. H. F. Polyspermic Fertilization in Pigs After Tubal Deposition of Excessive Numbers of Spermatozoa. *J. Exp. Zool.* **1973,** *183* (1), 57–62.

Hunter, R. H. F. Chronological and Cytological Details of Fertilization and Early Embryonic Development in the Domestic Pig, Sus scrofa. *Anat. Rec.* **1974,** *178* (2), 169–85.

Hunter, R.H.F. Sperm Transport and Reservoirs in the Pig Oviduct in Relation to the Time of Ovulation. *J. Reprod. Fertil.* **1981,** *63* (1), 109–117.

Hunter, R. H. F. Pre-Ovulatory Arrest and Peri-Ovulatory Redistribution of Competent Spermatozoa in the Isthmus of the Pig Oviduct. *J. Reprod. Fertil.* **1984,** *72* (1), 203–211.

Hunter, R. H. F. Fertilization of Pig Eggs *In Vivo* and *In Vitro*. *J. Reprod. Fertil.* **1990,** *Suppl. 40*, 211–226.

Hunter, R. H. F. Sperm Release from Oviduct Epithelial Binding is Controlled Hormonally by Peri-Ovulatory Graafian Follicles. *Mol. Reprod. Dev.* **2008,** *75* (1), 167–174.

Hunter, R. H. F.; Dziuk, P.J. Sperm Penetration of Pig Eggs in Relation to the Timing of Ovulation and Insemination. *J. Reprod. Fertil.* **1968,** *15* (2), 199–208.

Hunter, R. H. F.; Nichol, R. Capacitation Potential of the Fallopian Tube: a Study Involving Surgical Insemination and the Subsequent Incidence of Polyspermy. *Gamete Res.* **1988,** *21* (3), 255–266.

Hunter, R. H. F.; Rodriguez-Martinez, H. Analysing Mammalian Fertilisation: Reservations and Potential Pitfalls with an *In Vitro* Approach. *Zygote.* **2002,** *10* (1), 11–15.

Hunter, R. H. F.; Rodriguez-Martinez, H. Capacitation of Mammalian Spermatozoa *In Vivo*, with a Specific Focus on Events in the Fallopian Tubes. *Mol. Reprod. Dev.* **2004,** *67* (2), 243–250.

Joseph, A.; Yao, H.; Hinton, B. T. Development and Morphogenesis of the Wolffian/ Epididymal Duct, More Twists and Turns. *Dev. Biol.* **2009,** *325* (1), 6–14.

Kim, E.; Yamashita, M.; Kimura, M.; Honda, A.; Kashiwabara, S. I.; Baba, T. Sperm Penetration Through *Cumulus* Mass and Zona Pellucida. *Int. J. Dev. Biol.* **2008,** *52* (5–6), 677–682.

Kim, N. H.; Day, B. N.; Lim, J. G.; Lee, H. T.; Chung, K.S. Effects of Oviductal Fluid and Heparin on Fertility and Characteristics of Porcine Spermatozoa. *Zygote.* **1997,** *5* (1), 61–65.

Kim, N. H.; Funahashi, H.; Abeydeera, L. R.; Moon, S. J.; Prather, R. S.; Day, B. N. Effects of Oviductal Fluid on Sperm Penetration and Cortical Granule Exocytosis During Fertilization of Pig Oocytes *In Vitro. J. Reprod. Fertil.* **1996,** *107* (1), 79–86.

Kouba, A. J.; Abeydeera, L. R.; Alvarez, I. M.; Day, B. N.; Buhi, W. C. Effects of the Porcine Oviduct-Specific Glycoprotein on Fertilization, Polyspermy, and Embryonic Development *In Vitro. Biol. Reprod.* **2000,** *63* (1), 242–250.

Koziorowska-Gilun, M.; Koziorowski, M.; Strzeżek, J.; Fraser, L. Seasonal Changes in Antioxidant Defence Systems in Seminal Plasma and Fluids of the Boar Reproductive Tract. *Reprod. Biol.* **2011,** *11* (1), 37–47.

Langendijk, P.; Soede, N. M.; and Kemp, B. Uterine Activity, Sperm Transport, and the Role of Boar Stimuli Around Insemination in Sows. *Theriogenology.* **2005,** *63* (2), 500–513.

Leese, H. J. The Formation and Function of Oviduct Fluid. *J. Reprod. Fertil.* **1988,** *82* (2), 843–856.

Leese, H. J.; Tay, J. I.; Reischl, J.; Downing, S. J. Formation of Fallopian Tubal Fluid: Role of a Neglected Epithelium. *Reproduction.* **2001,** *121* (3), 339–346.

Li, Y.-H.; Ma, W.; Li, M.; Hou, Y.; Jiao, L.-H.; Wang, W.-H. Reduced Polyspermic Penetration in Porcine Oocytes Inseminated in a New *In Vitro* Fertilization (IVF) System: Straw IVF. *Biol. Reprod.* **2003,** *69* (5), 1580–1585

Lishko, P. V.; Botchkina, I. L.; Fedorenko, A.; Kirichok, Y. Acid Extrusion from Human Spermatozoa is Mediated by Flagellar Voltage-Gated Proton Channel. *Cell.* **2010,** *140* (3), 327–337.

Liu, Y.; Wang, D.-K.; Chen, L.-M. The Physiology of Bicarbonate Transporters in Mammalian Reproduction. *Biol. Reprod.* **2012,** *86* (4), 99.

Lodish, H.; Berk, A.; Zipursky, S.; Matsudaira, P.; Baltimore, D.; Darnell, J.*Molecular Cell Biology, 4th ed.*; New York, 2000.

López-Úbeda, R.; García-Vázquez, F.; Gadea, J.; Matás, C. Oviductal Epithelial Cells Selected Boar Sperm According to Their Functional Characteristics. *Asian J. Androl.* **2017,** *19* (4), 396–403.

Mann, T.; Lutwak-Mann, C. Male reproductive function and semen. In *Themes and Trends in Physiology, Biochemistry and Investigative Andrology.* Springer-Verlag: Berlin, 1981.

Matás, C.; Coy, P.; Romar, R.; Marco, M.; Gadea, J.; Ruiz, S. Effect of Sperm Preparation Method on *In Vitro* Fertilization in Pigs. *Reproduction.* **2000,** *125* (1), 133–141.

Matás, C.; Sansegundo, M.; Ruiz, S.; García-Vázquez, F. A.; Gadea, J.; Romar, R.; Coy, P. Sperm Treatment Affects Capacitation Parameters and Penetration Ability of Ejaculated and Epididymal Boar Spermatozoa. *Theriogenology.* **2010,** *74* (8), 1327–1340.

Matás, C.; Vieira, L.; García-Vázquez, F. A.; Avilés-López, K.; López-Úbeda, R.; Carvajal, J. A.; Gadea, J. Effects of Centrifugation Through Three Different Discontinuous Percoll Gradients on Boar Sperm Function. *Anim. Reprod. Sci.* **2011,** *127* (1–2), 62–72.

Matthijs, A.; Engel, B.; Woelders, H. Neutrophil Recruitment and Phagocytosis of Boar Spermatozoa after Artificial Insemination of Sows, and the Effects of Inseminate

Volume, Sperm Dose and Specific Additives in the Extender. *Reproduction.* **2003**, *125* (3), 357–367.

Mattioli, M.; Galeati, G.; Bacci, M. L.; Seren, E. Follicular Factors Influence Oocyte Fertilizability by Modulating the Intercellular Cooperation Between *Cumulus* Cells and Oocyte. *Gamete Res.* **1988**, *21* (3), 223–232.

Mattioli, M.; Lucidi, P.; Barboni, B. Expanded Cumuli Induce Acrosome Reaction in Boar Sperm. *Mol. Reprod. Dev.* **1998**, *51* (4), 445–453.

Mourad, N. I.; Gianello, P. Gene Editing, Gene Therapy, and Cell Xenotransplantation: Cell Transplantation Across Species. *Curr. Transplant. Reports.* **2017**, *4* (3), 193–200.

Nagai, T. Current Status and Perspectives in IVM-IVF of Porcine Oocytes. *Theriogenology.* **1994**, *41* (1), 73–78.

Nagai, T.; Moor, R. M. Effect of Oviduct Cells on the Incidence of Polyspermy in Pig Eggs Fertilized *In Vitro. Mol. Reprod. Dev.* **1990**, *26* (4), 377–382.

Nichol, R.; Hunter, R. H. F.; Gardner, D. K.; Leese, H. J.; Cooke, G. M. Concentrations of Energy Substrates in Oviductal Fluid and Blood Plasma of Pigs During the Peri-Ovulatory Period. *J. Reprod. Fertil.* **1992**, *96* (2), 699–707.

Nishigaki, T.; José, O.; González-Cota, A. L.; Romero, F.; Treviño, C. L.; Darszon, A. Intracellular pH in Sperm Physiology. *Biochem. Biophys. Res. Commun.* **2014**, *450* (3), 1149–1158.

Okamura, N.; Tajima, Y.; Soejima, A.; Masuda, H.; Sugita, Y. Sodium Bicarbonate in Seminal Plasma Stimulates the Motility of Mammalian Spermatozoa Through Direct Activation of Adenylate Cyclase. *J. Biol. Chem.* **1985**, *260* (17), 9699–9705.

Okazaki, T.; Akiyoshi, T.; Kan, M.; Mori, M.; Teshima, H.; Shimada, M. Artificial Insemination with Seminal Plasma Improves the Reproductive Performance of Frozen-Thawed Boar Epididymal Spermatozoa. *J. Androl.* **2012**, *33* (5), 990–998.

Orlowski, J.; Grinstein, S. Na$^+$/H$^+$ Exchangers. *Compr. Physiol.* **2011**, *1* (4), 2083–2100.

Park, C. H.; Lee, S. G.; Choi, D. H.; Lee, C. K. A Modified Swim-Up Method Reduces Polyspermy During *In Vitro* Fertilization of Porcine Oocytes. *Anim. Reprod. Sci.* **2009**, *115* (1–4), 169–181.

Parrish, J.J. Bovine *In Vitro* Fertilization: *In Vitro* Oocyte Maturation and Sperm Capacitation with Heparin. *Theriogenology.* **2014**, *81* (1), 67–73.

Pérez-Cerezales, S.; Boryshpolets, S.; Eisenbach, M. Behavioral Mechanisms of Mammalian Sperm Guidance. *Asian J. Androl.* **2015**, *17* (4), 628.

Petrunkina, A. M.; Gehlhaar, R.; Drommer, W.; Waberski, D.; Töpfer-Petersen, E. Selective Sperm Binding to Pig Oviductal Epithelium *In Vitro. Reproduction.* **2001**, *121* (6), 889–896.

Petrunkina, A. M.; Waberski, D.; Günzel-Apel, A. R.; Töpfer-Petersen, E. Determinants of Sperm Quality and Fertility in Domestic Species. *Reproduction.* **2007**, *134* (1), 3–17.

Quinn, P. Enhanced Results in Mouse and Human Embryo Culture Using a Modified Human Tubal Fluid Medium Lacking Glucose and Phosphate. *J. Assist. Reprod. Genet.* **1995**, *12* (2), 97–105.

Rath, D.; Long, C. R.; Dobrinsky, J. R.; Welch, G. R.; Schreier, L. L.; Johnson, L. A. *In Vitro* Production of Sexed Embryos for Gender Preselection: High-Speed Sorting of X-Chromosome-Bearing Sperm to Produce Pigs After Embryo Transfer. *J. Anim. Sci.* **1999**, *77* (12), 3346–3352.

Rath, D.; Schuberth, H. J.; Coy, P.; Taylor, U. Sperm Interactions from Insemination to Fertilization. *Reprod. Domest. Anim.* **2008**, *43* (s5), 2–11.

Rodriguez-Martinez, H. Role of the Oviduct in Sperm Capacitation. *Theriogenology.* **2007**, *68* (s1), 138–146.

Rodriguez-Martinez, H.; Ekstedt, E.; Einarsson, S. Acidification of Epididymal Fluid in the Boar. *Int. J. Androl.* **1990**, *13* (3), 238–243.

Rodriguez-Martinez, H.; Larsson, B.; Pertoft, H.; Kjellén, L. GAGs and Spermatozoon Competence *In Vivo* and *In Vitro*. In *Gametes: Development and Function*. Serono Symposia: Italy, pp. 239–274, 1998.

Rodríguez-Martínez, H.; Saravia, F.; Wallgren, M.; Tienthai, P.; Johannisson, A.; Vázquez, J. M.; Martínez, E.; Roca, J.; Sanz, L.; Calvete, J. J. Boar Spermatozoa in the Oviduct. *Theriogenology.* **2005**, *63* (2), 514–535.

Rodriguez-Martinez, H.; Tienthai, P.; Atikuzzaman, M.; Vicente-Carrillo, A.; Rubér, M.; Alvarez-Rodriguez, M. The Ubiquitous Hyaluronan: Functionally Implicated in the Oviduct?. *Theriogenology.* **2016**, *86* (1), 182–186.

Rodriguez-Martinez, H.; Tienthai, P.; Suzuki, K.; Funahashi, H.; Ekwall, H.; Johannisson, A. Involvement of Oviduct in Sperm Capacitation and Oocyte Development in Pigs. *Reprod. Suppl.* **2001**, *58*, 129–145.

Romar, R.; Funahashi, H.; Coy, P. *In Vitro* Fertilization in Pigs: New Molecules and Protocols to Consider in the Forthcoming Years. *Theriogenology.* **2016**, *85* (1), 125–134.

Rozeboom, K. J.; Troedsson, M. H. T.; Crabo, B. G. Characterization of Uterine Leukocyte Infiltration in Gilts After Artificial Insemination. *J. Reprod. Fertil.* **1998**, *114* (2), 195–199.

Sano, H.; Matsuura, K.; Naruse, K.; Funahashi, H. Application of a Microfluidic Sperm Sorter to the *In-Vitro* Fertilization of Porcine Oocytes Reduced the Incidence of Polyspermic Penetration. *Theriogenology.* **2010**, *74* (5), 863–870.

Schuberth, H. J.; Taylor, U.; Zerbe, H.; Waberski, D.; Hunter, R.; Rath, D. Immunological Responses to Semen in the Female Genital Tract. *Theriogenology.* **2008**, *70* (8), 1174–1181.

Setchell, B. P.; Sånchez-Partida, L. G.; Chairussyuhur, A. Epididymal Constituents and Related Substances in the Storage of Spermatozoa: A Review. *Reprod. Fertil. Dev.* **1993**, *5* (6), 601–612.

Smith, T. T. The Modulation of Sperm Function by the Oviductal Epithelium. *Biol. Reprod.* **1998**, *58* (5), 1102–4.

Soriano-Úbeda, C.; García-Vázquez, F. A.; Romero-Aguirregomezcorta, J.; Matás, C. Improving Porcine *In Vitro* Fertilization Output by Simulating the Oviductal Environment. *Sci. Rep.* **2017**, *7*, 1–12.

Soriano-Úbeda, C.; Romero-Aguirregomezcorta, J.; Matás, C.; García-Vázquez, F. A. Manipulation of Bicarbonate Concentration in Sperm Capacitation Media Improves *In Vitro* Fertilisation Output in Porcine Species. *J. Anim. Sci. Biotechnol.* **2019**, *10* (1), 19.

Suarez, S. S. Interactions of Spermatozoa with the Female Reproductive Tract: Inspiration for Assisted Reproduction. *Reprod. Fertil. Dev.* **2007**, *19* (1), 103–110.

Suarez, S. S. Mammalian Sperm Interactions with the Female Reproductive Tract. *Cell Tissue Res.*. **2016**, *363* (1), 185–194.

Suarez, S. S.; Dai, X.-B.; DeMott, R. P.; Redfern, K.; Mirando, M. A. Movement Characteristics of Boar Sperm Obtained from the Oviduct or Hyperactivated *In Vitro*. *J. Androl.* **1992**, *13* (1), 75–80.

Sullivan, R.; Saez, F.; Girouard, J.; Frenette, G. Role of Exosomes in Sperm Maturarion During the Transit Along the Male Reproductive Tract. *Blood Cells Mol Dis.* **2005**, *35*, 1–10.

Sumransap, P.; Tummaruk, P.; Kunavongkrit, A. Sperm Distribution in the Reproductive Tract of Sows After Intrauterine Insemination. *Reprod. Domest. Anim.* **2007**, *42* (2), 113–117.

Suzuki, K.; Asano, A.; Eriksson, B.; Niwa, K.; Nagai, T.; Rodriguez-Martinez, H. Capacitation Status and *In Vitro* Fertility of Boar Spermatozoa: Effects of Seminal Plasma, *Cumulus*-Oocyte-Complexes-Conditioned Medium and Hyaluronan. *Int. J. Androl.* **2002**, *25* (2), 84–93.

Suzuki, K.; Eriksson, B.; Shimizu, H.; Nagai, T.; Rodriguez-Martinez, H. Effect of Hyaluronan on Monospermic Penetration of Porcine Oocytes Fertilized *In Vitro*. *Int. J. Androl.* **2000**, *23* (1), 13–21.

Syntin, P.; Dacheux, F.; Druart, X.; Gatti, J. L.; Okamura, N.; Dacheux, J. L. Characterization and Identification of Proteins Secreted in the Various Regions of the Adult Boar Epididymis. *Biol. Reprod.* **1996**, *55* (5), 956–974.

Tajima, Y.; Okamura, N.; Sugita, Y. The Activating Effects of Bicarbonate on Sperm Motility and Respiration at Ejaculation. *Biochim. Biophys. Acta.* **1987**, *924* (3), 519–529.

Talevi, R.; Gualtieri, R. Molecules Involved in Sperm-Oviduct Adhesion and Release. *Theriogenology.* **2010**, *73* (6), 796–801.

Taylor, U.; Rath, D.; Zerbe, H.; Schuberth, H.J. Interaction of Intact Porcine Spermatozoa with Epithelial Cells and Neutrophilic Granulocytes During Uterine Passage. *Reprod. Domest. Anim.* **2008**, *43* (2), 166–175.

Taylor, U.; Schuberth, H. J.; Rath, D.; Michelmann, H. W.; Sauter-Louis, C.; Zerbe, H. Influence of Inseminate Components on Porcine Leucocyte Migration *In Vitro* and *In Vivo* After Pre- and Post-Ovulatory Insemination. *Reprod. Domest. Anim.* **2009**, *44*(2), 180–188.

Tienthai, P. The Porcine Sperm Reservoir in Relation to the Function of Hyaluronan. *J. Reprod. Dev.* **2015**, *61* (4), 245–50.

Tomlinson, M.; White, A.; Barratt, C.; Bolton, A.; Cooke, I. The Removal of Morphologically Abnormal Sperm Forms by Phagocytes: A Positive Role for Seminal Leykocytes? *Hum Reprod.* **1992**, *7* (4), 517–22.

Töpfer-Petersen, E.; Friess, A. E.; Nguyen, H.; Schill, W. B. Evidence for a Fucose-Binding Protein in Boar Spermatozoa. *Histochemistry.* **1985**, *83* (2), 139–145.

Töpfer-Petersen, E.; Henschen, A. Acrosin Shows Zona and Fucose Binding, Novel Properties for a Serine Proteinase. *FEBS Lett.* **1987**, *226* (1), 38–42.

Töpfer-Petersen, E.; Romero, A.; Varela, P. F.; Ekhlasi-Hundrieser, M.; Dostàlovà, Z.; Sanz, L.; Calvete, J. J. Spermadhesins: A New Protein Family. Facts, Hypotheses and Perspectives. *Andrologia.* **1998**, *30* (4–5), 217–224.

Töpfer-Petersen, E.; Wagner, A.; Friedrich, J.; Petrunkina, A.; Ekhlasi-Hundrieser, M.; Waberski, D.; Drommer, W. Function of the Mammalian Oviductal Sperm Reservoir. *J. Exp. Zool.* **2002**, *292* (2), 210–215.

Töpfer-Petersen, E.; Ekhlasi-Hundrieser, M.; Tsolova, M. Glycobiology of Fertilization in the Pig. *Int. J. Dev. Biol.* **2008**, *52* (5–6), 717–736.

Visconti, P. E. Understanding the Molecular Basis of Sperm Capacitation Through Kinase Design. *Proc. Natl. Acad. Sci.* **2009**, *106* (3), 667–668.

Visconti, P. E.; Bailey, J. L.; Moore, G. D.; Pan, D.; Olds-Clarke, P.; Kopf, G. S. Capacitation of Mouse Spermatozoa. I. Correlation Between the Capacitation State and Protein Tyrosine Phosphorylation. *Development.* **1995,** *121* (4), 1129–1137.

Visconti, P. E.; Kopf, G. S. Regulation of Protein Phosphorylation During Sperm Capacitation. *Biol. Reprod.* **1998,** *59* (1), 1–6.

Visconti, P. E.; Moore, G. D.; Bailey, J. L.; Leclerc, P.; Connors, S. A.; Pan, D.; Olds-Clarke, P.; Kopf, G. S. Capacitation of Mouse Spermatozoa. II. Protein Tyrosine Phosphorylation and Capacitation are Regulated by a cAMP-Dependent Pathway. *Development.* **1995,** *121* (4), 1139–1150.

Waberski, D.; Magnus, F.; Ardón, F.; Petrunkina, A. M.; Weitze, K. F.; Töpfer-Petersen, E. Binding of Boar Spermatozoa to Oviductal Epithelium *In Vitro* in Relation to Sperm Morphology and Storage Time. *Reproduction.* **2006,** *131* (2), 311–318.

Waberski, D.; Petrunkina, A. M.; Töpfer-Petersen, E. Can External Quality Control Improve Pig AI Efficiency? *Theriogenology,* **2008,** *70* (8), 1346–1351.

Wang, W.; Abeydeera, L. R.; Prather, R. S.; Day, B. N. Morphologic Comparison of Ovulated and *In Vitro*-Matured Porcine Oocytes, with Particular Reference to Polyspermy after *In Vitro* Fertilization. *Mol. Reprod. Dev.* **1998,** *49* (3), 308–316.

Watson, A. L.; Carlson, D. F.; Largaespada, D. A.; Hackett, P. B.; Fahrenkrug, S. C. Engineered Swine Models of Cancer. *Front. Genet.* **2016,** *7* (78), 1–16.

Watson, P. F.; Green, C. E. *Cooling and Capacitation of Boar Spermatozoa: What do They Have in Common?* Boar Semen Preservation IV; Lawrence: Allen Press, pp. 53–60, 2000.

Wennemuth, G.; Carlson, A. E.; Harper, A. J.; Babcock, D. F. Bicarbonate Actions on Flagellar and Ca^{2+}-Channel Responses: Initial Events in Sperm Activation. *Development.* **2003,** *130* (7), 1317–1326.

Wolf, D. P. *The Mammalian Egg's Block to Polyspermy. Fertilization and Embryonic Development In Vitro;* Plenum Press: New York, pp. 183–197, 1981.

Yanagimachi, R. Fertility of Mammalian Spermatozoa: Its Development and Relativity. *Zygote.* **1994a,** *2* (4), 371–372.

Yanagimachi, R. *Mammalian fertilization. The Physiology of Reproduction;* Raven Press: New York, pp. 189–317, 1994b.

Yeste, M.; Castillo-Martín, M.; Bonet, S.; Briz, M. D. Direct Binding of Boar Ejaculate and Epididymal Spermatozoa to Porcine Epididymal Epithelial Cells is Also Needed to Maintain Sperm Survival in *In Vitro* Co-Culture. *Anim. Reprod. Sci.* **2012,** *131* (3–4), 181–193.

Yeste, M.; Lloyd, R. E.; Badia, E.; Briz, M.; Bonet, S.; Holt, W. V. Direct Contact Between Boar Spermatozoa and Porcine Oviductal Epithelial Cell (OEC) Cultures is Needed for Optimal Sperm Survival *In Vitro. Anim. Reprod. Sci.* **2009,** *113* (1-4), 263–278.

Yoshioka, K.; Suzuki, C.; Onishi, A. Defined System for *In Vitro* Production of Porcine Embryos Using a Single Basic Medium. *J. Reprod. Dev.* **2008,** *54* (3), 208–213.

CHAPTER 10

Reproductive Biotechnologies Applied to Artificial Insemination in Swine

FRANCISCO ALBERTO GARCÍA-VÁZQUEZ[1,2,*], CHIARA LUONGO[1], GABRIELA GARRAPPA[1,3], and ERNESTO RODRÍGUEZ TOBÓN[1]

[1]Department of Physiology, Faculty of Veterinary Science, International Excellence Campus for Higher Education and Research "Campus Mare Nostrum", University of Murcia, Murcia, Spain

[2]Institute for Biomedical Research of Murcia (IMIB-Arrixaca), Murcia, Spain

[3]Institute of Animal Research of the Semi-Arid Chaco (IIACS), Agricultural Research Center (CIAP), National Institute of Agricultural Technology (INTA), Tucumán, Argentina

*Corresponding author. E-mail: fagarcia@um.es

ABSTRACT

Artificial insemination (AI) is the most widespread reproductive technique used in porcine. This chapter provides firstly relevant information about the workflow involved in porcine AI, from the collection of boar ejaculate and seminal doses preparation to the sperm deposition in the female by AI devices and spermatozoa journey toward the oocyte. Secondly, we summarize new issues and future perspectives trying to increase the porcine AI efficiency, such as new fertility biomarkers, improving the composition of extenders used for semen dilution, or studying new methods for sperm selection as the use of magnetic nanoparticles to remove damaged spermatozoa.

10.1   INTRODUCTION

Advances in reproductive biotechnologies have allowed the increase of efficiency in animal production in several species. Artificial insemination (AI) has been one of the most successful applied reproductive biotechnologies since its implementation several decades ago (reviewed by Soriano-Úbeda et al. 2013). In the case of porcine species, AI (porcine AI, pAI) is routinely used in most of the farms (Riesenbeck, 2011), which among other factors, has allowed to place pork production as one of the most important meat industries worldwide (Knox, 2014; Zhang et al. 2018).

The advantages of the pAI are innumerable (Knox, 2016), although to achieve considerable success, multiple factors must be properly geared. AI methodology *per se* is a simple technique which requires scarce material to perform, just a single plastic tube ending in a tip that fits within the cervix. AI device has changed slightly through the years, but these changes has also considerably improved its effectiveness (i.e. deeper deposition which reduces the number of sperm per seminal dose increasing the number of seminal doses produced per boar) (García-Vázquez et al. 2019a; Llamas-Lopez et al. 2019). However, AI is not only the process in which spermatozoa are deposited in the female genital tract. The great numbers reached in porcine reproductive performance (farrowing rates, litter sizes) in the last years are attributable to the improvement of different factors (Knox, 2016) (Fig. 10.1). Boars are one of the main pieces in pAI puzzle because they support the initial step in seminal doses production. Boars are usually confined in facilities known as AI-centers or boar studs. Then, sanitary status, genetic, semen collection training or housing in AI-centers are essential factors to contemplate for proficient semen production. After ejaculate collection, the processing of semen starts which includes an initial dilution in an extender, subsequently quality spermatozoa evaluation and packing in bags or bottles for further conservation and/or distribution. Once seminal doses are prepared, the other important piece to complete the pAI puzzle is the female. Even after having the best semen, it is useless if it is deposited into a female without an optimal moment of estrus. So, estrus detection and physiology knowledge of oestrus cycle are key factors for a successful AI. Finally, after seminal dose deposition, spermatozoa start a complicated journey in search of the oocyte. During insemination (natural or artificial) millions of spermatozoa are deposited but only a few of them are able to reach the place of fertilization (Tummaruk and Tienthai, 2010). Most of the mechanisms involved in this drastic reduction of spermatozoa within the female genital tract are still unknown.

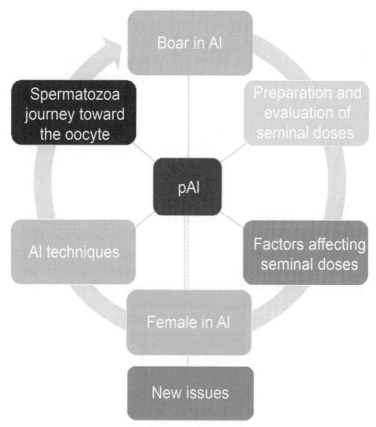

FIGURE 10.1   Scheme of the phases involved in porcine Artificial Insemination (pAI).

Although several reproductive biotechnologies associated with AI process have currently been applied in porcine, others are still under study and researchers are constantly trying to solve the reproductive porcine industry demands. Nowadays, some of these new investigations in pAI seems far to be applied but surely, they are the base to continue and increase the efficiency of this methodology even more in the future. These and other factors are going to be treated more extensively along the following sections.

10.2 THE ROLE OF THE BOAR IN ARTIFICIAL INSEMINATION

Over the years, the development of reproductive technologies has permitted an increase of farm size and the birth of specialized AI-centers (Knox, 2014). This scenario has allowed to raise the reproductive performance and, in consequence, the economic impact on productive efficiency of pAI (reviewed by Knox, 2016). AI-centers are in charge of producing seminal doses with enough quality to be used in AI programs. Then, seminal doses produced from a single ejaculate of a boar allow inseminating several sows (Maes et al., 2011). The total number of seminal doses generated varies depending on the type of AI used, cervical (CAI) or post-cervical artificial insemination (PCAI), because of the different number of sperm and volume needed. In general terms, the CAI-doses are composed of 3×10^9 sperm cells in a final volume of 90 ml, while the PCAI-doses are composed of 1.5×10^9 sperm cells in a final volume of 45 ml (Hernández-Caravaca et al., 2012; Bortolozzo et al., 2015). The number of doses obtained annually per boar is about 2000 for CAI method (Mezalira et al., 2005), and consequently approximately the double of seminal doses in the case of PCAI.

The quality of an ejaculate depends on multiple factors including animal welfare, environmental temperature, light exposure, feeding or housing. These conditions have been improved through the specialization of AI-centers, by using automatic systems for temperature, feeding and watering control (Knox, 2016). Moreover, the design of AI-centers is also focused on preventing the entry of pathogens. In this sense, AI-centers have two entries, one for vehicles and other for pedestrians. Once inside, each AI-center is divided into different areas such as an isolation area for boar (where health checks are performed), a boar housing area, a semen collection area, and a laboratory, in which semen samples are prepared, stored and shipped. Likewise, it is important to maintain a high level of hygiene since people can be carriers of diseases (Waberski and Weitze, 2010).

When new boars arrive at an AI-center, they should be isolated for 40–45 days before contact with other animals in order to check their health status (Althouse, 2007). Once this time has elapsed, boars are housed individually in pens (Knox, 2016), allowing visual contact and smell with other animals (Lopez-Rodriguez et al., 2017). The pens have an available area per boar of at least 6 m² according to the European legislation (Commission Directive 2001/93/EC). The type of boar housing can influence boar health and it must be safe and allow easy handling of the animals (Althouse, 2007).

In order to enter the collection rotation, 7 months old boars are subjected to a training period and selected based on good health and semen quality (Bortolozzo et al., 2015; Knox, 2016). The frequency of collection can influence the production and quality of ejaculate, and in this sense a maximum of 3 times in two weeks is considered optimal (Knox, 2016). Therefore, a period of rest between extractions is necessary to complete spermatozoa maturation within the epididymis (Pruneda et al., 2005).

The semen collection is performed in specific facilities that allow the operator to safely handle the boar (Althouse, 2007). A collection dummy is placed within the pen, equipped with two lateral supports on which the boar can position the front legs. Moreover, vertical galvanized pipes on 2 or 3 sides of the perimeter of the collection pen can be placed allowing the operator to escape easily when necessary (Althouse, 2007). Apart from the traditional pen, the *"Reicks collection pen"* is the most used collection method in AI-centers. This method is similar to the traditional collection facility, but with an additional small pen for the operator. By this way, the operator can handle the boar standing outside by a sliding gate during the collection process (Levis and Reicks, 2005). Additionally, some AI-centers have a warm-up pen to aid with sexual stimulation of the boar. Then, boars will require less time to mount the dummy and for semen output (Althouse, 2007). Once the boar is situated on the dummy, the process of semen collection starts. But before explaining the methods of semen collection it is necessary to talk briefly about the swine ejaculate. The whole boar ejaculate is about 200–300 ml with a concentration higher than 30 x 10^9 sperm cells per ml (Rodríguez-Martínez et al., 2005). Apart from sperm cells, the ejaculate is composed of seminal plasma (SP). The ejaculation can last up to 15 min divided in three fractions. The first fraction, called pre-spermatic fraction (10–15 ml), contains secretions from urethral and bulbourethral glands and prostate. It is characterized by the absence of sperm cells (or very poor number) and a high bacterial count, whereby it is discarded (Maes et al., 2011; Lopez-Rodriguez et al., 2017). The second fraction (70–100 ml), the spermatic-rich fraction, contains the majority of spermatozoa (80–90%) and SP, derived from testes, epididymis, and accessory reproductive glands (Garner and Hafez, 2000). The third fraction (120–200 ml) is called post-spermatic rich fraction and contains few sperm cells and more SP than the spermatic-rich fraction. As indicated, SP represents an important part of the whole ejaculate in porcine species. This male biological fluid is a complex milieu in which spermatozoa are immersed during the ejaculation and is mainly composed by inorganic and organic components, such as carbohydrates, lipids, amino acids and proteins (Sancho and Vilagran, 2013). Through the ejaculation, a gelatinous substance (called tapioca) is produced by bulbourethral glands, especially during the emission of the third fraction. Tapioca acts as a plug in the cervix of the sow during natural insemination, to seal the cervix reducing ejaculate backflow (Knox, 2001).

Returning to the methods of semen collection, these can be performed mainly by two methods (Fig. 10.2): 1) the manual method or also called gloved-hand technique; and 2) the automatic technique. Nowadays, the gloved-hand method is the main technique of choice in AI-centers (Knox et al., 2008). In any case, hygiene rules should be followed to avoid bacterial contamination (Lopez-Rodriguez et al., 2017). For this reason, the initial steps are the same for both methods and consist of cleaning the penis and the area surrounding the preputial orifice. During this process, the operator's hand is covered by a plastic glove to manipulate the boar penis, then is removed after cleaning (Althouse et al., 2000; Aneas et al., 2008). Then the operator can proceed with one of semen collection methods. During the gloved-hand technique, the collection continues using only the inner glove composed of polyvinyl, due to latex gloves provoke spermatozoa toxicity (Ko et al., 1989). The operator grabs the penis and exerts pressure imitating the pressure exerted by the cervix of the sow (Maes et al., 2011). The automatic method, unlike the manual method, does not allow collecting a single fraction, but the whole ejaculate is collected. In this case, once the penis is externalized, the operator connects the penis of the boar to a system with an artificial vagina. This system is equipped with a disposable sanitary sleeve that allows direct contact between the penis and artificial vagina and avoids ejaculate contamination. After that, the operator activates air pressure to close the artificial vagina with the aim of grabbing the penis (Waberski and Weitze, 2010). In both, manual and automatic methods, the ejaculate is collected in a plastic container equipped with a filter to discard the gelatinous fraction (Aneas et al., 2008). This container is pre-warmed (38 °C) to avoid damage caused by thermal shock, and then placed in warm water to keep the temperature constant (Maes et al., 2011).

The main difference between the two collection methods is that technician efficiency increases using the automatic method, allowing an increase in the number of ejaculates collected per hour (Aneas et al., 2008). Additionally, by the automatic method, bacterial contamination is reduced, and ejaculate volume and total number of sperm are higher than the manual method (Aneas et al., 2008). However, the automatic method is not widely used because the whole ejaculation is collected, including a high SP amount. In fact, it has been proved that better results were obtained when the post-spermatic rich fraction was discarded (Centurion et al., 2003; Okazaki and Shimada, 2012).

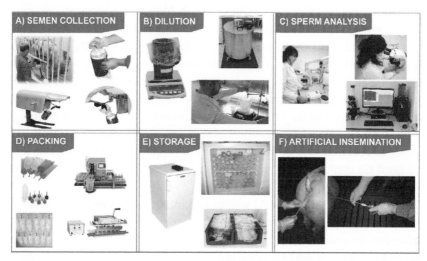

FIGURE 10.2   Procedure of seminal doses elaboration. (A) Semen collection: gloved-hand and automatic technique; (B) Dilution in an appropriate extender; (C) Sperm analyses: concentration determination by spectrophotometric, spermatozoa motility evaluation by microscope or computerized assisted sperm analysis system (CASA); (D) Packing: different package for seminal doses (bottles, tubes and bags/flat bags); automatic packing machines; (E) Storage: seminal doses conservation at 15–17 °C; (F) Artificial insemination procedure. (Images provided by Pedro José Llamas-López and Minitube).

10.3   PREPARATION AND EVALUATION OF THE SEMINAL DOSES

After collection, the ejaculate is placed at the laboratory of AI-center, where an initial qualitative evaluation is determined: color (gray-white to white), appearance (milky to creamy) and odor (Althouse, 2007). The different methods of semen collection and the environment where it is extracted can affect some parameters of the seminal sample.

Once the ejaculate is suitable for processing after this initial appreciation, the next step is the determination of spermatozoa concentration. Traditionally, the most used method to calculate the cell concentration has been the counting chambers such as *Neubauer*, *Bürker*, and *Thoma* (Althouse, 2007; Brito et al., 2016). Nowadays, this method has been surpassed by spectrophotometric techniques because manual counting is a slow process (Brito et al., 2016). In an ejaculate, the opacity depends on the number of cells among other elements of the SP that could interfere with the passage of the light through the sample. Therefore, it is recommendable to dilute a small sample for obtaining a more reliable result (depending extender, dilution rates from 1:4–1:25) (Althouse, 2007). Besides, errors in the evaluation can occur if the dilution is not correct or untimely reading (Althouse, 2007; Brito et al., 2016). CASA (Computerized Assisted Sperm Analysis) system can also be used to determine the concentration, although this system is more recommendable to assess sperm motility (Amann and Waberski, 2014; Brito et al., 2016), as will be explained later. Another method for cell counting is the flow cytometry, which allows rapid and automated counts of many cells. However, the use of flow cytometry is limited due to its high cost and the need for qualified personnel to manage the equipment and interpret the results (Brito et al., 2016).

Then, seminal doses for AI will be elaborated and stored. The first step is to dilute the ejaculate in an adequate extender to conserve the semen and drive the spermatozoa during AI (Fig. 10.2b). The different extenders for the preservation of spermatozoa are divided into three groups according to the storage period (short, medium and long-term based on their ability to preserve spermatozoa from 1 day up to 10 days after collection) (Karageorgiou et al., 2016; Pezo et al., 2019b). There are numerous extenders commercially available although the exact composition is not fully known due to economic interests. In general terms, extenders are composed by: (1) nutrients: to maintain cell metabolism, being the most common glucose and fructose; (2) pH controller: bicarbonate, sodium citrate, Tris or HEPES; (3) osmotic pressure controller: NaCl and KCl; (4) antibiotics: to inhibit bacterial growth (Yeste, 2017). Bacteriospermia is one of the main problems in AI worldwide (Yeste, 2017). Problems derived by the presence of bacteria affect directly the semen quality impacting fertility rates and causes endometritis in recipient females (Althouse et al., 2000; Maes et al., 2008; Bussalleu and Torner, 2013). Although antibiotics are frequently used in extenders, bacterial resistance has been reported in up to 90% (Schulze et al., 2014) of the seminal doses studied. Then, new alternatives to conventional antibiotics are on the light of researching (Schulze et al., 2014) (see Section 10.8.3.).

After dilution, a spermatozoa quality control is necessary to ensure that the process has been performed adequately. Spermatozoa quality parameters commonly evaluated in AI-centers are morphoanomalies (commonly classified as normal morphology, proximal and distal cytoplasmic droplet or tails defects, folded and coiled) (García-Vázquez et al., 2015) and motility (Brito et al., 2016). In the case of motility, there are several methods for its evaluation (Fig. 10.2): (1) light field or phase contrast microscopy: a subjective manner to evaluate total motility (values from 0 to 100%) and progressive motility (values from 0 to 5, where 5 score represents the highest level of progressivity), although this method has a high degree of inaccuracy; 2) CASA system: evaluates spermatozoa motility and kinetic parameters through a high-resolution camera mounted on a phase contrast microscope (Brito et al., 2016). The motility parameters offered by CASA system are the following: Total and progressive motility (%), curvilinear velocity (VCL), rectilinear velocity (VSL), average speed (VAP) (all of them expressed in μm/s), linearity Index (LIN, VSL/VCL in percentage), straightness Index (STR, VSL/VAP in percentage), oscillation Index (WOB, VAP/VCL in percentage), average amplitude of the lateral displacement of the head (ALH, μm), beat frequency (BCF, Hz) (Amann and Waberski, 2014). Although this method is the most objective and evaluates different parameters of sperm kinetics, some factors have to be considered to reduce variability during evaluation. Such factors are sample temperature, dilution factor, frequency and duration of mixing, or chamber depth (Broekhuijse et al., 2011).

Another technique for accurate assessments of sperm samples is the flow cytometry (Broekhuijse et al., 2015). This technique permits the evaluation of a huge number of cells in a short time determining special characteristics in the spermatozoa by using fluorochromes (Broekhuijse et al., 2015). Some of the evaluable parameters by flow cytometry are spermatozoa viability, DNA integrity, mitochondrial activity, membrane fluidity, and acrosome reaction (Broekhuijse et al., 2012).

However, most of the parameters evaluated for the quality of ejaculates have not been fully correlated with fertility (Broekhuijse et al., 2012). Thus, a multivariate analysis seems to be more efficient in determining a quality ejaculate (Knox, 2016). Nowadays, researchers are putting effort into looking for some new biomarkers for reliable determination of the fertility of a seminal dose (see Section 10.8.1).

Finally, the process of the individual seminal dose starts (Althouse, 2007). The volume and number of spermatozoa per seminal dose will depend on the type of AI that will be performed (see Section 10.6). Subsequently, the seminal dose will be packaged in its final container (bottles, tubes or bags/flat bags) (Fig. 10.2) made of non-toxic plastic material (Althouse, 2007; Nerin et al., 2014). In highly specialized AI-centers the laboratories have automatic packing machines, which optimizes the time and ensures the same volume in the doses (Yeste, 2017). After packing, seminal doses can be refrigerated for storage (15–17 °C) (Yeste, 2017) (Fig. 10.2).

10.4 FACTORS AFFECTING SEMINAL DOSES ELABORATION AND CONSERVATION

The elaboration and conservation of the seminal doses is not an extremely complex process. However, there are several factors that should be known during the procedure to get a final product of enough quality and guarantee of success during AI (Fig. 10.2). One of the main critical points during seminal doses elaboration is the dilution which involves temperature, steps of dilution and storage conditions.

Boar spermatozoa are very susceptible to cold shock; therefore, the temperature of the ejaculate and extender during mixing is a critical point. Drastic cooling from ejaculate temperature (~38°C) to refrigeration temperature (~15°C) reduces spermatozoa viability and motility (Johnson, 2000). Then, the procedure of dilution is focused on decreasing the temperature gradually. The protocol of dilution followed by AI-centers are mainly one-step or two-step dilution, and temperature plays a key role in both (Waberski, 2009). The one-step dilution consists in the mix of the ejaculate with the extender at ~33°C or room temperature. In the two-step protocol, ejaculate is diluted 1:1 (at ~33°C), followed by a second dilution. This second dilution could be carried out using a pre-heated extender (~33°C) or at room temperature (22–23°C) without differences between them in terms of motility and membrane/acrosome integrity (López-Rodríguez et al. 2012). There is also a three-step protocol dilution which consists in a first dilution (1:1, ~33°C), second dilution (adding 50% of the remaining extender volume at ~33°C) and third dilution (adding the remaining 50% of the extender at ~33°C) (Schulze et al., 2018). The one-step dilution at

~33°C is the most recommendable procedure due to less work labor, lower risk of mistakes because of simplicity, and better spermatozoa quality results (Schulze et al., 2018). The orders in which the semen and extender are mixed (extender to the semen or reverse) have not adverse effects on the spermatozoa quality (Schulze et al., 2017). Commonly, once the seminal doses are ready, a period of ~90 min at room temperature is necessary before being transferred to 15–17°C (Waberski, 2009).

Boar spermatozoa quality is impaired during storage and it is determined by the conditions and the length of this storage (Johnson et al., 2000; Waberski et al., 2011; Schulze et al., 2013; Yeste, 2017). Sperm motility and viability has been determined as the main parameters affected during refrigeration (Althouse et al., 1998). Boar sperm membrane alteration, showing as a change in permeability allowing the entry to stains, is considered a great indicator of spermatozoa storage-related damage (Johnson et al., 2000; Roca et al., 2005; Bielas et al., 2017). Spermatozoa DNA is also affected by refrigeration, alterations have been described after the first hour of storage (Bielas et al., 2017) and after a longer period of storage of 3 or 4 days (Fraser and Strzezek, 2004; Boe-Hansen et al., 2005; Pérez-Llano et al., 2009).

Supplementation of seminal doses just before AI has been suggested as a good practice to solve the detrimental effect of storage. In this sense, several hormones have been tested, such as oxytocin (Peña et al., 1998; Okazaki et al., 2014), relaxine (Feugang et al., 2015) or prostaglandin $F_2\alpha$ (Maes et al., 2003). On the other hand, a significant number of studies have focused their goals in the improvements of seminal doses storage conditions. One of the strategies used has been the supplementation of additives to the extender such as hyaluronic acid (tested to postponed premature capacitation; Yeste et al. 2008) or bovine serum albumin (BSA, used for long-term extender; Zhang et al., 2015; Yeste et al., 2017) among others. More information about new additives in extender will be found in Section 10.8.3.

Other approaches improving spermatozoa conservation conditions have been the rotation and homogenization of semen samples during their storage to prevent spermatozoa sedimentation. Contrary to initial thoughts, rotation of semen samples triggers an increase in pH with negative effects on spermatozoa quality during storage (Schulze et al., 2015). Similarly, the homogenization of doses during storage impaired mitochondrial activity, acrosome and plasma membrane integrity (Menegat et al., 2017).

Accordingly, rotation and homogenization may not be a recommendable action during the storage of seminal doses.

As aforementioned, the recommended temperature of storage ranges from 15 to 17 °C (Yeste, 2017) and storages temperatures below 12 °C induce cold shock with detrimental effects in boar spermatozoa (Althouse et al., 1998; Johnson et al., 2000). According to this, the need for maintaining the temperature in a limited range during shipping of seminal doses from AI-center to the farms represents a logistic problem (Riesenbeck, 2011). Besides keep constant the seminal dose temperature from its elaboration to its use, another aspect that should be considered during seminal doses transportation is vibration emission. It has been proposed that vibration might have a negative impact on pH values during transportation (Johnson et al., 1982). Therefore, vibration emission with 300 rpm frequencies for 6 h resulted in alkalization of semen extender (Schulze et al., 2018) which impairs sperm motility (Gatti et al., 1993; Vyt et al., 2007). Some others spermatozoa quality parameters such as mitochondrial activity, acrosome, plasma membrane integrity, and thermo-resistance showed a negative frequency-dependent effect of vibration emissions during simulated trans-portation (Schulze et al., 2018). In order to control this factor, a novel monitoring tool for boar semen transport has been developed. This device, established using mobile sensing, works as a data logger of vibration emission from seminal doses (Schulze et al., 2018). Thanks to this new technology, further studies aimed to find the optimal shipping packing for boar seminal doses may be attained.

Apart from refrigeration, there are other strategies for the long-term preservation of boar spermatozoa, such as cryopreservation or lyophiliza-tion. Cryopreservation is performed in the presence of cryoprotectants, to avoid cold shock. In fact, boar spermatozoa are subjected to changes at low temperature because of their plasmatic membrane composition, poor in cholesterol (Rodriguez-Martinez and Wallgren, 2010; Casas and Flores, 2013; Yeste, 2017). Cryopreservation may be performed in two ways: 1) *Slow freezing*: spermatozoa are freezing in an extender containing cryoprotectants, using controlled-rate freezers; in this case, the formation of ice crystals within the suspension, due to the flow of water between intracellular and extracellular space, can induce spermatozoa damage (Johnson et al., 2000; Watson, 2000; Holt and Van Look, 2004); 2) *Fast freezing* or *vitrification*: it is performed with very high cooling rates. By this method, water does not form ice crystals, but it reaches the vitreous state. Despite vitrification requires less time and costs than slow freezing, it is not currently used because of the osmotic effect due to high concentrations of cryoprotectants (Arraztoa et al., 2017). A possible solution could be an alternative vitrification method in the absence of cryoprotectants, called *spheres method* (Arraztoa et al., 2017). This method consists of using microdroplets of spermatozoa samples, dipping in liquid nitrogen and obtaining spheres. Otherwise, lyophilization consists of sperm cell dehydration by evaporation (*conventional heat-drying*) or by sublimation (*freeze-drying*) (Zăhan et al., 2014). One of the negative aspects of lyophilization is that spermatozoa lose motility after rehydration. However, the spermatozoa acrosome membrane remains intact, so intracytoplasmic sperm injection may be used (Zăhan et al., 2014).

Nowadays, there are ongoing research to improve long-term preservation method to increase spermatozoa survival. Actually, only 1% of pAI is performed using cryopreserved spermatozoa because of low fertilizing ability of spermatozoa after thawing (Yeste, 2017; García-Vázquez et al., 2019a).

10.5 THE ROLE OF THE FEMALE IN ARTIFICIAL INSEMINATION

After processing semen samples, the seminal doses are shipped to the farms (Maes et al., 2011) for further AI. Previously, it is necessary to keep in mind the different female populations existing at the farm. Females are classified based on the number of farrowing: 1) nulliparous (or gilts): females without any previous farrowing; 2) primiparous: sows with one farrowing; 3) multiparous: sows with more than one farrowing.

In order to proceed with AI, estrus detection, timing and number of inseminations per sow have to be considered (Maes et al., 2011). The gilts can receive the first insemination when they are 7–8 months old, weighing ~130–140 kg and preferably after the second or third detected estrus (Waberski and Weitze, 2010). The first step before perform AI is estrus detection. Most of the protocols at the farm estimate estrus detection twice-daily (in the morning and in the afternoon) (Langendijk et al., 2000).

Before illustrating the possible methods to perform estrus detection, it is important to understand the oestrus cycle in porcine females. The oestrus cycle lasts 21 days and it is divided into two stages: 1) the follicular phase which is split in proestrus and oestrus (1–3 days both of them); 2) the luteal phase divided in metoestrus and dioestrus (2–3 days and 13–18 days, respectively). The estrus stage can last from 36 to 90 h, depending mainly on the age of the sow (Steverink et al., 1999), and it is character-ized by hormonal changes, in particular, an increase in estrogen levels. Following the peak of estrogen (24–48 h before estrus) (Guthrie et al., 1972), vulvar edema is observed and, subsequently, 36–40 h after the first estrus signals, the ovulation occurs (Yeste and Castillo-Martín, 2013). The main rules that should be considered to perform the estrus detection are the following: 1) prefer the early hours of the morning and before feeding; 2) expose the sow to the presence and/or smell of a boar, because sows show a procreative behavior in presence of the male (de Jonge et al., 1994); 3) handle the sow calmly to allow relaxing (Sterle and Safranski, 2000).

For estrus detection, the sow should preferably be exposed to a mature boar. The sow in estrus stage will show a standing reflex (stiffness) being sexually receptive. The most widely used estrus detection method on farms is the manual method, also called *"back pressure test"* (reviewed by Cornou, 2006). The operator presses on the back of the sow and evaluates the response giving a score, based on length and strength of the stiffness (Willemse and Boender, 1966; Cronin et al., 1982). The parameters observed are vulvar reddening and swelling caused from blood inflow (Sterning, 1995; Langendijk et al., 2000), tilted ears, riding behavior, and vocalizing (Steverink et al., 1999). The manual method requires more animal handling time and physical labor by the staff, so it would be preferable to apply an automatic method. There are different techniques to perform estrus detection by an automatic manner. One of them is the *"infrared sensor"*. By this method, a sensor is placed 50 cm above the body of the sow to detect the level of physical activity, increased at the onset of the estrus (reviewed by Cornou, 2006). An alternative procedure for estrus detection is the *"electronic method"*, which consists of placing a boar in a closed pen, the sow on the outside of the facility, and monitoring how long the sow spends close to the boar pen (Ostersen et al., 2010). Additionally, the estrus may be detected measuring body temperature (ear base, vaginal or rectal), because of its change during the days of estrus, hormonal changes, and follicular growth (reviewed by Cornou, 2006). Measure of body temperature is not widely used, providing non-specific information, due to changes in temperature around the estrus. Instead, regarding hormonal changes and follicular growth, they are of limited applicability under field conditions, requiring specific trained technicians able to perform these techniques (reviewed by Cornou, 2006). Moreover, in the last few years, a new modern method of estrus detection is emerging, the called *"infrared thermography"*. It is a non-invasive method, able to detect changes in vulvar skin temperature by infrared radiation emission. This technique is performed by an infrared thermal camera placed at 1 m from the rear end of the sow by drawing a polygon around the vulva, to outline the area where the temperature needs to be measured (Simões et al., 2014).

Once the estrus has been detected, the AI can be performed (reviewed by Knox, 2016). It is important to carry out the AI at the onset of the estrus to deposit the semen into the uterus before ovulation occurs. By this way, spermatozoa have time to be capacitated and acquire fertilizing ability (Waberski and Weitze, 2010). The estrus does not have a defined duration, whereby the number of inseminations depends on the duration of estrus (reviewed by Knox, 2016). Usually, AI is performed twice per sow every 24 h during the estrus or, even three if the estrus period is extended (Knox et al., 2008).

10.6 ARTIFICIAL INSEMINATION TECHNIQUE

The first use of AI dates from the 14th century when an Arabic Chief used semen stolen from a rival to successfully inseminate his own mares (Bowen, 1969). It was not until many years later in 1678 that sperm cells were observed for the first time by Leeuwenhoek with an own created microscope (Leeuwenhoek, 1678). The next historic landmark took place a century later when Spallanzani performed the first insemination in a bitch with success giving birth to three pups, whereby was demonstrated the actual feasibility of AI (Spallanzani, 1784). Afterward, the contributions of Professor Ivanov from Russia by the end of the 19th century were central for the establishment of AI as a practical procedure in domestic animals (Ivanov 1907; 1922). The development of semen extenders by this author together with the design of artificial vaginas by Milovanov in 1964 opened a new era in animal AI (Broekhuijse et al., 2012; Soriano-Úbeda et al., 2013; Knox, 2015).

Thanks to Ivanov's work, pAI also started in the early 1900s in Russia (Ivanov 1970; 1922), having the biggest growth in the 1940s in the United States (McKenzie, 1931). Polge conducted more studies on pAI in Western Europe (Polge, 1956) and Niwa did the same in Japan (Niwa, 1958). The possibility of store semen for a long enough period that comes after the development of properly extenders (initiated by Ivanov in Russia in 1922 and Philips and Lardy in the United States in 1940) allowed the shipment and use in the field. Porcine AI was quickly spread worldwide (Salisbury et al., 1978) and by the 20th century, a standardized protocol was established for farmers and technicians.

Since the beginning, CAI was the technique performed widely. CAI is an easy and simple technique that can be done by any swine farm personnel. This method consists in depositing the semen dose within the cervix (Fig. 10.3) using a catheter that engages with the folds of the cervix and simulates the corkscrew tie of the boar's penis (Polge, 1956). At the beginning, AI was performed by means of a reusable catheter, or Melrose catheter, that mimicked the spiral shape of the boar penis (Melrose and O'Hagan, 1961). This was rapidly superseded by disposables supplies that facilitated safe insemination minimizing microbial contamination and limiting work by suppressing the needed for cleaning and sterilization after every use (Knox, 2015). Nowadays, several AI catheters with modified tips are commercially available; basically they consist of a simple polypropylene tube with an expanded polyurethane sponge tip which adopts basically three different forms: spiral, foam or multi-ring and that casts itself to the cervical folds (Watson and Behan, 2002; Soriano-Úbeda et al., 2013) (Fig. 10.3).

Most frequent CAI seminal dose consists of an ~90 ml dose with 3.0 × 10^9 sperm cells (García-Vázquez et al., 2019a). Several studies have been made in order to define the best concentration for a seminal dose, a wide range between 1.0–4.0 × 10^9 sperm cells in 20 to 200 ml of final volume have been tested (Soriano-Úbeda et al., 2013; Knox, 2015). The standard CAI procedure is done in the presence of a boar to induce the necessary myometrial contraction for spermatozoa transport through the cervical canal (Langendijk et al., 2005) and the semen flow using gravity and gentle pressure. Also, backpressure needs to be applied by the AI operator or using a backpack with weight to mimic the boar compression (Knox, 2015).

The basic outlines of the process of pAI have remained unchanged over time, although many details have varied considerably. The advance of AI technologies in porcine has been mainly based on the place of semen deposition, meaning that the deeper the deposition less spermatozoa is needed with the consequent economical savings.

In this sense, one of the first improvements to AI technique based on a non-surgical deposition of semen into the uterus was described in the late 1950s by Hancock (Hancock, 1959) but was not commercially reported until the 2000s (Watson and Beham, 2002). In this case, a non-traumatic catheter device, consisting of a catheter (outer tube)- cannula (inner tube), was developed and allow to deposit the spermatozoa into the uterus body, closer to the site of fertilization than CAI (Watson and Beham, 2002; Hernández-Caravaca et al., 2012). The main objective of this new AI methodology (PCAI or intrauterine insemination), was to achieve a high reduction on the sperm cell and volume used per dose avoiding any nega-tive effect on reproductive performance (Fig. 10.3) (Watson and Behan, 2002; Rozeboom et al., 2004; Mezalira et al., 2005; Roberts and Bilkei, 2005; Hernández-Caravaca et al., 2012).

The use of PCAI technique provides several advantages on the field such as the increased number of seminal doses produced per boar which allow a faster improvement in genetics and the number of males per farm could be reduced, all of which represent an economic improvement. More-over, PCAI technique is faster than CAI, when in CAI normally needs 2.76 ± 0.63 min per inseminated sow, PCAI is made in 1.12 ± 0.05 min (Hernández-Caravaca et al., 2012). This is mainly explained because this technique saved one of the main physical barriers, the cervix, and allowed a quick introduction of the semen doses releasing sperm cells closer to the fertilization place. Many different sperm cells concentration and dose volume had been testing for PCAI, and are still controversial, but there is an agreement about the use on the field of a 40–45 ml dose with a concen-tration of approximately 1.5×10^9 sperm cells with the same or also better results than CAI (Watson and Behan, 2002; Hernández-Caravaca et al., 2012; García-Vázquez et al., 2019a).

CAI has been substituted by PCAI worldwide during the last years, but the success was restricted to multiparous sows (García-Vazquez et al., 2019b). Primiparous and nulliparous females suppose a limitation for PCAI, with success rates of technique application close to 86% and 20% respectively (Sbardella et al., 2014; Hernández-Caravaca et al., 2017). The main cause of this variance could be explained because of the differences in the cervix that difficult the progression of the cannula (Behan and Watson, 2005; Araujo et al., 2009; Hernández-Caravaca et al., 2017). In this sense, significant differences have been found in the morphology of the cervix when the cervix of multiparous and nulliparous females was compared (García-Vázquez et al., 2019b). These authors report that multiparous sows present a longer cervix, a greater content of connective tissue and lower muscle fibers compared to nulliparous females. The amount of connective tissue is highly correlated with cervix distension capacity, whereby, it was proposed that these differences might be partly responsible for the low performance of PCAI in gilts (Rodriguez-Antolin et al., 2012).

In order to solve these anatomic limitations, a new device was developed by Behan and Watson in 2005 allowing a greater penetration of the cervix of the gilt and the use of a lower concentration of spermatozoa but with similar reproductive performance than traditional CAI. Moreover, a new PCAI device specially designed for nulliparous supposed, a successful application in 60% of the inseminated gilts (Hernández-Caravaca et al., 2017). A new approach for AI in gilts has emerged as the denomination of Deep cervical AI (Dp-CAI). This new method is based on the use of a novel AI device (Fig. 10.3) which gets deeper into the cervical funnel, allowing to reduce conventional sperm concentration and volume of semen dose without impairing reproductive parameters, achieving success insemination in almost 90% of the gilts (Llamas-López et al., 2019).

As mentioned, the site of semen deposition has been the main target to get improvement on AI technology. According to this, a new protocol for AI was developed with the main goal of release sperm cells deeper into the uterus named deep intrauterine insemination (DUI). First trails in DUI were made in 1999 (Krueger et al., 1999) when performed a successful surgical deep intrauterine insemination releasing a small amount of semen (0.5 ml) close to the utero-tubal junction. Despite being a breakthrough by minimizing the dose, the impossibility of their use in field condition inspires other authors to keep trying to improve it. Two years later, a non-surgical deep uterine insemination which deposits the semen into uterine horns, performed by an optic fiber endoscope was developed, achieving normal farrowing rates and litter sizes using a low seminal dose (5–20 x 10^7 sperm cells in 10 ml) (Martinez et al., 2001). In this study, DUI was performed by the insertion of a commercial AI catheter on the cervix and after that, the endoscope was inserted through the catheter and propelled forward along the uterine horn which adopted a spiral shape (Martinez et al., 2001; Vázquez et al., 2005). DUI allowed a reduction of 20-fold and 6-fold in sperm concentration of fresh and frozen semen respectively (Vázquez et al., 2008). Although this supposed a great advance in AI procedure, still represented an expensive and fragile instrument unsuitable for use under field conditions (Martinez et al., 2001). In this sense, the same group developed a new inexpensive device (Fig. 10.3) for DUI performed based on the propulsion force and flexibility of the endoscope (Martinez et al., 2002). In this new technique, the flexible catheter was inserted into one uterine horn in 95.4% of the sows in 3–5 minutes but gestations were in both uterine horns (Martinez et al., 2002).

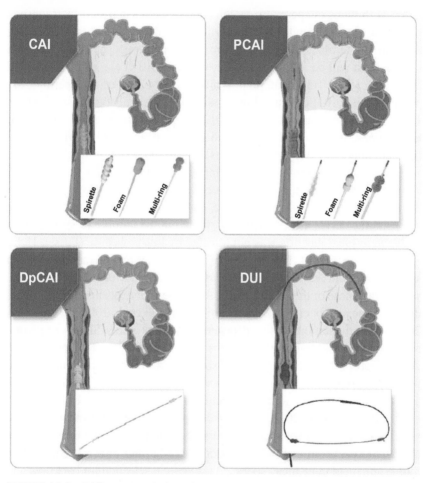

FIGURE 10.3   Different AI techniques in swine. CAI: cervical AI; PCAI: in post-cervical AI semen is deposited in the uterine body; DpCAI: in deep cervical AI the semen is deposited in the anterior section of the cervix (especially indicated for nulliparous females); DUI: in deep intrauterine insemination the semen is deposited in one of the uterine horns. (Images of CAI and PCAI devices were provided by Import-Vet S.A. Spain).

10.7   SPERMATOZOA JOURNEY WITHIN THE FEMALE GENITAL TRACT

After AI, billions of spermatozoa colonize the uterus and start their journey within the female genital tract, crossing the uterine horns until reaching the site of fertilization (the oviduct). However, not all the deposited spermatozoa will be able to attain the oviduct (First et al., 1968; Viring and Einarsson, 1981; Tummaruk and Tienthai, 2010). Part of the spermatozoa population is lost in the backflow (loss through the vulva) (Steverink et al., 1998; Hernández-Caravaca et al., 2012; García-vázquez et al., 2015a,b; I. Hernández-Caravaca et al., 2015) and by the influx of polymorphonuclear (PMN) granulocytes (by phagocytosis) within the uterus lumen during the first 3–4 h after insemination (Matthijs et al., 2003; Taylor et al., 2009), among other mechanisms. Some strategies have been developed to reduce the backflow during AI. For example, placing a cotton tampon or a plastic plug into the cervix after semen deposition, but the number of spermatozoa at the utero-tubal junction was not affected by this procedure (Pursel, 1982; Steverink et al., 1998). The PMN influx occurs after the interaction between spermatozoa and female uterine tissues and it depends on different factors, such as the phase of the oestrus cycle, the number of deposited spermatozoa, dose volume and extender composition (Schuberth et al., 2008; Taylor et al., 2009). Once the seminal dose is deposited within the uterus, SP plays a pivotal role in spermatozoa transport, survival and fertilizing ability (Rozeboom et al., 2000). Transport is facilitated by the stimulation of uterine contractions due to its estradiol content (Claus, 1990; Langendijk et al., 2005). Moreover, SP aids spermatozoa survival by modulating the immune response (Rozeboom et al., 1998; Katila, 2012), due to the presence of SP-proteins, mostly spermadhesins, that coat spermatozoa surface and reduce the uterine influx of PMN (Rozeboom et al., 1998; Rodriguez-Martinez et al., 2010). Viable, motile and membrane intact spermatozoa prevent selection for backflow and PMN influx, through a binding between sperm and uterine epithelial cells by protein interactions, such as spermadhesins, lectin and lectin-like (Töpfer-Petersen et al., 1998; Rath et al., 2008; Taylor et al., 2008). The reduction in PMN influx may increase the number of spermatozoa able to reach the fertilization site (Yamaguchi et al., 2013). However, it should be considered that, during AI, SP components are reduced because of semen dilution by the extender. Thus, the immune response within the uterus will be low modulated by the SP. To solve this problem, new strategies are being developed such as the addition of caffeine and calcium chloride ($CaCl_2$) to the semen extender (Matthijs et al., 2003; Yamaguchi et al., 2009).

The SP is not only implicated in the uterine immune response. This male fluid contains molecules, termed decapacitation factors, able to stimulate or inhibit sperm capacitation (Piehl et al., 2013), a process that modifies sperm membrane making spermatozoa able to fertilize. Within the uterus, before reaching the oviduct, SP-decapacitation factors, such as spermadhesins AQN-3 and AWN-1, coat spermatozoa to avoid early capacitation, allowing spermatozoa continue their journey toward the oocyte (Leahy and Gadella, 2011). Spermatozoa will be gradually decoated by SP-factors in order to allow the onset of capacitation and acquire fertilizing ability (Garner and Hafez, 2000).

During sperm transport within the uterus, spermatozoa are not only in contact with SP but with other reproductive fluids from the female such as the uterine and oviductal fluids (UF and OF, respectively). The UF is composed by ions, growth factors, cytokines, proteins, proteolytic enzymes, as shown in different species (Iritani et al., 1969; Iritani et al., 1971; Gardner et al., 1996). The UF has a double effect on spermatozoa, aiding their transport towards the site of fertilization (Casado-Vela et al., 2009) and at the same time attacks unprotected spermatozoa from SP affecting motility and viability, as shown in mice (Kawano et al., 2014).

After crossing the hostile uterine environment, surviving spermatozoa reach the oviduct where interacting with the OF, a biological fluid containing inorganic and organic molecules, such as the bicarbonate that allows spermatozoa capacitation, a physiological process that makes them able to fertilize the oocyte (Rodríguez-Martínez et al., 2005). Within the oviduct, spermatozoa meet a suitable microenvironment that aids them to reach the ampullary-isthmic junction, the site of fertilization in porcine species (Hunter, 1981; Yeste, 2013). The oviduct is also involved in sperm transport towards the oocyte, but spermatozoa must colonize the oviduct before ovulation. Thus, spermatozoa have a strategy binding to oviductal cells in the isthmus, where constitute the sperm reservoir (Rodríguez-Martínez et al., 2005). During this phase, OF aids spermatozoa to stay in a state of quiescence, preventing sperm capacitation up to ovulation (Mburu et al., 1996). Later, spermatozoa are exposed to post-ovulatory OF that allows the onset of capacitation (Yeste, 2013), after that, they move towards the ampullar-isthmic junction.

10.8   NEW ISSUES AND FUTURE PERSPECTIVES IN PORCINE ARTIFICIAL INSEMINATION

Porcine industry constantly demands improvements for maximizing efficiency and research effort are constant underway to find new strategies to solve them. As described throughout the previous sections reproductive biotechnologies applied in AI have been increasing progressively and spread on improve reproductive issues. However, there are some not fully efficient aspects that need to be amended to make the "reproductive area" more profitable.

Since several years ago, the research is oriented in several ways. In this sense, the selection of boars with the highest reproductive efficiency and genetic merit is crucial for ensuring faster progress (Dyck et al., 2011). Research is also focused to obtain better extender composition and accomplish longer preservation time as possible, without detrimental effects on spermatozoa quality. Furthermore, the development of new accessible technology for sperm selection available for its use on farm conditions and improvement on AI protocols are other working branches in which swine industry is expending effort. This section provides an overview of the current and future strategies focused to enhance pAI technology.

10.8.1   FERTILITY BIOMARKERS

A single boar can service about 2000 sows yearly, so it is worth to note the significant genetic and economic impact of that single boar semen has on the productivity of the swine industry (Feugang, 2017). Current semen analysis in AI-centers, which includes parameters of sperm motility and morphology measurements, are useful to indicate semen quality but still unable to predict boar fertility and reproductive performance (Dyck et al., 2011; Kwon et al., 2015a). Researcher efforts are concentrated in genomics and proteomics approaches, aimed at the goal of identified biomarkers for assessing male fertility. Advances in molecular techniques can now be used for selection of boars based on a direct comparison of gene (Lin et al., 2006; Kaewmala et al., 2011; Zhang et al., 2018; Kim et al., 2019) and/ or protein expression between semen, SP and/or spermatozoa of boars of known high and low fertility (Dyck et al., 2011; Kwon et al., 2014, 2015, 2017; Rahman et al., 2017).

In a proteomic approach, differences in protein expression have been detected when spermatozoa from superior boar (high litter size) were compared with spermatozoa from inferior boar (low litter size) (Kwon et al., 2015a). According to this, positive fertility markers in superior boars (Kwon et al., 2015a) and negative biomarkers in inferior boar spermatozoa were recognized (Kwon et al., 2015b). Besides, the same authors proposed that differential expressed proteins in spermatozoa before and after capacitation can help to differentiate males with high fertility (Kwon et al., 2015c; Rahman et al., 2017). Fertility-related biomarkers can be used to predict male fertility in different breeds but an efficient selection of markers for the breed of interest is recommended to be considered for more precise conclusions (Kwon et al., 2017, 2018).

Otherwise, studies of potential fertility biomarkers were also performed in porcine SP (Dyck et al., 2011). SP-proteins have a fundamental role during spermatozoa protection and capacitation, and therefore in fertilization (reviewed by Dyck et al., 2011). According to that, differences in SP-proteins expression were analyzed to find a feasible biomarker related to boar fertility using high-through-put proteomics techniques. Several SP-proteins were identified as possible markers. In this sense, differences in protein expression were observed related to sperm capacitation (May et al., 2015), oxidative stress (Novak et al., 2010; May et al., 2015) and farrowing rate and litter size (Pérez-Patiño et al., 2018) among others.

Additionally, gene marker candidates to predict boar fertility have been proposed. Polymorphisms (Lin et al., 2005) and alternative splicing or genetic variation (Zhang et al., 2018) of some candidate genes were considered as feasible markers for improving spermatozoa quality traits and boar reproductive performance. A transcriptomic approach in combination with proteomic information was also applied for biomarker discovery related to spermatozoa quality and fertility traits (Kaewmala et al., 2011). Furthermore, a negative correlation of a gene connected to sperm ion channel regulation with boar litter size was observed and proposed as a specific marker for male fertility evaluation (Kim et al., 2019).

In summary, the general idea of a single test to predict spermatozoa quality and/or boar better fertility between groups of boars may be feasible in a short future (Novak et al., 2010). The incorporation of genomic and proteomic biomarkers into the boar selection process in the future may significantly improve reproductive efficiency.

10.8.2 SPERMATOZOA PHOTO-STIMULATION

Phototherapy for medical treatment has been successfully applied in different areas such as rheumatology, surgery, and dermatology (reviewed by Yeste et al., 2018). The main effect of low-level light irradiation on the cell, also called photobiomodulation, appears to be related to an increase of ATP level, a highly necessary molecule for sperm motility and egg maturation. So, this discipline has gained followers in the reproduction area (Abdel-Salam and Harith, 2015; Yeste et al., 2018).

In this sense, photo-stimulation of boar semen has been tested either *in vitro* or *in vivo* conditions without any negative effect on DNA integrity (Yeste et al., 2016, 2018). Briefly, the photo-stimulation protocol used was 10 min LED stimulation (L-phase), 10 min darkness (D-phase) and another 10 min of LED stimulation (L-phase) (Yeste et al., 2016). A significantly increased in farrowing rates and in the number of total and live-piglets born per parturition was achieved with this pre-treatment, showing a better success when the initial fertility rate of the farm is low (Yeste et al., 2016). Moreover, the positive effect of photo-stimulation on motility was demonstrated in spermatozoa after exposure to short-term thermal stress (Pezo et al., 2019a). Likewise, in a later study, the effect of LED light chamber exposure was examined on the *in vitro* quality of boar sperm (Luther et al., 2018). However, and in contrast with previous results, no differences were found in sperm kinematic parameters, neither in mitochondria function nor membrane integrity between untreated and treated doses. Therefore, the authors conclude that previous improvements achieved might be due to other parameters not tested in the mentioned work (Luther et al., 2018).

Despite the promising results that this technique represents, it is still necessary to continue researching this topic (Abdel-Salam and Harith, 2015; Yeste et al., 2018).

10.8.3 BOAR EXTENDER IMPROVEMENTS

Efforts in extender improvements are focused on reaching preservation of boar semen in the best conditions, with the main goal of achieving spermatozoa quality after a long time of preservation. The progress of the research in this area is addressed in different strategies that delve into the crucial points of the preservation technique, including the restriction of bacterial contamination (Bussalleu and Torner, 2013; Morrell and Wallgren, 2014; Schulze et al., 2014), conservation temperature (López Rodríguez et al., 2012), extender components (Pezo et al., 2019b), and use of additives (Bresciani et al., 2017; Cavalleri et al., 2018; Wang et al., 2018). It is worth notice that the higher the production intensity in the pig industry became, the higher the technology for semen processing and preservation will be required.

One of the indispensable components in the porcine semen extender is the antibiotic. Currently, antibiotics must be added to semen extender to control possible contaminations and it is regulated by national and international guidelines. Despite, global policies are aimed at reducing the development of bacterial resistance and general use of antibiotics in semen extender could be avoided or strictly limited in the next years (Morrell and Wallgren, 2014). In addition, some studies have proved that an extraordinary percentage of bacteria present in seminal doses are resistant to regular antibiotics (Maroto Matín et al., 2010; Bussalleu and Torner, 2013; Morrell and Wallgren, 2014). In this sense, some alternatives to antibiotics are being proposed. The addition of antimicrobial peptides (AMP), potent peptides part of innate immune response which acts as broad-spectrum antibiotics, has been tested and achieving a good performance decreasing bacterial growth without prejudicial effects on semen quality (Busalleu et al., 2016; Sancho et al., 2017). Also, a cationic AMP has been proved to be potential molecules to replace the common antibiotics (Schulze et al., 2014, 2016). Although it is not an additive to extend, other methods have also been proposed to reduce the bacterial load as the use of colloids. Single layer centrifugation (SLC) is a novel technology that could be easily used in the field and a feasible alternative to antibiotics. Briefly, semen amount is poured into a centrifuge tube with a single layer of colloid and centrifuged for 20 min (Morrell and Wallgren, 2011). The results obtained after the centrifugation indicated a reduction of bacterial similar that achieve with the use of antibiotics. A similar strategy had been applied in sperm selection with the aim of improves spermatozoa cryopreservation quality (Macías-García et al., 2008; Van Wienen et al., 2010; Martinez-Alborcia et al., 2012). Further research is needed to define the effects of this method in semen with longer storage periods and subjected to different temperatures.

Otherwise, it is well known that spermatozoa quality and fertilizing capacity is affected by oxidative stress (by the generation of reactive oxygen species-ROS) during preservation in many species (Alvarez and Storey, 1983; Storey, 1997; Zhang et al., 2016; López-Rodríguez et al., 2017). Glutathione antioxidant function in semen against oxidative stress has been proposed (Gadea et al., 2004). According to this, the addition of L-glutamine, glutathione and/or cysteine to semen extender has been demonstrated to have a protective effect on sperm cells exposed to oxidative stress during liquid preservation (Funahashi and Sano, 2005; Wang et al., 2008; Zang et al., 2016).

Beside the antioxidant, other alternative has been proved to reduce or suppress negative effects of oxidative stress on boar semen as the addition of *Astragalus polysaccharide* (APS) (Fu et al., 2017), natural antioxidants as Rooibos (*Asparalathus linearis*) (Ros-Santella and Pintus, 2017) and aminoguanidine (Pintus et al., 2018) achieving a good performance in sperm protection.

Although results obtained by inseminating with liquid semen stored at 15–17 °C are like those obtained in natural mating, the lifespan of spermatozoa is limited and can only be preserved in average for 5 days (Michael et al., 2008). Despite the existence of good quality boar extenders, studies of newly improved formulations are incessant. There is a growing interest in improved long-term extender composition to achieve optimal storage conditions (Vyt et al., 2004; Funahashi and Sano, 2005; Lee and Park, 2015a,b; Bielas et al., 2017). In this sense, an improved in sperm membrane protection was accomplished when the extender was flowed through a neodymium magnet (Lee and Park, 2015a,b). These results suggest that magnetized semen extender before dilution could increase the longevity of spermatozoa preservation. A novel long-term semen extender was developed by Brescani et al., which allowed to stored doses for 12 days at 17 °C. Its formulation was based on the incorporation of new molecules, as the energy precursor, a disaccharide (sucrose) and an enzymatic agent (invertase) (Bresciani et al., 2017).

10.8.4 NANOTECHNOLOGY: CONTRIBUTIONS TO REPRODUCTION ENHANCEMENT

Nanotechnology has emerged in the last years as a very useful tool in different areas (Angelakeris, 2017). This new technology allows innovative applications in a wide range of disciplines, including agriculture (Hill and Li, 2017), biotechnology/biomedicine, magnetic resonance imaging and environmental remediation (Lu et al., 2007). Nanotechnology is also acquiring importance and is already being used within the field of reproductive biology (Feugang, 2017).

Magnetic nanoparticles (MNPs) offer the opportunity to specifically target spermatozoa and allow detecting and removing damaged or abnormal spermatozoa from an ejaculate (Odhiambo et al., 2014; Feugang et al., 2015, Durfey et al., 2017; Feugang, 2017). In this sense, a protocol for subtraction of apoptotic spermatozoa has been developed and applied in many species such as human (Grunewald et al., 2001), mice (Green et al., 2006), bull (Odhiambo et al., 2014), boar (Feugang et al., 2015) and rabbit (Vasicek et al., 2010). Briefly, MNPs are conjugated with Annexin-V, which target with externalized phosphatidylserine residues of early apoptotic spermatozoa surface membrane. Then, when MNPs and fresh semen are co-incubated, abnormal sperms link to MNPs are separated and trapping through a magnetic field (Durfey et al., 2019). Using the same principle, other molecules such as lectin to recognize acrosome-reacted spermatozoa, had been conjugated with MNPs to obtain a population of selected sperm (Feugang et al., 2015).

Otherwise, a novel sex-sorted semen technique was developed with nanoparticles technology, employing functionalized gold nanoparticles to identify Y-chromosome (Rath et al., 2013). Briefly, these authors designed a bivalent nanoparticle conjugated with a cell penetrating peptide and allow nanoparticles to penetrate the spermatozoa membrane to hybridizing nucleic acid. These hybridizations are selective at the Y-chromosome and can be recognized by optical detection due to its specific aggregation pattern. The result is a sex-specific sorting in the spermatozoa population trapping only the sperm with the determined sex of interest (Rath et al., 2013).

10.8.5 FIXED-TIME ARTIFICIAL INSEMINATION

Fixed-time artificial insemination (FTAI) allows inseminating sows and gilts with a single semen dose by the induction of ovulation at a fixed time (Bortolozzo et al., 2015; De Rensis and Kirkwood, 2016). The main benefits of FTAI are the reduction in labour costs and requirements due to the possibility of inseminating without the need for estrus detection. At the same time, achieve faster genetic progress by the increase and optimize the use of better boars (Baroncello et al., 2017).

Principal ovulation inducers used in FTAI protocol for weaned sows are two GnRH analogues, buserelin or triptorelin acetate (De Rensis and Kirkwood, 2016). Briefly, buserelin protocol consists of the administration of this hormone 86–89 h post-weaning followed by single insemination after 30–33 h of hormone injection. This protocol only can be applied in sows showing estrus behavior, which represents a limitation of this procedure (Driancourt et al., 2013; Baroncello et al., 2017). On the other hand, in triptorelin protocol, hormone administration must be done 96 h after weaning and insemination is performed 22–24 h later. In this case, all sows can be inseminated, without the need of estrus detection (Knox et al., 2014, 2017). However, the use of FTAI in gilts is more complicated because it requires previous estrus cycle synchronization by progestogen for several days prior to ovulation induction (Bortolozzo et al., 2005; Martinat-Botté et al., 2010). This makes the commercial use of FTAI in gilts more expensive and complex. Therefore, nowadays FTAI use is limited to weaned sows and only in specific situations for gilts (García-Vázquez et al., 2019a).

ACKNOWLEDGMENTS

The authors would like to thank Import-Vet S.A., Minitube and Pedro José Llamas-López for providing the images to illustrate the chapter.

KEYWORDS

- **biomarkers**
- **post-cervical insemination**
- **reproductive fluids**
- **semen processing and handling**

REFERENCES

Abdel-Salam, Z.; Harith, M. A. Laser Researches on Livestock Semen and Oocytes: A Brief Review. *J. Adv. Res.* **2015,** *6* (3), 311–317.

Althouse, G. C. Artificial Insemination in Swine: Boar Stud Management. Current Therapy in Large Animal. *Theriogenology.* **2007,** 731–738.

Althouse, G. C.; Wilson, M. E.; Kuster, C.; Parsley, M. Characterization of Lower Temperature Storage Limitations of Fresh-Extended Porcine Semen. *Theriogenology.* **1998,** *50* (4), 535–543.

Althouse, G. C.; Kuster, C. E.; Clark, S. G.; Weisiger, R. M. Field Investigations of Bacterial Contaminants and their Effects on Extended Porcine Semen. *Theriogenology.* **2000,** *53* (5), 1167–1176.

Alvarez, J. G., and Storey, B. T. Role of Superoxide Dismutase in Protecting Rabbit Spermatozoa from O2 Toxicity Due to Lipid Peroxidation. *Biol Reprod.* **1983,** *28*,1129–1136.

Amann, R. P., and Waberski, D. Computer-Assisted Sperm Analysis (CASA): Capabilities and Potential Developments. *Theriogenology.* **2014,** *81,* 5–17.e3.

Aneas, S. B.; Gary, B. G.; Bouvier, B. P. Collectis® Automated Boar Collection Technology. *Theriogenology.* **2008,** *70* (8), 1368–1373.

Angelakeris, M. Magnetic Nanoparticles: A Multifunctional Vehicle for Modern Theranostics. *Biochimica et Biophysica Acta* (BBA)-General Subjects. **2017,** *1861* (6), 1642–1651.

Araujo, E. B.; Costa, E. P.; Costa, A. H. A.; Lopes, F. G.; Macedo, G. G.; Paula, T. A. R. Reproductive Performance of Sows Submitted to Intrauterine Insemination. *Braz. J. Vet. Res. Anim. Sci.* **2009,** *38* (8):1460–1467.

Arraztoa, C. C.; Miragaya, M. H.; Chaves, M. G.; Trasorras, V. L.; Gambarotta, M. C.; Neild, D. M. Porcine Sperm Vitrification II: Spheres Method. *Andrologia.* **2017,** *49* (8), 1–8.

Baroncello, E.; Bernardi, M. L.; Kummer, A. D.; Wentz, I.; Bortolozzo, F. P. Fixed-Time Post-Cervicalartificial Insemination in Weaned Sows Following Buserelin Use Combined With/Without eCG. *Reprod Domest Anim.* **2017,** *52*, 76–82.

Barone, F.; Ventrella, D.; Zannoni, A.; Forni, M.; Bacci, M. L. Can Microfiltered Seminal Plasma Preserve the Morphofunctional Characteristics of Porcine Spermatozoa in the Absence of Antibiotics? A Preliminary Study. *Reprod. Domest. Anim.* **2016,** *51* (4), 604–610.

Behan, J. R.; and Watson, P. F. The Effect of Managed Boar Contact in the Post-Weaning Period on the Subsequent Fertility and Fecundity of Sows. *Anim. Reprod. Sci.* **2005,** *88* (3–4), 319–324.

Bielas, W.; Nizański, W.; Partyka, A.; Rzasa, A.; Mordak, R. Effect of Long-Term Storage in Safe Cell+ Extender on Boar Sperm DNA Integrity and Other Key Sperm Parameters. *Acta Veterinaria Scandinavica.* **2017,** *59* (1), 1–12.

Boe-Hansen, G. B.; Ersbøll, A. K.; Greve, T.; Christensen, P. Increasing Storage Time of Extended Boar Semen Reduces Sperm DNA Integrity. *Theriogenology.* **2005,** *63* (7), 2006–2019.

Bortolozzo, F. P.; Menegat M. B.; Mellagi, A. P. G.; Bernardi, M. L.; Wentz, I. New Artificial Insemination Technologies for Swine. *Reprod. Domest. Anim.*. **2015,** *50*, 80–84. Bortolozzo, F. P.; Uemoto, D. A.; Bennemann, P. E.; Pozzobon, M. C.; Castagna, C. D.; Peixoto, C. H.; Barioni, W.; Wentz, I. Influence of Time of Insemination Relative to Ovulation and Frequency of insemination on Gilt Fertility. *Theriogenology.* **2005,** *64* (9), 1956–1962.

Bowen, J. M. Artificial Insemination in the Horse. *Equine Vet. J.* **1969**, *1* (3), 98–110.

Bresciani, C.; Bianchera, A.; Bettini, R.; Buschini, A.; Marchi, L.; Cabassi, C. S.; Alberto Sabbioni, A.; Righi, F.; Mazzoni, C.; Parmigiani, E. Long-Term Liquid Storage and Reproductive Evaluation of an Innovative Boar Semen Extender (Formula12®) Containing a Non-Reducing Disaccharide and an Enzymatic Agent. *Anim. Reprod. Sci.* **2017**, *180*, 10–16.

Brito, L. F. C.; Althouse, G. C.; Aurich, C.; Chenoweth, P. J.; Eilts, B. E.; Love, C. C.; Luvoni, G. C.; Mitchell, J. R.; Peter, A. T.; Pugh, D. G.; Waberski, D. Andrology Laboratory Review: Evaluation of Sperm Concentration. *Theriogenology.* **2016**, *85*, 1507–1527.

Broekhuijse, M. L.; Gaustad, A. H.; Bolarin Guillen, A.; Knol, E. F. Efficient Boar Semen Production and Genetic Contribution: The Impact of Low-Dose Artificial Insmeination on Fertility. *Reprod. Domest. Anim.* **2015**, *suppl 2*, 103–109.

Broekhuijse, M. L.; Sostaric, E.; Feitsma, H.; Gadella, B. M. Additional Value of Computer Assisted Semen Analysis (CASA) Compared to Conventional Motility Assessments in Pig Artificial Insemination. *Theriogenology.* **2011**, *76*, 1473–1486.

Broekhuijse, M. L.; Feitsma, H.; Gadella, B. M. Artificial Insemination in Pigs: Predicting Male Fertility. *Vet. Q.* **2012**, *32*(3–4), 151–157.

Bussalleu, E.; Sancho, S.; Briz, M. D.; Yeste, M.; Bonet, S. Do Antimicrobial Peptides PR-39, PMAP-36 and PMAP-37 Have Any Effect on Bacterial Growth and Quality of Liquid-Stored Boar Semen? *Theriogenology.* **2017**, *89*, 235–243.

Bussalleu, E.; Torner, E. Quality Improvement of Boar Seminal Doses. In *Boar Reproduction: Fundamentals and New Biotechnological Trends*; Bonet S.; Casas I.; Holt W. V.; Yeste M.; Eds., Heidelberg: Springer, **2013**; p. 517–550.

Casado-Vela, J.; Rodriguez-Suarez, E.; Iloro, I.; Ametzazurra, A.; Alkorta, N.; García-Velasco, J. A.; Matorras, R.; Prieto, B.; González, S.; Nagore, D.; Elortza F. Comprehensive Proteomic Analysis of Human Endometrial Fluid Aspirate research articles. *J. Proteome Res.* **2009**, 4622–4632.

Casas, I.; Flores, E. *Gene Banking: The Freezing Strategy.* In *Boar Reproduction: Fundamentals and New Biotechnological Trends.* Bonet S.; Casas I.; Holt W. V.; Yeste M.; Eds.; Heidelberg: Springer, **2013**, p. 551–588.

Cavalleri, R.; Becker, J. S.; Pavan, A. M.; Bianchetti, P.; Goettert, M. I.; Ethur, E. M.; Bustamante-Filho, I. C. Essential Oils Rich in Monoterpenes are Unsuitable as Additives to Boar Semen Extender. *Andrologia.* **2018**, *50* (8), e13074.

Centurion, F.; Vazquez, J. M.; Calvete, J. J.; Roca, J.; Sanz, L.; Parrilla, I.; Garcia, E. M.; Martinez, E. A. Influence of Porcine Spermadhesins on the Susceptibility of Boar Spermatozoa to High Dilution. *Biol Reprod.* **2003**, *69* (2),640–6.

Claus, R. Physiological Role of Seminal Components in the Reproductive Tract of the Female pig. *J. Reprod. Fertil. Suppl. Supplement.* **1990**, *40*, 117–131. Retrieved from

Colenbrander, B.; Feitsma, H.; Grooten, H. J. Optimizing Semen Production For Artificial Insemination in Swine. *J Reprod Fertil Suppl.* **1993**, *48*, 207–15.

Cornou, C. Automated Oestrus Detection Methods in Group Housed Sows: Review of the Current Methods and Perspectives for Development. *Livest. Sci.* **2006**, *105* (1-3), 1–11.

Cronin, G. M.; Hemsworth, P. H.; Winfield, C. G. Oestrous Behaviour in Relation to Fertility and Fecundity Of Gilts. *Animal Reproduction Science.* **1982**, *5* (2), 117–125.

De Jonge, F. H.; Mekking, P.; Abbott, K.; Wiepkema, P. R. Proceptive and Receptive Aspects of Oestrus Behaviour in Gilts. *Behavioural Processes.* **1994**, *31* (2–3), 157–166.

De Rensis, F.; Kirkwood, R. N. Control of Estrus and Ovulation: Fertility to Timed Insemination of Gilts and Sows. *Theriogenology.* **2016,** *86,* 1460–1466.

Driancourt, M. A.; Cox, P.; Rubion, S.; Harnois-Milon, G.; Kemp, B.; Soede, N. M. Induction of an LH Surge and Ovulation by Buserelin (as Receptal) Allows Breeding of Weaned Sows with a Single Fixed-Time Insemination. *Theriogenology.* **2013,** *80,* 391–399.

Durfey, C. L.; Burnett, D. D.; Liao, S. F.; Steadman, C. S.; Crenshaw, M. A.; Clemente, H. J.; Willard, S. T.; Ryan, P. L.; Feugang, J. M. Nanotechnology-Based Selection of Boar Spermatozoa: Growth Development and Health Assessments of Produced Offspring. *Livest. Sci.* **2017,** *205,* 137–142.

Durfey, C. L.; Swistek, S. E.; Liao, S. F.; Crenshaw, M. A.; Clemente, H. J.; Thirumalai, R. V.; Steadman, C. S.; Ryan, P. L.; Willard, S. T.; Feugang, J. M. Nanotechnology-Based Approach for Safer Enrichment of Semen with Best Spermatozoa. *J. Anim. Sci. Biotechnol.* **2019,** *10* (1), 14.

Dyck, M. K.; Foxcroft, G. R.; Novak, S.; Ruiz-Sanchez, A.; Patterson, J.; Dixon, W. T. Biological Markers of Boar Fertility. *Reprod. Domest. Anim.* **2011,** *46* (SUPPL. 2), 55–58.

Feugang, J. M. Novel agents for sperm purification, sorting, and imaging. *Mol. Reprod. Dev.* **2017,** *84* (9), 832–841.

Feugang, J. M.; Liao, S.; Crenshaw, M.; Clemente, H.; Willard, S.; Ryan, P. Lectin-functionalized magnetic iron oxide nanoparticles for reproductive improvement. *JFIV Reprod Med Genet.* **2015,** *3* (145), 17–19.

Feugang, J. M.; Rodríguez-Muñoz, J. C.; Dillard, D. S.; Crenshaw, M. A.; Willard, S. T.; Ryan, P. L. Beneficial effects of relaxin on motility characteristics of stored boar spermatozoa. *Reprod. Biol. Endocrinol.* **2015,** *13* (1), 24.

First, N. L.; Short, R. E.; Peters, J. B.; Stratman, F. W. Transport and Loss of Boar Spermatozoa in the Reproductive Tract of the Sow. *J. Anim. Sci.* **1968,** *27,* 1037–1040.

Flowers, W. L. Management of Boars for Efficient Semen Production. *J Reprod Fertil Suppl.* **1997,** *52,* 67–78.

Fraser, L., and Strzezek, J. The Use of Comet Assay to Assess DNA Integrity of Boar Spermatozoa Following Liquid Preservation at 5 Degrees C and 16 Degrees C. *Folia Histochemica et Cytobiologica.* **2004,** *42* (1), 49–55.

Fu, J.; Yang, Q.; Li, Y.; Li, P.; Wang, L.; Li, X. A Mechanism by Which Astragalus Polysaccharide Protects Against ROS Toxicity Through Inhibiting the Protein Dephosphorylation of Boar Sperm Preserved at 4 C. *J. Cell. Physiol.* **2018,** *233* (7), 5267–5280.

Funahashi, H., and Sano, T. Select Antioxidants Improve the Function of Extended Boar Semen Stored at 10 Degrees C. *Theriogenology.* **2005,** *63* (6):1605–1616.

Gadea, J.; Sellés, E.; Marco, M. A.; Coy, P.; Matás, C.; Romar, R.; Ruiz, S. Decrease in Glutathione Content in Boar Sperm After Cryopreservation: Effect of the Addition of Reduced Glutathione to the Freezing and Thawing Extenders. *Theriogenology.* **2004,** *62,* 690–701.

García-Vázquez, F. A.; Hernández-Caravaca, I.; Matás, C.; Soriano-Úbeda, C.; Abril-Sánchez, S.; Izquierdo-Rico, M. J. Morphological Study of Boar Sperm During Their Passage through the Female Genital Tract. *J Reprod. Dev.* **2015,** *61* (5), 407–413.

García-Vázquez, F. A.; Llamas-López, P. J.; Jacome, M. A.; Sarrias-Gil, L.; Albors, O. L. Morphological Changes in the Porcine Cervix: A Comparison Between Nulliparous and

Multiparous Sows with Regard to Post-Cervical Artificial Insemination. *Theriogenology.* **2019b,** *127,* 120–129.

García-Vázquez, F. A.; Mellagi, A. P. G.; Ulguim, R. R.; Hernández-Caravaca, I.; Llamas-López, P. J.; Bortolozzo, F. P. Post-Cervical Artificial Insemination in Porcine: The Technique that Came to Stay. *Theriogenology.* **2019a,** *129,* 37–45.

Gardner, D. K.; Lane, M.; Calderon, I.; Leeton, J. Environment of the Preimplantation Human Embryo *In Vivo*: Metabolite Analysis of Oviduct and Uterine Fluids and Metabolism of *Cumulus* Cells. *Fertil. Steril.* **1996,** *65* (2), 349–353. Retrieved from

Garner, D. L. Hafez, E. S. E. *Spermatozoa and Seminal Plasma.* In *Reproduction in Farm Animals* Hafez, B. E S E Hafez, E. S. E. Ed.; **2000;** pp. 96–109,

Gatti, J. L.; Chevrier, C.; Paquignon, M.; Dacheux, J. L. External Ionic Conditions, Internal pH and Motility of Ram and Boar Spermatozoa. *J. Reprod. Fertil.* **1993,** *98,* 439–449.

Geens, M.; Van de Velde, H.; De Block, G.; Goossens, E.; Van Steirteghem, A.; Tournaye, H. The Efficiency of Magnetic-Activated Cell Sorting and Fluorescence-Activated Cell Sorting in the Decontamination of Testicular Cell Suspensions in Cancer Patients. *Hum. Reprod.* **2006,** *22*(3), 733–742.

Grunewald, S.; Paasch, U.; Glander, H. J. Enrichment of Non–Apoptotic Human Sperma-tozoa After Cryopreservation by Immunomagnetic Cell Sorting. *Cell Tissue Bank.* **2001,** *2*(3), 127–133.

Guthrie, H. D.; Henricks, D. M.; Handlin, D. L. Plasma Estrogen, Progesterone and Luteinizing Hormone Prior to Estrus and During Early Pregnancy in Pigs 1. *Endocrinology.* **1972,** *91* (3), 675–679.

Hamonic, G.; Pasternak, J. A.; Kaser, T.; Meurens, F.; Wilson, H. L. Extended Semen for Artificial Insemination in Swine as a Potential Transmission Mechanism for Infectious Chlamydia suis. *Theriogenology.* **2016,** *86,* 949–956.

Hancock, J. L. Pig insemination technique. *Vet. Rec.* **1959,** *71,* 26, 523.

Hernández-Caravaca, I.; Izquierdo-Rico, M. J.; Matás, C.; Carvajal, J. A.; Vieira, L.; Abril, D.; Soriano-Úbeda, C.; García-Vázquez, F. A. Reproductive Performance and Backflow Study in Cervical and Post-Cervical Artificial Insemination in Sows. *Anim. Reprod. Sci.* **2012,** *136* (1–2), 14–22.

Hernández-Caravaca, I.; Soriano-Úbeda, C.; Matás, C.; Izquierdo-Rico, M. J.; García-Vázquez, F. A. Boar Sperm with Defective Motility are Discriminated in the Backflow Moments after Insemination. *Theriogenology.* **2015,** *83* (4), 655–661.

Hernández-Caravaca, I.; Llamas-López, P. J.; Izquierdo-Rico, M. J.; Soriano-Úbeda, C.; Matás, C.; Gardón, J. C.; García-Vázquez, F. A. Optimization of Post-Cervical Artificial Insemination in Gilts: Effect of Cervical Relaxation Procedures and Catheter Type. *Theriogenology.* **2017,** *90,* 147–152.

Hill, E. K.; Li, J. Current and Future Prospects for Nanotechnology in Animal Production. *J. Anim. Sci. Biotechnol.* **2017,** *8* (1), 1–13.

Holt, W. V, Van Look, K. J. W. Concepts in Sperm Heterogeneity, Sperm Selection and Sperm Competition as Biological Foundations for Laboratory Tests of Semen Quality. *Reprod.* **2004,** *127* (5), 527–535.

Hunter, R. H. F. Sperm transport and reservoirs in the pig oviduct in relation to the time of ovulation. *J. Reprod. Fertil.* **1981,** *63* (1), 109–117.

Iritani, A.; Gomes, W. R.; Vandemark, N. L. Secretion Rates and Chemical Composition of Oviduct and Uterine Fluids in Ewes. *Biol. Reprod.* **1969,** *1* (1), 72–76. Retrieved from http://www.ncbi.nlm.nih.gov/pubmed/5408687.

Iritani, A.; Nishikawa, Y.; Gomes, W. R.; VanDemark, N. L. Secretion Rates and Chemical Composition of Oviduct and Uterine Fluids in Rabbits. *J. Anim. Sci.* **1971,** *33* (4), 829–835.

Ivanov, E. I. De la fécondation artificielle chez les mammifères. *Arch Sci Biol.* **1907,** *12,* 377-511.

Ivanov, E. I. On the Use of Artificial Insemination for Zootechnical Purposes in Russia. *J Agric Sci.* **1922,** *12,* 244–256.

Johnson, L. A.; Aalbers, J. G.; Willems, C. M.; Rademaker, J. H.; Rexroad Jr.; C. E. Use of Boar Spermatozoa for Artificial Insemination. III. Fecundity of Boar Spermatozoa Stored in Beltsville Liquid and Kiev Extenders for Three Days at 18 C. *J. Anim. Sci.* **1982,** *54,* 132–136.

Johnson, L. A.; Weitze, K. F.; Fiser, P.; Maxwell, W. M. Storage of Boar Semen. *Anim Reprod Sci.* **2000,** *62,* 143–172.

Kaewmala, K.; Uddin, M. J.; Cinar, M. U.; Große-Brinkhaus, C.; Jonas, E.; Tesfaye, D.; Phatsara, C.; Tholen, E.; Looft, C.; Schellander, K. Association Study and Expression Analysis of CD9 as Candidate Gene for Boar Sperm Quality and Fertility Traits. *Anim. Reprod. Sci.* **2011,** *125*(1–4), 170–179.

Karageorgiou, M. A.; Tsousis, G.; Boscos, C. M.; Tzika, E. D.; Tassis, P. D.; Tsakmakidis, I. A. A Comparative Study of Boar Semen Extenders with Different Proposed Preservation Times and Their Effect on Semen Quality and Fertility. *Acta Veterinaria Brno.* **2016,** *85,* 23–31.

Katila, T. Post-Mating Inflammatory Responses of the Uterus. *Reprod. Domest. Anim.* **2012,** *47* (SUPPL. 5), 31–41.

Kawano, N.; Araki, N.; Yoshida, K.; Hibino, T.; Ohnami, N.; Makino, M.; Kanai, S.; Hasuwa, H.; Yoshida, M.; Miyado, K.; Akihiro U. Seminal Vesicle Protein SVS2 is Required for Sperm Survival in the Uterus. *Proc. Natl. Acad. Sci.* **2014,** *111* (11), 4145–4150.

Kim, K. U.; Pang, W. K.; Kang, S.; Ryu, D. Y.; Song, W. H.; Rahman, M. S.; Kwon, W. S.; Pang, M. G. Sperm Solute Carrier Family 9 Regulator 1 is Correlated with Boar Fertility. *Theriogenology.* **2019,** *126,* 254–260.

Knox R. V. Impact of Swine Reproductive Technologies on Pig and Global Food Production. *Adv Exp Med Biol.* **2014,** *752,* 131–160.

Knox, R. V. Semen Processing, Extending and Storage for Artificial Insemination in Swine. *Swine Reproductive Extension Specialist.* **2011.**

Knox, R. V. Artificial insemination in pigs today. *Theriogenology.* **2016,** *85* (1), 83–93.

Knox, R.; Levis, D.; Safranski, T.; Singleton, W. An Update on North American Boar Stud Practices. *Theriogenology.* **2008,** *70* (8), 1202–1208.

Knox, R. V.; Esparza-Harris, K. C.; Johnston, M. E.; Webel, S. K. Effect of Numbers of Sperm and TIMING of A Single, Post-Cervical Insemination on the Fertility of Weaned Sows Treated with OvuGel®. *Theriogenology.* **2017,** *92,* 197–203.

Knox, R. V.; Taibl, J. N.; Breen, S. M.; Swanson, M. E.; Webel, S. K. Effects of Altering the Dose and Timing of Triptorelin When Given as an Intravaginal Gel for Advancing and Synchronizing Ovulation in Weaned Sows. *Theriogenology.* **2014,** *82,* 379–86.

Ko, J. C.; Evans, L. E.; Althouse, G. C. Toxicity Effects of Latex Gloves on Boar Spermatozoa. *Theriogenology.* **1989,** *31* (6), 1159–1164.

Kwon, W. S.; Rahman, M. S.; Ryu, D. Y.; Khatun, A.; Pang, M. G. Comparison of Markers Predicting Litter Size in Different Pig Breeds. *Andrology.* **2017,** *5* (3), 568–577.

Kwon, W. S.; Shin, D. H.; Ryu, D. Y.; Khatun, A.; Rahman, M. S.; Pang, M. G. Applications of Capacitation Status for Litter Size Enhancement in Various Pig Breeds. *Asian-australas. J. Anim. Sci.* **2018,** *31* (6), 842.

Kwon, W. S.; Pang, M. G.; Rahman, M. S.; Kim, Y. J.; Oh, S. A.; Park, Y. J. Proteomic Approaches for Profiling Negative Fertility Markers in Inferior Boar Spermatozoa. *Sci. Rep.* **2015b,** *5* (1), 1–10.

Kwon, W. S.; Rahman, M. S.; Lee, J. S.; Yoon, S. J.; Park, Y. J.; Pang, M. G. Discovery of Predictive Biomarkers for Litter Size in Boar Spermatozoa. *Mol. Cell Proteomics* **2015a,** *14* (5), 1230–1240.

Kwon, W. S.; Rahman, M. S.; Ryu, D. Y.; Park, Y. J.; Pang, M. G. Increased Male Fertility Using Fertility-Related Biomarkers. *Sci. Rep.* **2015c,** *5* (1), 1–11.

Langendijk, J. A.; Slotman, B. J.; van der Waal, I.; Doornaert, P.; Berkof, J.; Leemans, C. R. Risk-Group Definition by Recursive Partitioning Analysis of Patients with Squamous Cell Head and Neck Carcinoma Treated with Surgery and Postoperative Radiotherapy. *Cancer.* **2005,** *104* (7), 1408–1417.

Langendijk, P.; Soede, N.; Kemp, B. Uterine Activity, Sperm Transport, and The Role Of Boar Stimuli Around Insemination in Sows. *Theriogenology.* **2005,** *63,* 500–513.

Langendijk, P.; van den Brand, H.; Soede, N. M.; Kemp, B. Effect of Boar Contact on Follicular Development and on Estrus Expression after Weaning in Primiparous Sows. *Theriogenology.* **2000,** *54* (8), 1295–1303. Retrieved from http://www.ncbi.nlm.nih.gov/pubmed/11192188.

Leahy, T.; and Gadella, B. M. Capacitation and Capacitation-Like Sperm Surface Changes Induced by Handling Boar Semen. *Reprod. Domest. Anim.* **2011,** *46* (Suppl 2), 7–13.

Lee, S. H.; and Park, C. K. Antioxidative Effects of Magnetized Extender Containing Bovine Serum Albumin on Sperm Oxidative Stress During Long-Term Liquid Preservation of Boar Semen. *Biochem. Biophys. Res. Commun.* **2015b,** *464* (2), 467–472.

Lee, S. H.; and Park, C. K. Effect of Magnetized Extender on Sperm Membrane Integrity and Development of Oocytes *In Vitro* Fertilized with Liquid Storage Boar Semen. *Anim. Reprod. Sci.* **2015a,** 154, 86–94.

Leeuwenhoek, A. De natis è semine genitali animalculis. *R Soc (Lond) Philos Trans.* **1678,** *12,*1040–1043.

Levis, D. G., and Reicks, D. L. Assessment of Sexual Behavior and Effect of Semen Collection Pen Design and Sexual Stimulation of Boars on Behavior and Sperm Output—A Review. *Theriogenology.* **2005,** *63* (2), 630–642.

Li, J.; Zhang, J.; Li, Q.; Li, Y.; Wei, G. Effects of Negative Pressure on Boar Semen Quality During Liquid Storage at 17°C. *Indian J. Anim. Res.* **2017,** (B-791), 1–5.

Lin, C. L.; Ponsuksili, S.; Tholen, E.; Jennen, D. G. J.; Schellander, K.; Wimmers, K. Candidate Gene Markers for Sperm Quality and Fertility of Boar. *Anim. Reprod. Sci.* **2006,** *92* (3–4), 349–363.

Llamas-López, P. J.; López-Úbeda, R.; López, G.; Antinoja, E.; García-Vázquez, F. A. A New Device for Deep Cervical Artificial Insemination in Gilts Reduces the Number of Sperm Per Dose Without Impairing Final Reproductive Performance. *J. Anim. Sci. Biotechnol.* **2019,** *10* (1).

López Rodríguez, A.; Rijsselaere, T.; Vyt, P.; Van Soom, A.; Maes, D. Effect of Dilution Temperature on Boar Semen Quality. *Reprod. Domest. Anim.* **2012**, *47* (5), e63–e66.

Lopez Rodriguez, A.; Van Soom, A.; Arsenakis, I.; Maes, D. Boar Management and Semen Handling Factors Affect the Quality of Boar Extended Semen. *Porcine Health Manag.* **2017**, *3*, 15.

Lu, A. H.: Salabas, E. L.; Schüth, F. Magnetic Nanoparticles: Synthesis, Protection, Functionalization, and Application. *Angewandte Chemie—International Edition.* **2007**, *46* (8), 1222–1244.

Luther, A.; Le Thi, X.; Schäfer, J.; Schulze, M.; Waberski, D. Irradiation of Semen Doses with LED-Based Red Light in a Photo Chamber Does Not Improve *In Vitro* Quality of Thermically Stressed Boar Spermatozoa. *Reprod. Domest. Anim.* **2018**, *53* (4), 1016–1019.

Macías-García, B. M.; Morrell, J. M.; Ortega-Ferrusola, C.; González-Fernández, L.; Tapia, J. A.; Rodriguez-Martinez, H.; Peña, F. J. Centrifugation on a single layer of colloid selects improved quality spermatozoa from frozen-thawed stallion semen.*Anim. Reprod. Sci.* **2009**,*114*(1–3), 193–202.

Maes, D. G.; Mateusen, B.; Rijsselaere T.; De Vliegher, S.; Van Soom, A.; de Kruif, A. Motility Characteristics of Boar Spermatozoa After Addition of Prostaglandin F₂. *Theriogenology.* **2003**, *60*,1435–43.

Maes, D.; Lopez Rodriguez, A.; Rijsselaere, T.; Vyt, P.; Van Soom, A. Artificial Insemination in Pigs. In *Artificial Insemination in Farm Animals.* **2011**.

Maes, D.; Nauwynck, H.; Rijsselaere, T.; Mateusen, B.; Vyt, P.; De Kruif, A.; Van Soom, A. Diseases in Swine Transmitted by Artificial Insemination: An Overview. *Theriogenology.* **2008**, *70*, 1337–45.

Maroto Martin, L. O.; Munoz, E. C.; de Cupere, F.; van Driessche, E.; Echemendia-Blanco, D.; Rodriguez, J. M.; Beeckmans, S. Bacterial Contamination of Boar Semen Affects the Litter Size. *Anim. Reprod. Sci.* **2010**, *120*, 95–104.

Martinat-Botté, F.; Venturi, E.; Guillouet, P.; Driancourt, M. A.; Terqui, M. Induction and Synchronization of Ovulations of Nulliparous and Multiparous Sows with an Injection of Gonadotropin-Releasing Hormone Agonist (Receptal). *Theriogenology* **2010**, *73*, 332–342.

Martinez, E.; Vazquez, J. M.; Roca, J.; Lucas, X.; Gil, M.; Parrilla, I.; Vazquez, J. L.; Day, B. Successful Non-Surgical Deep Intrauterine Insemination with Small Numbers of Spermatozoa in Sows. *Reprod.* **2001**, *122* (2), 289–296.

Martinez, E. A; Vazquez, J. M; Roca, J; Lucas, X; Gil, M. A; Parrilla, I; Vazquez, J.L; Day, B. N. Minimum Number of Spermatozoa Required For Normal Fertility after Deep Intrauterine Insemination in Non-Sedated Sows. *Reproduction.* **2002**, *123*(1), 163–170.

Martinez-Alborcia, M. J.; Morrell, J. M.; Parrilla, I.; Barranco, I.; Vázquez, J. M.; Martinez, E. A.; Roca, J. Improvement of Boar Sperm Cryosurvival by Using Single-Layer Colloid Centrifugation Prior Freezing. *Theriogenology.* **2012**, *78* (5), 1117–1125.

Matás, C.; Vieira, L.; García-Vázquez, F. A.; Avilés-López, K.; López-Úbeda, R.; Carvajal, J. A.; Gadea, J. Effects of Centrifugation Through Three Different Discontinuous Percoll Gradients on Boar Sperm Function. *Anim. Reprod. Sci.* **2011**, *127* (1–2), 62–72.

Matthijs, A.; Engel, B.; Woelders, H. Neutrophil Recruitment and Phagocytosis of Boar Spermatozoa After Artificial Insemination of Sows, and the Effects of Inseminate Volume, Sperm Dose and Specific Additives in the Extender. *Reproduction.* **2003**, *125* (3), 357–367.

May, N.; Patterson, J. L.; Pinilla, J. C.; Carpenter, A.; Werner, T.; Triemert, E.; Holden, N.; Foxcroft, G. R.; Dixo, W. T.; Dyck, M. K. Seminal Plasma Proteins Associated with Boar Fertility. *Reprod Dom Anim.* **2015,** *50,* 110–8.

Mburu, J. N.; Einarsson, S.; Lundeheim, N.; Rodriguez-Martinez, H. Distribution, Number And Membrane Integrity of Spermatozoa in the Pig Oviduct in Relation to Spontaneous Ovulation. *Anim. Reprod. Sci.* **1996,** *45* (1–2), 109–121.

McKenzie, F. F. A Method for Collection of Boar Semen. *J Am Vet Assoc.* 1931, *78,* 244–246.

Medrano, A.; Pena, A.; Rigau, T. and Rodriguez-Gil, J. E. Variations in the Proportion of Glycolytic/Non-Glycolytic Energy Substrates Modulate Sperm Membrane Integrity and Function in Diluted Boar Samples Stored at 15-17 Degrees C. *Reprod Domest Anim.* **2005,** *40,* 448–53.

Melrose, D. R., O'Hagan, C. Investigations into the Technique of Artificial Insemination in the Pig. In: *Proceedings of the Fourth International Congress on the Animal Reproduction,* vol. 4. *The Hague.* **1961,** p. 855–859.

Menegat, M. B.; Mellagi, A. P.; Bortolin, R. C.; Menezes, T. A.; Vargas, A. R.; Bernardi, M. L.; Wentz, I.; Gelain, D. P.; Moreira, J. C.; Bortolozzo, F. P. Sperm Quality and Oxidative Status as Affected by Homogenization of Liquid-Stored Boar Semen Diluted in Short- and Long-Term Extenders. *Anim. Reprod. Sci.* **2017,** *179,* 67–79.

Mezalira, A.; Dallanora, D.; Bernardi, M.; Wentz, I.; Bortolozzo, F. Influence of Sperm Cell Dose and Post-Insemination Backflow on Reproductive Performance of Intrauterine Inseminated Sows. *Reprod. Domest. Anim.* **2005,** 40, 1–5.

Michael, A. J.; Alexopoulos, C.; Pontiki, E. A.; Hadjipavlou-Litina, D. J.; Saratsis, P.; Ververidis, H. N.; Boscos, C. M. Quality and Reactive Oxygen Species of Extended Canine Semen After Vitamin C Supplementation. *Theriogenology.* **2008,** *70* (5),827–835.

Morrell, J.; Wallgren, M. Alternatives to Antibiotics in Semen Extenders: A Review. *Pathogens.* **2014,** *3* (4), 934–946.

Morrell, J. M., and Wallgren, M. Control of Bacterial Contamination in Boar Semen Doses. In *Science and Technology against Microbial Pathogens; Research, Development and Evaluation*; Mendez-Vilas, A.; Ed.; World Scientific Publishing Co.; Pte. Ltd.: Singapore, Singapore. 2011, pp. 303–308.

Nerin, C.; Ubeda, J. L.; Alfaro, P.; Dahmani, Y.; Aznar, M.; Canellas, E.; Ausejo, R. Compounds from Multilayer Plastic Bags Cause Reproductive Failures in Artificial Insemination. *Sci. Rep.* **2014,** *4,* 4913.

Niwa, T. *Artificial insemination with swine in Japan.* 1958, pp.13.

Novak, S.; Ruiz-Sanchez, A.; Dixon, W. T.; Foxcroft, G. R.; Dyck, M. K. Seminal Plasma Proteins as Potential Markers of Relative Fertility in Boars. *J. Androl.* **2010,** *31* (2), 188–200.

Odhiambo, J. F.; DeJarnette, J. M.; Geary, T. W.; Kennedy, C. E.; Suarez, S. S.; Sutovsky, M.; Sutovsky, P. Increased Conception Rates in Beef Cattle Inseminated with Nanopurified Bull Semen.*Biol. Reprod.* **2014,** *91* (4), 97.

Okazaki, T.; Ikoma, E.; Tinen, T.; Akiyoshi, T.; Mori, M.; Teshima, H. Addition of Oxytocin to Semen Extender Improves Both Sperm Transport to the Oviduct and Conception Rates in Pigs Following AI. *Anim. Sci. J.* **2014,** *85* (1), 8–14.

Okazaki, T., Shimada, M. New Strategies of Boar Sperm Cryopreservation: Development of Novel Freezing and Thawing Methods with a Focus on the Roles of Seminal Plasma. *Anim. Sci. J.* **2012,** *83* (9), 623–629.

Ostersen, T.; Cornou, C.; Kristensen, A. R. Detecting Oestrus by Monitoring Sows' Visits to a Boar. *Comput. Electron. Agric.* **2010**, *74* (1), 51–58.

Peña, F. J.; Dominguez, J. C.; Carbajo, M.; Anel, L.; Alegre, B. Treatment of Swine Summer Infertility Syndrome by Means of Oxytocin Under Field Conditions. *Theriogenology.* **1998**, *49* (4), 829–836.

Pérez-Llano, B.; Sala, R.; Reguera, G.; García-Casado, P. Changes in Subpopulations of Boar Sperm Defined According to Viability and Plasma and Acrosome Membrane Status Observed During Storage at 15°C. *Theriogenology.* **2009**, *71* (2), 311–317.

Pérez-Patiño, C.; Parrilla, I.; Barranco, I.; Vergara-Barberán, M.; Simó-Alfonso, E. F.; Herrero-Martínez, J. M.; Rodríguez-Martínez H.; Martinez, E.; Roca, J. New In-Depth Analytical Approach of the Porcine Seminal Plasma Proteome Reveals Potential Fertility Biomarkers. *J. Proteome Res.* **2018**, *17* (3), 1065–1076.

Pezo, F.; Romero, F.; Zambrano, F.; Sánchez, R. S. Preservation of boar semen: An update. *Reprod. Domest. Anim.*2019b, 1-12.

Pezo, F.; Zambrano, F.; Uribe, P.; Ramírez-Reveco, A.; Romero, F.; Sanchéz, R. LED-Based Red Light Photostimulation Improves Short-Term Response of Cooled Boar Semen Exposed to Thermal Stress at 37°C. *Andrologia.* **2019a**, e13237.

Philips, P. H.; Lardy, H. A. A Yolk-Buffer Pabulum for the Preservation of Bull Semen. *J Dairy Sci.* **1940**, *23*,399–404.

Piehl, L. L.; Fischman, M. L.; Hellman, U.; Cisale, H.; Miranda, P. V. Boar Seminal Plasma Exosomes: Effect on Sperm Function and Protein Identification by Sequencing. *Theriogenology.* **2013**, *79* (7), 1071–1082.

Pinart, E.; Domènech, E.; Bussalleu, E.; Yeste, M.; Bonet, S. A Comparative Study of the Effects of Escherichia coli and Clostridium perfringens Upon Boar Semen Preserved in Liquid Storage. *Anim. Rep. Sci.* **2017**, *177*, 65–78.

Pintus, E.; Kadlec, M.; Jovičić, M.; Sedmíková, M.; Ros-Santaella, J. Aminoguanidine Protects Boar Spermatozoa against the Deleterious Effects of Oxidative Stress. *Pharmaceutics.* **2018**, *10* (4), 212.

Polge, C. The Development of Artificial Insemination Service for Pigs. *Anim. Breed Abstr.* **1956**, *24*,209–217.

Pruneda, A.; Pinart, E.; Dolors Briz, M.; Sancho, S.; Garcia-Gil, N.; Badia E, Kádár E, Bassols J, Bussalleu E, Yeste M, Bonet S. Effects of a High Semen-Collection Frequency on the Quality of Sperm from Ejaculates and from Six Epididymal Regions in Boars. *Theriogenology.* **2005**, *63* (8), 2219–2232.

Pursel, V. G. Effect of Uterine Ligation and Cervical Plugs on Retention of Frozen-Thawed Boar Sperm. *J.Anim. Sci.* **1982**, *54* (1), 137–141.

Rahman, M. S.; Kwon, W. S.; Pang, M. G. Prediction of Male Fertility Using Capacitation-Associated Proteins in Spermatozoa. *Mol. Reprod. Dev.* **2017**, *84* (9), 749–759.

Rath, D.; Barcikowski, S.; de Graaf, S.; Garrels, W.; Grossfeld, R.; Klein, S.; Knabe, W.; Knorr, C.; Kues, W.; Meyer, H.; Michl, J.; Moench-Tegeder, G.; Rehbock, C.; Taylor, U.; Washausen, S. Sex Selection of Sperm in Farm Animals: Status Report and Developmental Prospects. *Reprod.* **2013**, *145* (1), R15-R30.

Rath, D.; Schuberth, H. J.; Coy, P.; Taylor, U. Sperm Interactions from Insemination to Fertilization. *Reprod. Domest. Anim.* **2008**, *43* (SUPPL. 5), 2–11.

Riesenbeck A. Review on International Trade with Boar Semen. *Reprod Domest Anim.* **2011**, *46* (Suppl. 2),1–3.

Riesenbeck, A.; Schulze, M.; Rüdiger, K.; Henning, H.; Waberski, D. Quality Control of Boar Sperm Processing: Implications from European AI Centres and Two Spermatology Reference Laboratories. *Reprod. Domest. Anim.* **2015**, *50*, 1–4.

Roberts, P. K.; Bilkei, G. Field Experiences on Post-Cervical Artificial Insemination in the Sow. *Reprod. Domest. Anim.* **2005**, *40*(5), 489–491

Roca, J.; Parrilla, I.; Bolarin, A.; Martinez, E. A.; Rodriguez-Martinez, H. Will AI in Pigs Become More Efficient? *Theriogenology.* **2016**, *86*, 187–193.

Roca, J.; Rodríguez, M. J.; Gil, M. A.; Carvajal, G.; Garcia, E. M.; Cuello, C.; Martinez, E. A. Survival and *In Vitro* Fertility of Boar Spermatozoa Frozen in the Presence of Superoxide Dismutase and/or Catalase. *J. Androl..* **2005**, *26* (1), 15–24.

Rodriguez, A. L.; Rijsselaere, T.; Vyt, P.; Van Soom, A.; Maes, D. Effect of Dilution Temperature on Boar Semen Quality. *Reprod. Domest. Anim.* **2012**, *47* (5), e63–e66.

Rodríguez-Antolín, J.; Nicolás, L.; Cuevas, E.; Bravo, I.; Castelán, F.; Martínez-Gómez, M. Morphological Characteristics of the Cervix in Domestic Sows. *Anat Sci Int.* **2012**, *87*,195–202.

Rodriguez-Martinez, H.; Saravia, F.; Wallgren, M.; Martinez, E. A.; Sanz, L.; Roca, J.; Vázquez, J.M, Calvete, J. J. Spermadhesin PSP-I/PSP-II Heterodimer Induces Migration of Polymorphonuclear Neutrophils into the Uterine Cavity of the Sow. *J. Reprod. Immunol.* **2010**, *84* (1), 57–65.

Rodríguez-Martínez, H.; Saravia, F.; Wallgren, M.; Tienthai, P.; Johannisson, A.; Vázquez, J. M.; Martinez, E. A.; Roca, J.; Sanz, L.; Calvete, J. J. Boar Spermatozoa in the Oviduct. *Theriogenology.* **2005**, *63*(2 SPEC. ISS.), 514–535.

Rodriguez-Martinez, H., and Wallgren, M. Advances in Boar Semen Cryopreservation. *Vet. Med. Int.* **2010**.

Ros-Santaella, J. L.; Pintus, E. Rooibos (Aspalathus linearis) Extract Enhances Boar Sperm Velocity up to 96 Hours of Semen Storage. *PloS one.* **2017**, *12* (8), e0183682.

Rozeboom, K. J.; Troedsson, M. H. T.; Hodson, H. H.; Shurson, G. C.; Crabo, B. G. The Importance of Seminal Plasma on the Fertility of Subsequent Artificial Inseminations in Swine. *J. Anim. Sci.* **2000**, *78* (2), 443–448.

Rozeboom, K. J.; Troedsson, M. H.; Crabo, B. G. Characterization of Uterine Leukocyte Infiltration in Gilts after Artificial Insemination. *J. Reprod. Fertil.* **1998**, *114* (2), 195–199.

Rozeboom, K.; Reicks, D.; Wilson, M. The Reproductive Performance and Factors Affecting On-Farm Application of Low-Dose Intrauterine Deposit of Semen in Sows. *J. Anim. Sci.* **2004**, *82*, 2164–2168.

Rueff, L. Diagnostic Approaches to Reproductive Failure in Pigs. *J Swine Health Prod.* **2000**, *8*, 285–287.

Salisbury, G. W.; VanDemark, N. L.; Lodge, J. R. Physiology of Reproduction and Artificial Insemination of Cattle. WH Freeman and Company, **1978**, Ed. 2.

Sancho, S.; Briz, M.; Yeste, M.; Bonet, S.; Bussalleu, E. Effects of the Antimicrobial Peptide Protegrine 1 on Sperm Viability and Bacterial Load of Boar Seminal Doses. *Reprod. Domest. Anim.* **2017**, *52*, 69–71.

Sancho, S., and Vilagran, I. The Boar Ejaculate: Sperm Function and Seminal Plasma Analyses. In *Boar Reproduction.* Berlin, Heidelberg: Springer Berlin Heidelberg, **2013**, (pp. 471–516).

Sbardella P. E.; Ulguim R. R.; Fontana D. L.; Ferrari C. V.; Bernardi M. L.; Wentz I.; Bortolozzo F. P. The Post-Cervical Insemination Does Not Impair the Reproductive Performance of Primiparous Sows. *Reprod Domest Anim.* **2014,** *49*, 59e64.

Schuberth, H. J.; Taylor, U.; Zerbe, H.; Waberski, D.; Hunter, R.; Rath, D. Immunological Responses to Semen in the Female Genital Tract. *Theriogenology.* **2008,** *70* (8), 1174–1181.

Schulze, M.; Ammon, C.; Schaefer, J.; Luther, A. M.; Jung, M.; Waberski, D. Impact of Different Dilution Techniques on Boar Sperm Quality and Sperm Distribution of the Extended Ejaculate. *Anim Reprod Sci.* **2017,** *182*, 138–145.

Schulze, M.; Bortfeldt, R.; Schäfer, J.; Jung, M.; Fuchs-Kittowski, F. Effect of Vibration Emissions During Shipping of Artificial Insemination Doses on Boar Semen Quality. *Anim. Reprod. Sci.* **2018,** *192*, 328–334.

Schulze, M.; Dathe, M.; Waberski, D.; Müller, K. Liquid Storage of Boar Semen: Current and Future Perspectives on the Use of Cationic Antimicrobial Peptides to Replace Antibiotics in Semen Extenders. *Theriogenology.* **2016,** *85* (1), 39–46.

Schulze, M.; Henning, H.; Rüdiger, K.; Wallner, U.; Waberski, D. Temperature Management During Semen Processing: Impact on Boar Sperm Quality Under Laboratory and Field Conditions. *Theriogenology.* **2013,**. *80* (9), 990–998.

Schulze, M.; Jakop, U.; Jung, M.; Cabezón, F. Influences on thermo-resistance of boar spermatozoa. *Theriogenology.* **2019,** *127*, 15–20.

Schulze, M.; Junkes, C.; Mueller, P.; Speck, S.; Ruediger, K.; Dathe, M.; Mueller, K. Effects of Cationic Antimicrobial Peptides on Liquid-Preserved Boar Spermatozoa. *PloS one.* **2014,** *9* (6), e100490.

Schulze, M.; Kuster, C.; Schafer, J.; Jung, M.; Grossfeld, R. Effect of Production Management on Semen Quality During Long-Term Storage in Different European Boar Studs. *Anim Reprod Sci.* **2018,** *190*, 94–101.

Schulze, M.; Rüdiger, K.; Waberski, D. Rotation of Boar Semen Doses During Storage Affects Sperm Quality.*Reprod. Domest. Anim.* **2015,** *50* (4), 684–687.

Simões, V. G.; Lyazrhi, F.; Picard-Hagen, N.; Gayrard, V.; Martineau, G. P.; Waret-Szkuta, A. Variations in the Vulvar Temperature of Sows During Proestrus and Estrus as Determined by Infrared Thermography and its Relation to Ovulation. *Theriogenology.* **2014,** *82* (8), 1080–1085.

Soriano-Úbeda, C.; Matás, C.; García-Vázquez, F. A. An Overview of Swine Artificial Insemination: Retrospective, Current and Prospective Aspects. *J. Exp. Appl. Anim. Sci.* **2013,** *1* (1), 67.

Spallanzani, L. Dissertations Relative to the Natural History of Animals and Vegetables. (Trans. By T. Beddoes). *Dissertations Relative to the Natural History of Animals and Vegetables. J. Murray, London.* **1784,** 195–199.

Sterle, J. and Safranski, T. Artificial Insemination in Swine: Breeding the Female. *The Pig Site.* 2000. https://thepigsite.com/articles/artificial-insemination-in-swine-breeding-the-female.

Sterning, M. Oestrous symptoms in primiparous sows. 2. Factors influencing the duration and intensity of external oestrous symptoms. *Anim. Reprod. Sci.* **1995,** *40* (1–2), 165–174.

Steverink, D. W.; Soede, N. M.; Bouwman, E. G.; Kemp, B. Semen Backflow after Insemination and its Effect on Fertilisation Results in Sows. *Anim. Reprod. Sci.* **1998,** *54* (2), 109–119.

Steverink, D. W.; Soede, N. M.; Groenland, G. J.; van Schie, F. W.; Noordhuizen, J. P.; Kemp, B. Duration of Estrus in Relation to Reproduction Results in Pigs on Commercial Farms. *J. Anim. Sci.* **1999,** *77* (4), 801–809. Retrieved from

Storey, B. T. Biochemistry of the Induction and Prevention of Lipoperoxidative Damage in Human Spermatozoa. *Mol Hum Reprod.* **1997,** *3,*203–13.

Strzezek, J.; Wysocki, P.; Kordan, W.; Kuklinska, M.; Mogielnicka, M.; Soliwoda, D.; Fraser, L. Proteomics of Boar Seminal Plasma–Current Studies and Possibility of Their Application in Biotechnology of Animal Reproduction. *Reprod Biol.* **2005,** *5* (3), 279–290.

Taylor, U.; Rath, D.; Zerbe, H.; Schuberth, H. J. Interaction of Intact Porcine Spermatozoa with Epithelial Cells and Neutrophilic Granulocytes During Uterine Passage. *Reprod. Domest. Anim.* **2008.**

Taylor, U.; Schuberth, H. J.; Rath, D.; Michelmann, H. W.; Sauter-Louis, C.; Zerbe, H. Influence of Inseminate Components on Porcine Leucocyte Migration *In Vitro* and *In Vivo* After Pre- and Post-Ovulatory Insemination. *Reprod. Domest. Anim.* **2009,** *44* (2), 180–188.

Töpfer-Petersen, E.; Romero, A.; Varela, P. F.; Ekhlasi-Hundrieser, M.; Dostàlovà, Z.; Sanz, L.; Calvete, J. J. Spermadhesins: A New Protein Family. Facts, Hypotheses and Perspectives. *Andrologia.* **1998,** *30* (4–5), 217–224.

Tummaruk, P., and Tienthai, P. Number of Spermatozoa in the Crypts of the Sperm Reservoir at About 24   h After a Low-Dose Intrauterine and Deep Intrauterine Insemination in Sows. *Reprod. Domest. Anim.* **2010,** *45* (2), 208–213.

Van Wienen, M.; Johannisson, A.; Wallgren, M.; Parlevliet, J.; Morrell, J. M. Single Layer Centrifugation with Androcoll-P can be Scaled-Up to Process Larger Volumes of Boar Semen. *ISRN Vet. Sci.,* **2011.**

Vasicek, J.; Parkanyi, V.; Ondruska, Ľ.; Makarevich, A.; Chrenek, P. The Potential Use of Magnetic Activated Cell Sorting for Elimination of Rabbit Apoptotic Spermatozoa. *Slovak J. Anim. Sci.* **2010,** *43,* 205–209.

Vazquez, J. M.; Martinez, E. A.; Roca, J.; Gil, M. A.; Parrilla, I.; Cuello, C.; Carvajala, G.; Lucasa, X.; Vazquez, J. L. Improving the Efficiency of Sperm Technologies in Pigs: The Value of Deep Intrauterine Insemination. *Theriogenology.* **2005,** *63*(2 SPEC. ISS.), 536–547.

Vazquez, J. M.; Roca, J.; Gil, M. A.; Cuello, C.; Parrilla, I.; Vazquez, J. L.; Martínez, E. A. New Developments in Low-Dose Insemination Technology. *Theriogenology.* **2008,** *70*(8), 1216–1224.

Viring, S.; Einarsson, S. Sperm Distribution Within the Genital Tract of Naturally Inseminated Gilts. *Nordisk Veterinaermedicin,* **1981,** *33* (3), 145–149.

Vyt, P.; Maes, D.; Dejonckheere, E.; Castryck, F.; Van Soom, A. Comparative Study on Five Different Commercial Extenders for Boar Semen. *Reprod. Domest. Anim.* **2004,** *39*(1), 8–12.

Vyt, P.; Maes, D.; Sys, S. U.; Rijsselaere, T.; Van Soom, A. Air Contact Influences the pH of Extended Porcine Semen. *Reprod. Domest. Anim.* **2007,** *42,* 218–220.

Waberski D. In *Critical steps from Semen Collection to Insemination.* Proceedings of the Annual Meeting of the EU-AI-Vets, Ghent, Belgium. **2009,** *66–69.*

Waberski, D.; and Weitze, K. F. Inseminaciòn artificial de la cerda. In *Manual de inseminaciòn artificial de los animales domésticos y de explotaciòn zootécnica.* D. Busch, Walter and Waberski Ed. **2010.**

Waberski, D.; Henning, H.; Petrunkina, A. Assessment of Storage Effects in Liquid Preserved Boar Semen. *Reprod. Domest. Anim.* **2011**, *46*, 45–48.

Wang, S.; Sun, M.; Wang, N.; Yang, K.; Guo, H.; Wang, J.; Zhang, Y.; Yue, S. Zhou, J. Effects of L-Glutamine on Boar Sperm Quality During Liquid Storage at 17° C. *Anim. Reprod. Sci.* **2018**, *191*, 76-84

Watson, P. F. The Causes of Reduced Fertility with Cryopreserved Semen. *Anim. Reprod. Sci.* **2000**, *60–61*, 481–492.

Watson, P. F.; Behan, J. R. Intrauterine Insemination of Sows with Reduced Sperm Numbers: Results of a Commercially Based Field Trial. *Theriogenology.* **2002**, *57*, 1683–1693.

Willemse, A. H., and Boender, J. A Quantitative and Qualitative Analysis of Oestrus in Gilts. **1966**.

Willenburg, K. L.; Miller, G. M.; Rodriguez-Zas, S. L.; Knox, R. V. Influence of Hormone Supplementation to Extended Semen on Artificial Insemination, Uterine Contractions, Establishment of a Sperm Reservoir, and Fertility in Swine. *J. Anim. Sci.* **2003**, *81* (4), 821–829.

Yamaguchi, S.; Funahashi, H.; Murakami, T. Improved Fertility in Gilts and Sows After Artificial Insemination of Frozen-Thawed Boar Semen by Supplementation of Semen Extender with Caffeine and CaCl2. *J. Reprod. Dev.* **2009**, *55* (6), 645–649.

Yamaguchi, S.; Suzuki, C.; Noguchi, M.; Kasa, S.; Mori, M.; Isozaki, Y.; Ueda S, Funahashi H, Kikuchi K, Nagai T, Yoshioka K. Effects of Caffeine on Sperm Characteristics After Thawing and Inflammatory Response in the Uterus after Artificial Insemination with Frozen-Thawed Boar Semen. *Theriogenology.* **2013**, *79* (1), 87–93.

Yeste, M. Boar Spermatozoa Within the Oviductal Environment (I): Sperm Reservoir. In *Boar Reproduction.* 2013, pp. 257–346. Springer Berlin Heidelberg.

Yeste, M. State-of-The-Art of Boar Sperm Preservation in Liquid and Frozen State. *Anim. Reprod.* **2017**, *14* (1), 69–81.

Yeste, M.; Briz, M.; Pinart, E.; Sancho, S.; Garcia-Gil, N.; Badia, E.; Bassols, J.; Pruneda, A.; Bussalleu, E.; Casas, I.; Bonet, S. Hyaluronic Acid Delays Boar Sperm Capacitation after 3 Days of Storage at 15 Degrees C. *Anim Reprod Sci.* **2008**, *109*,236–250.

Yeste, M.; Castillo-Martín, M.; Bonet, S.; Rodríguez-Gil, J. E. Impact of Light Irradiation on Preservation and Function of Mammalian Spermatozoa. *Anim. Reprod. Sci.* **2018**, *194*, 19–32.

Yeste, M.; Codony, F.; Estrada, E.; Lleonart, M.; Balasch, S.; Peña, A.; Bonet, S.; Rodríguez-Gil, J. E. Specific LED-Based Red-Light Photo-Stimulation Procedures Improve Overall Sperm Function and Reproductive Performance of Boar Ejaculates. *Sci. Rep.* **2016**, *6* (1), 1–13.

Zăhan, M.; Moldovan, C.; Dascăl, A. S.; Hettig, A.; Miclea, I.; Orlovschi, D.; Miclea, V. Boar sperm preservation by freeze-drying. *Porcine Res.4,* **2014**.

Zhang, J.; Chai, J.; Luo, Z.; He, H.; Chen, L.; Liu, X.; Zhou, Q. Meat and Nutritional Quality Comparison of Purebred and Crossbred Pigs. *Anim. Sci. J.* **2018**, *89* (1), 202–210.

Zhang, X. G.; Liu, Q.; Wang, L. Q.; Yang, G. S.; Hu, J. H. Effects of Glutathione on Sperm Quality During Liquid Storage in Boars. *Anim. Sci. J.* **2016**, *87*, 1195–1201.

Zhang, X. G.; Yan, G. J.; Hong, J. Y.; Su, Z. Z.; Yang, G. S.; Li, Q. W.; Hu, J. H. Effects of Bovine Serum Albumin on Boar Sperm Quality During Liquid Storage at 17°C. *Reprod Domest Anim.* **2015**, *50*, 263–269.

Index

Printed and bound by CPI Group (UK) Ltd, Croydon, CR0 4YY

23/10/2024

01777702-0008